Handbook of Experimental Pharmacology

Volume 128

Springer
Berlin
Heidelberg
New York
Barcelona
Budapest
Hong Kong
London
Milan
Paris
Santa Clara
Singapore
Tokyo

Pharmacotherapeutics of the Thyroid Gland

Contributors

J.W. Barlow, A.G. Burger, V.K.K. Chatterjee, T.C. Crowe
J.A. Franklyn, E. Gaitan, G. Hennemann, J.H. Lazarus
C-F. Lim, A.M. McGregor, C.A. Meier, E. Milgrom
M. Misrahi, S. Nagataki, M.F. Scanlon, M. El Sheikh
J.R. Stockigt, A.D. Toft, D.J. Topliss, T.J. Visser
A.P. Weetman, W.M. Wiersinga, N. Yokoyama

Editors

A.P. Weetman and A. Grossman

Springer

PROFESSOR DR. A.P. WEETMAN
Sir Arthur Hall
Professor of Medicine
The University of Sheffield
Department of Medicine
Clinical Sciences Centre
Northern General Hospital
Sheffield S5 7AU
United Kingdom

PROFESSOR DR. A. GROSSMAN
St. Bartholomew's Hospital
Department of Endocrinology
West Smithfield
London EC1A 7BE
United Kingdom

With 63 Figures and 29 Tables

ISBN-13:978-3-642-64519-8

Library of Congress Cataloging-in-Publication Data

Pharmacotherapeutics of the thyroid gland / contributors, J.W. Barlow ... [et al.]: editors, A.P. Weetman and A. Grossman.
p. cm. — (Handbook of experimental pharmacology; v. 128)
Includes bibliographical references and index.
ISBN-13:978-3-642-64519-8 e-ISBN-13:978-3-642-60709-7
DOI: 10.1007/978-3-642-60709-7

1. Thyroid gland—Effect of drugs on. 2. Thyroid hormones—Physiological effect. 3. Thyroid antagonists—Physiological effect. I. Barlow, J.W. II. Weetman, Anthony P. III. Grossman, Ashley. IV. Series.
[DNLM: 1. Thyroid Gland—drug effects. 2. Thyroid Hormones—physiology. 3. Antithyroid Agents—pharmacology. W1 HAB1L v. 128 1997/wk 202 p538 1997)
QP905.H3 vol. 128
[QP188, T54)
615¢.74]
DNLM/DLC
for Library of Congress 96-54721
CIP

Cover design: *design & production* GmbH, Heidelberg

Typesetting: Best-set Typesetter Ltd., Hong Kong

SPIN: 10503822 27/3020 – 5 4 3 2 1 0 – Printed on acid-free paper

Preface

We were a little bemused when asked to edit this volume in the series *Handbook of Experimental Pharmacology*. Carbimazole for an overactive thyroid (sometimes requiring substitution with propylthiouracil) and thyroxine for hypothyroidism hardly seemed to warrant a monograph in this extensive and well established series of books. Further reflection on the scope of the series, however, suggested that there was a place for a volume which dealt with the broader range of drug effects on the thyroid gland, particularly now we have learned so much more about the molecular mechanisms underlying thyroid hormone synthesis and intracellular action. This is, therefore, *not* a book on how to treat thyroid disorders (although we believe that it will still be of interest to the practising endocrinologist). We have, instead, aimed to bring together as much information as possible on the effects of drugs and other agents on the thyroid.

The first six chapters provide the physiological and pathological background necessary to understand the pharmacology contained in the later chapters of the book. Clinical aspects of thyroid diseases and their treatment are succinctly reviewed by Toft in Chap. 1. Scanlon has summarised the regulation of TRH and TSH secretion, so vital to the control of thyroid hormone production, in Chap. 2, and the recent spate of knowledge on the structure and function of the TSH receptor is reviewed by Misrahi and Milgrom in Chap. 3. This receptor could soon be an important target for pharmacological intervention.

Hennemann and Visser consider the physiology of thyroid hormone synthesis and metabolism in Chap. 4, and Stockigt and colleagues have reviewed how thyroid hormones are transported in Chap. 5. Important aspects of drug interference are dealt with in these chapters. At the end of this section, in Chap. 6, Franklyn and Chatterjee have provided an update on the interaction of thyroid hormones with their intracellular receptors, a topic which is essential for an understanding of the development of thyroid hormone antagonists, covered later in Chap. 13.

The remaining chapters concentrate on various pharmacological agents and their effects on thyroid function. Iodine is essential to thyroid hormone synthesis but also has important pharmacological effects which are discussed by Nagataki and Yokoyama in Chap. 7. Next El Sheikh and McGregor have summarised the mechanism of action of antithyroid drugs, agents which, after

50 years use, are still used as first line treatment by many endocrinologists dealing with Graves' disease. Chapter 9 by Lazarus deals with the effects of lithium on the thyroid gland, a topic of considerable importance given the number of patients receiving lithium as treatment for manic depression. Perhaps even more important numerically are the problems associated with amiodarone use, which are extensively reviewed by Wiersinga in Chap. 10. Meier and Burger have summarised in Chap. 11 the effects of other pharmacological agents on thyroid function, to complete the discussion of the key drugs which act on the thyroid gland.

Next, in Chap. 12, Gaitan considers the effects of a variety of environmental agents on thyroid function. It is likely that such agents are still underestimated as a cause of goitre and other thyroid problems. Developments in the production of thyroid hormone antagonists are reviewed by Barlow in Chap. 13, highlighting the potential that such agents may have in treatment in the future. Finally, one of us (Weetman) has discussed the effects of a variety of immunomodulatory agents in autoimmune thyroid disease: again, future developments in our ability to treat Graves' disease are likely to come from such forms of treatment.

Our thanks are due to all of the authors who have contributed these splendid reviews and who have provided manuscripts of such clarity that our editorial job has been a pleasure. We hope that you will enjoy reading these chapters as much as we did. We are also grateful to Springer-Verlag for supporting this venture, especially Doris Walker, whose ever ready help and skill has guided this book through its production and to Kathryn Watson in Sheffield and William Shufflebotham at Springer-Verlag for excellent secretarial and editorial assistance.

Sheffield and London, U.K. ANTHONY WEETMAN
August 1997 ASHLEY GROSSMAN

List of Contributors

BARLOW, J.W., Department of Endocrinology and Diabetes, Ewen Downie Metabolic Unit, Alfred Hospital, Commercial Road, Melbourne, Vic 3181, Australia

BURGER, A.G., Département de Médecine, Hôpital Cantonal, Division d'Endocrinologie et Diabétologie, Unité de Thyroïde, Rue Micheli-du-Crest 24, CH-1211 Genève 14, Switzerland

CHATTERJEE, V.K.K., University of Cambridge, Department of Medicine, Addenbrooke's Hospital, Cambridge CB2 2QQ, United Kingdom

CROWE, T.C., Department of Endocrinology and Diabetes, Ewen Downie Metabolic Unit, Alfred Hospital, Commercial Road, Melbourne, Vic 3181, Australia

FRANKLYN, J.A., Department of Medicine, University of Birmingham, Queen Elizabeth Hospital, Edgbaston, Birmingham B15 2TH, United Kingdom

GAITAN, E., VA Endocrinology Section, Department of Medicine, The University of Misissippi Medical Center, 2500 North State Street, Jackson, MS 39216-4505, USA

HENNEMANN, G., Department Internal Medicine III, University Hospital Dijkzigt, Dr. Molewaterplein 40, 3015 GD Rotterdam, The Netherlands

LAZARUS, J.H., University of Wales College of Medicine, Department of Medicine, Llandough Hospital, Penarth, Cardiff CF64 2XX, United Kingdom

LIM, C-F., Department of Endocrinology and Diabetes, Ewen Downie Metabolic Unit, Alfred Hospital, Prahran, Commercial Road, Melbourne, Vic 3181, Australia

MCGREGOR, A.M., Department of Medicine, King's College School of Medicine and Dentistry, Bessemer Road, London SE5 9PJ, United Kingdom

MEIER, C.A., Département de Médecine, Hôpital Cantonal, Division d'Endocrinologie et Diabétologie, Unité de Thyroïde, Rue Micheli-du-Crest 24, CH-1211 Genève 14, Switzerland

MILGROM, E., INSERM U 135, Faculté de Médecine de Bicêtre, Université Paris-Sud, 78, rue du Général Leclerc, F-94275 Le Kremlin-Bicêtre Cedex, France

MISRAHI, M., INSERM U 135, Faculté de Médecine de Bicêtre, Université Paris-Sud, 78, rue du Général Leclerc, F-94275 Le Kremlin-Bicêtre Cedex, France

NAGATAKI, S., The First Department of Internal Medicine, Nagasaki University School of Medicine, Nagasaki 852, Japan

SCANLON, M.F., University of Wales College of Medicine, Department of Medicine, Section of Endocrinology, Diabetes and Metabolism, Heath Park, Cardiff CF4 4XN, Wales, United Kingdom

SHEIKH, M. El, Department of Medicine, King's College School of Medicine and Dentistry, Bessemer Road, London SE5 9PJ, United Kingdom

STOCKIGT, J.R., Department of Endocrinology and Diabetes, Ewen Downie Metabolic Unit, Alfred Hospital, Commercial Road, Melbourne, Vic 3181, Australia

TOFT, A.D., Endocrine Clinic, Royal Infirmary, Edinburgh EH3 9YW, United Kingdom

TOPLISS, D.J., Department of Endocrinology and Diabetes, Ewen Downie Metabolic Unit, Alfred Hospital, Commercial Road, Melbourne, Vic 3181, Australia

VISSER, T.J., Erasmus Universiteit Rotterdam, Medical School, Department of Internal Medicine, Postbus 1738, NL-3000 DR Rotterdam, The Netherlands

WEETMAN, A.P., The University of Sheffield, Department of Medicine, Clinical Sciences Centre, Northern General Hospital, Sheffield S5 7AU, United Kingdom

WIERSINGA, W.M., Academisch Ziekenhius bij de Universiteit van Amsterdam, Academisch Medisch Centrum, Meibergdreef 9, Afd. Endocrinologie, Secretariaat F5-171, NL-1105 AZ Amsterdam Zuidoost, The Netherlands

YOKOYAMA, N., The First Department of Internal Medicine, Nagasaki University School of Medicine, Nagasaki 852, Japan

Contents

CHAPTER 3

The TSH Receptor

CHAPTER 4

Thyroid Hormone Synthesis, Plasma Membrane Transport and Metabolism

CHAPTER 5

Thyroid Hormone Transport

CHAPTER 6

Molecular Biology of Thyroid Hormone Action

CHAPTER 1

Introduction: Clinical Aspects of Thyroid Treatment

A.D. Toft

A. Introduction

Graves' disease is the most common cause of hyperthyroidism in the United Kingdom, accounting for some 70% of cases. The natural history of the hyperthyroidism in the majority is one of repeated episodes of relapse and remission each lasting several months. It is the minority, probably about 25%, who experience a single episode of hyperthyroidism followed by prolonged remission, and even the spontaneous development of hypothyroidism 10–20 years later (Irvine et al. 1977). If it were possible to predict the future behaviour of the hyperthyroidism when the patient presented, it would be appropriate to prescribe an antithyroid drug for 18–24 months for those destined for a single episode, and to advise surgery or radioiodine therapy for the remainder. However, despite many ingenious efforts based on factors such as HLA status, presence of thyroid-stimulating hormone (TSH)-receptor antibodies (TRAB) and goitre size, it has not been possible to categorize patients with Graves' disease in respect of outcome with any degree of accuracy and treatment remains empirical.

Standard teaching has been that the initial treatment in patients under 40–45 years of age is with an antithyroid drug with a recommendation for surgery should relapse occur. Older patients are treated with iodine-131. Of course, management varies from centre to centre and between countries and these differences have been highlighted in recent surveys of practice in Europe and in the United States. For example, the preferred treatment of a 43-year-old female presenting with hyperthyroidism of moderate severity due to Graves' disease who did not plan further pregnancies was antithyroid drugs (77%) by European physicians but iodine-131 (69%) by their North American counterparts. There was an even greater contrast in choice of therapy when the index case was changed to that of a 19-year-old female. One-third of physicians in the United States regarded iodine-131 as most appropriate, whereas the corresponding figure in Europe was only 4% (Glinoer et al. 1987; Solomon et al. 1990). The more liberal use of iodine-131 is finding favour with an increasing number of physicians (Franklyn and Sheppard 1992), but is permanent hypothyroidism the only significant adverse effect? At the same time there are claims that high remission rates can be achieved by the use of an unusual combination of antithyroid drugs and thyroxine (Hashizume et al. 1991). Surgery would seem to be the loser in the face of these two developments.

There is little or no debate about the management of toxic nodular goitre, which is with surgery or iodine-131 depending upon the age of the patient and the presence of significant mediastinal compression. The use of antithyroid drugs should be restricted to preoperative preparation.

It is perhaps surprising that any problems are perceived with the treatment of primary hypothyroidism, which is usually both gratifying and simple. Even the therapeutic difficulties in the patient with concomitant symptomatic ischaemic heart disease have been largely overcome as both angioplasty and coronary artery bypass surgery can be safely undertaken in the presence of untreated or partially treated hypothyroidism. Controversy, however, has arisen following the development of increasingly sensitive assays for TSH, which have raised the question of whether a low serum TSH concentration (<0.01 mU/l) is an indication of overtreatment when recorded in asymptomatic patients with normal serum concentrations of thyroid hormones. And what are the indications for treatment of subclinical hypothyroidism?

B. Choices of Treatment for the Hyperthyroidism of Graves' Disease

I. Iodine-131 Therapy

Those in favour of the more widespread use of iodine-131 therapy would argue that it is cheap, easy to administer and effective as a single dose in the majority of cases. By giving a relatively large dose of 400 MBq, patients will be hypothyroid within a year and subsequent management can pass to the primary care physician. The initial anxieties about an increase in incidence of post-treatment thyroid carcinoma and leukaemia have evaporated. Furthermore, the gonadal irradiation averages 0.8–1.4 rem, similar to that for a barium enema or intravenous pyelogram, and it has not been possible to show an association between incidental or therapeutic irradiation with iodine-131, even in children and adolescents, and congenital abnormalities in subsequent offspring – although the series are small. So why not advocate a policy of iodine-131 therapy for all non-pregnant patients with Graves' disease? Simply because there are anxieties about this treatment modality which cannot entirely be dismissed, particularly when there are other effective treatment options.

1. Acceptability of Irradiation

There is a heightened public awareness of the dangers of radioactivity as a result of widely reported accidents at nuclear power stations. Of the radionuclides used in diagnostic and therapeutic nuclear medicine, iodine-131 provides the greatest radiation hazard to other individuals who come into contact with the patient. The UK Ionizing Radiation Regulations of 1985 are designed to minimize their exposure (National Radiological Protection Board 1985) and other similar bodies exist. Because of the resultant disruption socially, domestically and at the workplace, albeit temporary, a significant minority, even among those over the age of 40–45 years for whom iodine-131 has always been the first choice of treatment, are refusing such an option. Disaffection with radioactive iodine is likely to increase if the recommendations of the International Commission on Radiological Protection are implemented, limiting the annual dose of radiation for members of the public to 1 mSv (International Comission on Radiological Protection 1990). In this circumstance, the patient treated for hyperthyroidism with 400 MBq iodine-131 will be advised to spend less than $1^1/_2$ h on public transport in the 1st week, to take 3 days off work, to sleep apart from his or her partner for 20 days and to avoid contact closer than 1.0 m with children aged 11 or less for up to 3 weeks (O'Doherty et al. 1993). This is hardly a practical treatment for active men and women in their twenties and early thirties with young families.

2. Gastric Carcinoma

A recent Swedish report analysed cancer mortality in more than 10000 patients with an average age of 56 years at the time of treatment with iodine-131, and found that there was a significant increased risk of death from cancer of the stomach more than 10 years after exposure (Hall et al. 1992). The probability of a radiation-induced cancer is proportional to the radiation dose received by the organ in question. It is perhaps not surprising, therefore, that an excess mortality from gastric carcinoma has been demonstrated, as after the thyroid, the stomach receives the greatest amount of radiation following a therapeutic dose of iodine-131 for hyperthyroidism; thyroid cancer does not develop because a relatively large radiation dose either kills or sterilizes the follicular cells.

The latest methods for predicting excess cancer risks following radiation exposure indicate that, for most radiosensitive organs, there will be an increasing risk of attributable cancer with time. This is because, after a latent period of a few years, the pattern of appearance of radiation-induced cancer is thought to follow a constant multiple of the "natural" baseline rates which themselves invariably increase with age. If people are young at the time of exposure, they have simply more life ahead of them in which radiation-induced cancer can be expressed, so that the cumulative lifetime risk is higher than for someone exposed at an older age. This view, taken together with the Swedish study, provides a cogent argument against reducing the long-established age threshold for radioiodine treatment for hyperthyroidism in Europe of 40–45 years.

3. Ophthalmopathy

Although a large retrospective study has shown no influence of the type of treatment of the hyperthyroidism of Graves' disease on the clinical course of the ophthalmopathy (SRIDAMA and DEGROOT 1989), most clinicians will cite anecdotal evidence that the eye disease will worsen most often after iodine-131. This clinical suspicion has been supported by a recent prospective study in which ophthalmopathy developed for the first time or was exacerbated in one-third of patients treated with iodine-131 and was twice as frequent, and of more severity, than in those treated with antithyroid drugs or surgery (TALLSTEDT et al. 1992). However, serum TSH concentrations were more often raised in the iodine-131-treated patients and subsequently it has been shown that the development of subclinical or overt hypothyroidism following iodine-131 is associated with the onset or exacerbation of ophthalmopathy (KUNG et al. 1994). Surprisingly, more patients in this study developed ophthalmopathy than experienced an exacerbation of pre-existing disease; and inhibition of the post-radioiodine surge in serum TRAB concentrations with methimazole and thyroxine as "block and replacement therapy" did not influence the natural history of the ophthalmopathy, although corticosteroids have been shown to be beneficial in this respect if given for 3–4 months (BARTALENA et al. 1989).

Unless the ophthalmopathy is severe, when even slight deterioration might result in the need for orbital decompression, the presence of eye disease is not a contraindication to treatment with iodine-131. However, it may be sensible to consider corticosteroids following iodine-131 therapy for 3–4 months in those with mild or moderate ophthalmopathy and to ensure in all patients that prolonged periods of thyroid failure do not occur in the early months after treatment. This would require closer supervision than the normal pattern for review in most centres. It would also be appropriate to advise that smoking is stopped as this is an established risk factor for ophthalmopathy (SHINE et al. 1990).

4. Calcitonin Deficiency

Although intrathyroidal C-cells do not concentrate radioactive iodine, they could be damaged indirectly due to their contiguity to follicular cells. Indeed, both basal and intravenous calcium-stimulated calcitonin concentrations are reduced in patients in whom hyperthyroidism has been treated with iodine-131 (TZANELA et al. 1993). The consequences of long-term calcitonin deficiency are not known but may include osteoporosis. This is particularly relevant as most patients treated with iodine-131 will develop hypothyroidism, and thyroxine replacement in a dose sufficient to suppress serum TSH concentrations may be a factor in reducing bone mineral density.

II. Thyroid Surgery

One year after subtotal thyroidectomy for Graves' disease, undertaken by an experienced surgeon, 80% of patients will be euthyroid, 15% will have permanent thyroid failure and in 5% operation will have failed to cure the hyperthyroidism (TOFT et al. 1978). These figures flatter to deceive as 50% will be hypothyroid after 25 years (FRANKLYN 1994), and even later recurrence of thyrotoxicosis is well recognized (KALK et al. 1978). Published figures for hypothyroidism may be overestimated unless it has been recognized that thyroid failure occurring in the first 6 months after operation may be temporary. Neither of the other two treatments for Graves' hyperthyroidism is associated with a scar or a 1% chance of permanent hypoparathyroidism or vocal cord palsy. Even in the absence of damage to a recurrent laryngeal nerve, significant changes in voice quality may be recorded after subtotal thyroidectomy (KARK et al. 1984), making surgery an inadvisable option for those who depend upon their voice for a living. Surgery does promise the longest period of euthyroidism and is probably the most appropriate treatment for young patients who are poorly compliant with antithyroid drugs, the hope being that if and when thyroid failure or recurrent hyperthyroidism occurs they will be sufficiently mature to adhere to treatment. The consensus is that surgery is indicated as the primary treatment in severely hyperthyroid young patients with large goitres in whom relapse is almost certain after a course of antithyroid drugs.

III. Antithyroid Drug Therapy

Drugs such as carbimazole and its active metabolite, methimazole, are effective in controlling hyperthyroidism because they inhibit thyroid hormone production. In patients with hyperthyroidism caused by Graves' disease, these drugs may also have an immunosuppressive action, causing a fall in the serum concentrations of TRAB (WEETMAN et al. 1984). The main disadvantage of antithyroid drug therapy is that the recurrence rate after treatment is stopped varies widely from 25% to 90% (SUGRUE et al. 1980; FRANKLYN 1994). Factors affecting the recurrence rate include dosage and duration of treatment (ALLANIC et al. 1990). One reason for using high doses of antithyroid drugs, which must be combined with thyroid hormone to avoid hypothyroidism, is the belief that their postulated immunosuppressive effect may be dose related. For example, in one study the recurrence rate was 55% in patients treated with an antithyroid drug alone and 25% in patients given combined therapy (ROMALDINI et al. 1983). However, in a large prospective multicentre European trial (REINWEIN et al. 1993), combination therapy was no more effective.

It is the dissatisfaction with these high recurrence rates, following prolonged treatment with antithyroid drugs for 18–24 months, which have led many physicians to begin to favour a more liberal age policy for the use of iodine-131. Against this background, the report that in Japanese patients the rate of relapse of hyperthyroidism could be reduced from 35% to less than 2% by treatment with methimazole for 18 months, to which thyroxine was added after the first 6 months and continued for 3 years after the antithyroid drug was stopped, could be regarded as the single most important development in the management of Graves' hyperthyroidism for many years (HASHIZUME et al. 1991). The explanation provided for these remarkable results was that by suppressing endogenous TSH secretion with thyroxine, thyroid antigen release would be inhibited and the serum concentration of TRAB, the cause of the hyperthyroidism of Graves' disease, would fall. If confirmed in other ethnic groups, combined antithyroid drug T_4 therapy would become the initial treatment of choice in all patients with Graves' hyperthyroidism, surgery and radioiodine being reserved for that small proportion of patients who relapse. Unfortunately when the study was repeated in a large number of Caucasian patients not only was there no difference in the rate of fall of serum TRAB concentrations between the antithyroid drug alone group and that taking combined therapy, but also rates of recurrence of hyperthyroidism were identical (McIver et al. 1996).

So on the one hand patients with Graves' disease are fortunate in that they have a choice of treatments, each of which is usually effective in controlling the hyperthyroidism, but on the other hand none is perfect and there is no overall frontrunner. The treatment offered and accepted will continue to depend upon the prejudices of the physician and of the patient and upon the local circumstances such as availability of isotope facilities and the services of an experienced surgeon. The author's prejudice is to reserve iodine-131 therapy for older patients and to favour prolonged courses of antithyroid drugs in younger patients repeated, if necessary, if surgery is declined. It is perfectly reasonable to maintain patients on small doses of an antithyroid drug for many years, recognizing that adverse effects may occur at any time, although usually within 3–6 weeks of starting treatment.

C. Subclinical Hyperthyroidism

Patients with normal serum concentrations of thyroid hormones but suppressed TSH in the context of Graves' disease in remission and nodular goitre have tended to be observed until overt hyperthyroidism develops, often after several years. However, there is now evidence that a low serum TSH concentration of itself is a risk factor for atrial fibrillation (Forfar et al. 1981; Sawin et al. 1994) and, particularly in the elderly, a case can be made for "nipping it in the bud" by administering iodine-131 and preventing the possibility of future morbidity or even mortality (Parker and Lawson 1973).

D. Correct Dose of Thyroxine in Primary Hypothyroidism

The advice of the American Thyroid Association in the management of primary hypothyroidism is that "the goal of therapy is to restore most patients to the euthyroid state and to normalize serum T_3 and T_4 concentrations" (Surks et al. 1990). This stance is a consequence of studies which have shown that doses of thyroxine which suppress TSH secretion have more widespread effects such as increasing nocturnal heart rate, shortening the systolic time interval, increasing urinary sodium excretion and serum enzyme activities in liver and muscle and decreasing the serum cholesterol concentration (LESLIE and TOFT 1988). These effects are similar to, but less marked than, those in overt hyperthyroidism. The greatest concern, however, is the possible deleterious effect on bone of over-replacement. Significant decreases in bone mineral density at various sites have been found in some but in no means all studies of pre- and postmenopausal women receiving long-term thyroxine therapy in doses sufficient to suppress TSH concentrations (TOFT 1994). It is difficult to reconcile the results of the various studies, many of which were small and poorly controlled for important risk factors for osteoporosis such as smoking, insufficient exercise, relative calcitonin deficiency due to thyroidectomy or iodine-131 treatment, previous hyperthyroidism and inadequate dietary intake of calcium and vitamin D. The current consensus is that a little too much thyroxine is likely to be only a minor aetiological factor in the development of osteoporosis, if it is a factor at all. Indeed there are those who would question the relevance of minor changes in target organ function in individuals who are asymptomatic, the more so when a recent retrospective study failed to demonstrate an increase in morbidity or mortality in thyroxine-treated patients with suppressed serum TSH compared to those with normal serum TSH (LEESE et al. 1992), nor is there any evidence of an increased fracture rate (SOLOMON et al. 1993). There is also the important clinical observation that some patients prefer taking a daily dose of thyroxine of 50 μg in excess of that required to normalize the serum TSH response to thyrotrophin-releasing hormone (CARR et al. 1988), and there is some evidence for tissue adaptation to thyroid hormone excess (NYSTRÖM et al. 1989). For practical purposes, therefore, it would seem reasonable to modify the advice of the American Thyroid Association to cater for those patients in whom there will only be a sense of well-being when the serum TSH concentration is undetectable, using an assay with a lower limit of detection of 0.01–0.05 mU/l. In this circumstance serum free T_4 is unlikely to exceed 30 pmol/l and T_3 will be unequivocally normal.

E. Subclinical Hypothyroidism: Treatment or Not?

Subclinical hypothyroidism is the rather unsatisfactory term used to describe asymptomatic patients in whom serum thyroid hormone concentrations are normal but TSH elevated. Developing spontaneously and due to autoimmune thyroid disease, it is present in 3% of the population and in 10% of postmenopausal women. It is commonly found after treatment of hyperthyroidism by surgery, iodine-131 or antithyroid drugs, but may result from the use of medication such as lithium carbonate or amiodarone.

There has been great interest in the effect of subclinical hypothyroidism and its treatment with thyroxine on circulating lipid concentrations because of the association of overt hypothyroidism with hyperlipidaemia and increased risk of ischaemic heart disease. The results of studies have been conflicting and no clear message emerges (Franklyn 1995; Kung et al. 1995).

Those favouring a pragmatic approach to the management of subclinical hypothyroidism will be most influenced by the knowledge that between 25% and 50% of such patients feel better while taking thyroxine (Cooper et al. 1984; Nyström et al. 1988) and by the fact that the annual rate of evolution from subclinical to overt hypothyroidism is approximately 5% (Tunbridge et al. 1981) and may be as high as 20% in patients over 65 years of age (Rosenthal et al. 1987). In those patients with minor elevations of serum TSH (<10 mU/l) and no goitre, history of thyroid disease or antithyroid peroxidase antibodies, the measurement should be repeated in 3–6 months to determine whether long-term treatment with thyroxine is necessary, because the initial raised concentration may simply reflect recovery from non-thyroidal illness or transient thyroid injury.

References

Allanic R, Fauchet R, Orgiazzi J, Madec AM, Genetet B, Lorcy Y, Le Guerrier AM, Delambre C, Derennes V (1990) Antithyroid drugs in Graves' disease: a prospective randomised evaluation of the efficacy of treatment duration. J Clin Endocrinol Metab 70:675–679

Bartelena L, Marcocci C, Bogazzi F, Panicucci K, Lepri A, Pinchera A (1989) Use of corticosteroids to prevent progression of Graves' ophthalmopathy after radioiodine therapy for hyperthyroidism. N Engl J Med 321:1349–1352

Carr D, McLeod DT, Parry G, Thorner HM (1988) Fine adjustment of thyroxine replacement dosage: comparison of the thyrotrophin releasing hormone test using a sensitive thyrotrophin assay with measurement of free thyroid hormones and clinical assessment. Clin Endocrinol (Oxf) 28:325–333

Cooper DS, Halpern R, Wood LC, Levin AA, Ridgway ED (1984) L-Thyroxine therapy in subclinical hypothyroidism: a double-blind, placebo-controlled trial. Ann Intern Med 101:18–24

Forfar JC, Feek CK, Miller HC, Toft AD (1981) Atrial fibrillation and isolated suppression of the pituitary-thyroid axis: response to specific antithyroid therapy. Int J Cardiol 1:43–48

Franklyn JA (1994) The management of hyperthyroidism. N Engl J Med 330:1731–1738

Franklyn J (1995) Subclinical hypothyroidism: to treat or not to treat, that is the question. Clin Endocrinol (Oxf) 43:443–444

Franklyn J, Sheppard M (1992) Radioiodine for hyperthyroidism. Br Med J 305:727–728

Glinoer D, Hesch D, Lagasse R, Laurberg P (1987) The management of hyperthyroidism due to Graves' disease in Europe in 1986. The results of an international survey. Acta Endocrinol (Copenh) 115 [Suppl 285]

Hall P, Berg G, Bjelkengren G, Boice JD, Ericsson U-B, Hallquist A, Lidberg K, Lundell G, Tennvall J, Wiklund K, Holm L-E (1992) Cancer mortality after iodine-131 therapy for hyperthyroidism. Int J Cancer 50:886–890

Hashizume K, Ichikawa K, Sakurai A, Suzuki S, Takeda T, Kobayashi M, Miyamoto T, Arai M, Nagasawa T (1991) Administration of thyroxine in treated Graves' disease – effects on the level of antibodies to thyroid-stimulating hormone receptors and on the risk of recurrence of hyperthyroidism. N Engl J Med 324:947–953

International Commission on Radiological Protection (1991) Recommendations of the International Commission on Radiological Protection. Ann ICRP 21:1–3 (ICRP publication 60)
Irvine WJ, Gray RS, Toft AD, Seth J, Lidgard GP, Cameron EHD (1977) Spectrum of thyroid function in patients remaining in remission after antithyroid drug therapy for thyrotoxicosis. Lancet ii:179–181
Kalk WJ, Durbach D, Kantor S, Levin J (1978) Post-thyroidectomy thyrotoxicosis. Lancet i:291–293
Kark AE, Kissin MW, Auerbach R, Meikle M (1984) Voice changes after thyroidectomy: role of the external laryngeal nerve. Br Med J 289:1412–1415
Kung AWC, Yau CC, Cheng A (1994) The incidence of ophthalmopathy after radioiodine therapy for Graves' disease: prognostic factors and the role of methimazole. J Clin Endocrinol Metab 79:542–546
Kung AWC, Pang RWC, Janus ED (1995) Elevated serum lipoprotein (a) in subclinical hypothyroidism. Clin Endocrinol (Oxf) 43:445–449
Leese GP, Jung RT, Guthrie C, Waugh N, Browning MCK (1992) Morbidity in patients on L-thyroxine: a comparison of those with a normal TSH to those with a suppressed TSH. Clin Endocrinol (Oxf) 37:500–503
Leslie PJ, Toft AD (1988) The replacement therapy problem in hypothyroidism. Ballieres Clin Endocrinol Metab 2:653–659
McIver B, Rae P, Beckett G, Wilkinson E, Gold A, Toft A (1996) Lack of effect of thyroxine in patients with Graves' disease treated with an antithyroid drug. N Engl J Med 334:220–224
National Radiological Protection Board (1985) Guidance notes for the protection of persons against ionising radiations arising from medical and dental use. EMSO, London, p 57
Nyström E, Caidahl K, Fager G, Wikkelso C, Lundberg P-A, Lindstedt G (1988) A double-blind cross-over 12-month study of L-thyroxine treatment of women with "subclinical" hypothyroidism. Clin Endocrinol 29:63–75
Nyström E, Lundberg P-A, Petersen K, Bergtsson C, Lindstedt G (1989) Evidence for a slow tissue adaptation to circulating thyroxine in patients with chronic L-thyroxine treatment. Clin Endocrinol (Oxf) 31:143–150
O'Doherty MJ, Kettle AG, Eustance CNP, Mountford PJ, Coakley AJ (1993) Radiation dose rates from adult patients receiving ^{131}I therapy for thyrotoxicosis. Nucl Med Commun 14:160–168
Parker JLW, Lawson DH (1973) Death from thyrotoxicosis. Lancet ii:894–895
Reinwein D, Benker G, Lazarus JH (1993) A prospective randomised trial of antithyroid drug dose in Graves' disease therapy. J Clin Endocrinol Metab 76: 1516–1521
Romaldini JH, Bromberg N, Werner RS, Tanaka LM, Rodrigues HF, Werner MC, Farah CS, Reis LCF (1983) Comparison of effects of high and low dosage regimens of antithyroid drugs in the management of Graves' hyperthyroidism. Clin Endocrinol Metab 57:563–570
Rosenthal MJ, Hunt WC, Garry PJ, Goodwin JS (1987) Thyroid failure in the elderly: microsomal antibodies as discriminant for therapy. JAMA 258:209–213
Sawin CT, Geller A, Wolf PA, Belanger AJ, Baker E, Bacharach P, Wilson PWF, Benjamin EJ, D'Agostino RB (1994) Low serum thyrotropin concentrations as a risk factor for atrial fibrillation in older persons. N Engl J Med 331:1249–1252
Shine B, Fells P, Edwards OM, Weetman AP (1990) Association between Graves' ophthalmopathy and smoking. Lancet ii:1261–1263
Solomon B, Glinoer D, Lagasse R, Wartofsky L (1990) Current trends in the management of Graves' disease. J Clin Endocrinol Metab 70:1518–1524
Solomon BL, Wartofsky L, Burman KD (1993) Prevalence of fractures in post-menopausal women with thyroid disease. Thyroid 3:17–23
Sridama V, DeGroot LJ (1989) Treatment of Graves' disease and the course of ophthalmopathy. Am J Med 87:70–73

Sugrue D, McEvoy M, Feely J, Drury MI (1980) Hyperthyroidism in the land of Graves: results of treatment by surgery, radioiodine and carbimazole in 837 cases. Q J Med 49:51–61

Surks MI, Chopra IJ, Mariash CN, Nicoloff JT, Solomon DH (1990) American Thyroid Association guidelines for use of laboratory tests in thyroid disorders. JAMA 263:1529–1532

Tallstedt L, Lundell G, Torring O, Wallin G, Ljunggren J-G, Blomgren H, Taube A (1992) Occurrence of ophthalmopathy after treatment for Graves' hyperthyroidism. N Engl J Med 326:1733–1738

Toft AD (1994) Thyroxine therapy. N Engl J Med 331:174–180

Toft AD, Irvine WJ, Sinclair I, McIntosh D, Seth J, Cameron EHD (1978) Thyroid function after surgical treatment of thyrotoxicosis. A report of 100 cases treated with propranolol before operation. N Engl J Med 198:643–647

Tunbridge WMJ, Brewis M, French JM, Appleton D, Bird T, Clark F, Evered DC, Evans JG, Hall R, Smith P, Stephenson J, Young E (1981) Natural history of autoimmune thyroiditis. Br Med J 282:258–262

Tzanela M, Thalassinos NC, Nikou A, Philokiproud (1993) Effect of ^{131}I treatment on the calcitonin response to calcium infusion in hyperthyroid patients. Clin Endocrinol (Oxf) 38:25–28

Weetman AP, McGregor AM, Hall R (1984) Evidence for an effect of antithyroid drugs on the natural history of Graves' disease. Clin Endocrinol (Oxf) 21:163–172

CHAPTER 2

Control of TRH and TSH Secretion

M.F. Scanlon

A. Introduction

The hypothalamus stimulates thyroid function via thyroid-stimulating hormone (TSH) since hypothyroidism occurs if the hypothalamus is lesioned or diseased, or if the pituitary stalk is transected. This stimulatory hypothalamic control is exerted by thyrotrophin-releasing hormone (TRH), a tripeptide produced by peptidergic neurons and transported along their axons to specialised nerve terminals in the median eminence of the hypothalamus where it is released into hypophyseal portal blood and hence transported to the anterior pituitary gland (Jackson 1982). Circulating thyroid hormones exert powerful negative feedback inhibitory actions on the thyrotrophs and also on TRH-producing hypothalamic neurons (Fig. 1). In addition, several secondary modulators exert lesser degrees of control over TSH secretion, the net result of which is the maintenance of a steady output of TSH and therefore of thyroid hormones. The neuroregulation of TSH secretion has recently been reviewed in depth (Scanlon and Toft 1995) which forms the basis for this chapter. The most important secondary modulators are somatostatin and dopamine, both of which inhibit the function of the thyrotrophs, and α-adrenergic pathways, which are, in general, stimulatory. Other modulators of thyroid function include glucocorticoid hormones, various cytokines and other inflammatory mediators.

B. Negative Feedback Action of Thyroid Hormones

Serum TSH in rats is rapidly suppressed to 10% of pretreatment concentrations within 5h of T_3 administration. Further TSH suppression occurs more slowly and only after chronic treatment with T_3. The rapid phase of TSH suppression is paralleled by an increase in nuclear T_3 content, and serum TSH concentrations rise as nuclear T_3 levels decline (Silva et al. 1978). There is an inverse relationship between nuclear T_3 receptor occupancy and serum TSH concentrations after acute administration of T_3. About half of pituitary nuclear T_3 is derived from the intracellular 5′-monodeiodination of thyroxine (T_4), which is a greater fraction than in other tissues; this monodeiodination may be the mechanism by which the thyrotrophs respond to changes in serum T_4 concentrations (Silva and Larsen 1978).

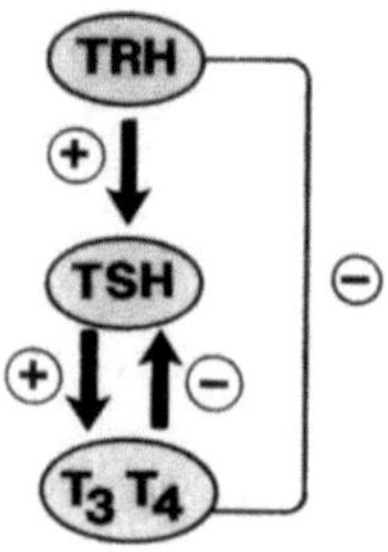

Fig. 1. Central pathways in the feedback regulation of TSH secretion. (From SCANLON and TOFT 1995, with permission)

The major actions of thyroid hormones are to regulate gene expression after binding to specific nuclear receptors. Thyroid hormone receptors are structurally related to the viral oncogene v-*erb* A and, together with steroid, vitamin D and retinoic acid receptors, form a family of receptor proteins with important structural similarities. Several cDNAs that encode different thyroid hormone receptors (α and β) have been described. Binding of T_3 to a site on the carboxyl-terminal end of the receptor activates the receptor so that the T_3-receptor complex binds to specific nucleotide sequences on target genes (EVANS 1988). In thyrotrophs, the activated T_3 receptor inhibits transcription of the α-subunit and TSH-β-subunit genes in proportion to nuclear T_3-receptor occupancy.

In addition to this action, thyroid hormones also modulate the expression of the TRH-receptor gene (YAMADA et al. 1992). The number of TRH receptors on thyrotrophs increases in hypothyroidism and can be reduced by thyroid hormone replacement (HINKLE et al. 1981). Conversely, in rat pituitary tumour cells, TRH itself reduces T_3-receptor gene expression (JONES and CHIN 1991), receptor number and T_3 responsiveness (KAJI and HINKLE 1987), which may represent a further site of feedback interaction between T_3 and TRH at the level of the pituitary. Thyroid hormones exert negative feedback actions on the hypothalamus (KAKUCSKA et al. 1992). TRH mRNA increases in the paraventricular nuclei in hypothyroidism and is reduced by thyroid hormone treatment. Furthermore, rats with bilateral lesions of the paraventricular nuclei do not show a normal rise of serum TSH and TSH-subunit mRNA after induction of primary hypothyroidism (TAYLOR et al. 1990), an effect that presumably reflects depletion of TRH. These results indicate that the paraventricular nuclei are a target for the action of thyroid hormones in the control of TRH gene expression and release, providing an additional mechanism for thyroidal regulation of TSH secretion (TAYLOR et al. 1990; KANUCSKA et al. 1992; GREER et al. 1993).

C. Structure and Actions of TRH

TRH is a weakly basic tripeptide, pyro-Glu-His-Pro-amide which, like other more complex peptides, is derived from post-translational cleavage of a larger precursor molecule (LECHAN et al. 1986). The cDNA sequence of the rat TRH precursor encodes a protein with a molecular size of 29000 daltons that contains five copies of the sequence Glu-His-Pro-Gly (JACKSON 1989). Rat pro-TRH is processed at paired basic residues to a family of peptides that include TRH and flanking and intervening sequences. These peptides may exert important intracellular or extracellular actions (WU 1989), in particular prepro-TRH-(160–169), which stimulates TSH gene expression (CARR et al. 1992, 1993). There may be preferential processing of pro-TRH to produce different peptides in different brain regions (LECHAN et al. 1986).

Immunoreactive TRH is widely distributed in the hypothalamus with highest concentrations in the median eminence and the so-called "thyrotrophic area" or paraventricular nuclei (JACKSON 1982). Lesions of the paraventricular nuclei reduce circulating TSH levels and prevent the increase in serum TSH that occurs in primary hypothyroidism (TAYLOR et al. 1990). TRH and pro-TRH perikarya are present in the parvicellular division of this nucleus (JACKSON and LECHAN 1985), which is the major site of origin of the immunoreactive TRH in the median eminence as opposed to other brain regions such as the tractus solitarius (SIAUD et al. 1987). The TRH gene is also expressed in the anterior pituitary (BRUHN et al. 1994; CROISSANDEAU et al. 1994) and TRH-positive axons are present in posterior pituitary tissue. However, lesions of the paraventriclar nuclei reduce the content of TRH in both anterior and posterior pituitary tissue, indicating that the hypothalamus is a source of some of the immunoreactive TRH in these areas.

The dominant stimulatory role of the hypothalamus in the control of the thyrotroph is mediated by TRH (JACKSON 1982). The pituitary TRH receptor belongs to the family of seven transmembrane domain, G-protein-coupled receptors. TRH is present in hypophyseal portal blood at physiologically relevant concentrations (SHEWARD et al. 1983) and administration of antibodies to TRH to animals can cause hypothyroidism. Intravenous administration of 15–500 μg TRH to normal humans causes a dose-related release in TSH. In normal subjects serum TSH levels increase within 2–5 min, are maximal at 20–30 min and return to basal by 2–3 h. Peak serum T_3 and T_4 levels occur about 3 and 8 h, respectively, after TRH administration. In addition to stimulating TSH release, TRH also stimulates TSH synthesis by promoting transcription and translation of the TSH subunit genes, actions that involve calcium influx, activation of phosphatidyl-inositol pathways and protein kinase C (CARR et al. 1991; SHUPNIK et al. 1992; HAISENLEDER et al. 1993). These actions are modulated by cAMP and the pituitary-specific transcription factor, Pit-1 (STEINFELDER et al. 1992; MASON et al. 1993; KIM et al. 1994) (Fig. 2).

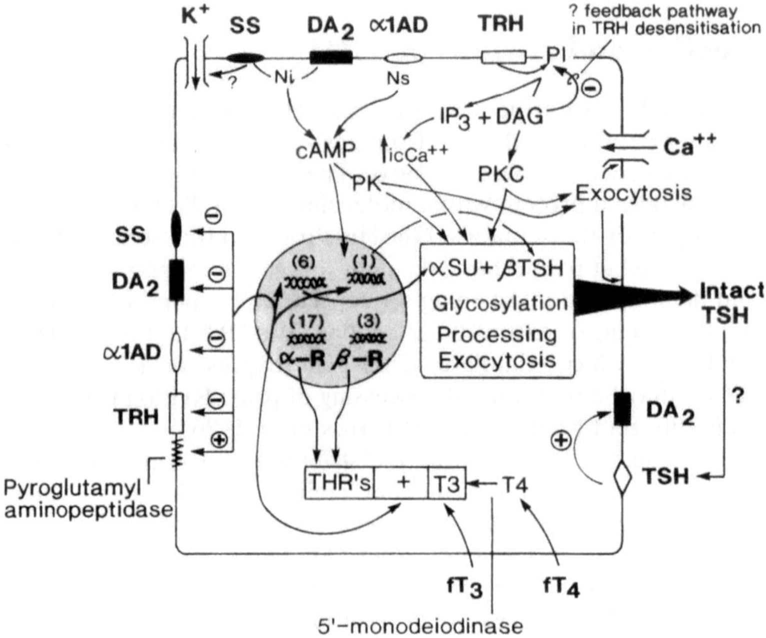

Fig. 2. Receptor-mediated actions on the thyrotroph T_3 reduces the actions of SS, DA, adrenaline and TRH probably via reduced number of corresponding receptors. These actions and the activation of pyroglutamyl aminopeptidase are probably due to binding of the activated thyroid hormone receptor (*THR*) to relevant parts of the genome. *Numbers in parentheses* indicate the chromosomal location of the genes for the α and β THRs and the α- and β-subunits of TSH. (From SCANLON and TOFT 1995, with permission)

TRH plays an important role in the post-translational processing of the oligosaccharide moieties of TSH, and hence exerts an important influence on the biological activity of TSH (MAGNER 1990). Full glycosylation of TSH is required for complete biological activity. This provides an explanation for the clinical observation that some patients with central hypothyroidism and slightly elevated basal serum TSH concentrations secrete TSH with reduced biological activity that increases after TRH administration. It is likely that alterations in both hypothalamic TRH secretion and in the response of thyrotrophs to TRH contribute to the variable biological activity of the TSH secreted by patients with different thyroid disorders (MIURA et al. 1989), and those with TSH-secreting pituitary adenomas (GESUNDHEIT et al. 1989).

D. Structure and Actions of Somatostatin

Somatostatin (SS) was originally isolated from ovine hypothalamic tissue because it inhibits GH release from anterior pituitary tissue. Subsequently, SS was found to inhibit TSH secretion in both animals and humans. The structure of the gene encoding SS in both humans (SHEN et al. 1982) and rats (MONTMINY et al. 1984) is now known. SS-producing hypothalamic neurons are found mainly in the anterior periventricular region. About half the SS in the median eminence arises from the preoptic region while the remainder arises from the suprachiasmatic and retrochiasmatic regions. A lower density of SS-producing neurons is present in the ventromedial and arcuate nuclei and also in the lateral hypothalamus (HALASZ 1986). SS is also widely distributed throughout the extrahypothalamic nervous system and other body tissues, where it exerts a wide array of inhibitory actions. It is secreted in two principal forms: a 14-amino-acid peptide and an N-terminal extended peptide (somatostatin-28). Its precursor, preproSS, is a 116-amino-acid peptide (SHEN et al. 1982; GOODMAN et al. 1983) that undergoes differential post-translational processing in different tissues to yield varying amounts of the 14- and 28-amino-acid forms of the hormone. Each of these forms is secreted into hypophyseal portal blood in physiologically relevant concentrations (MILLAR et al. 1983).

SS inhibits basal and TRH-stimulated TSH release from rat anterior pituitary cells (VALE et al. 1975), suggesting a dual control system for TSH, stimulation by TRH and inhibition by SS, analogous to that demonstrated for growth hormone: its physiological relevance was established in studies using antisera against SS. Incubation of anterior pituitary cells with anti-SS serum causes increased secretion of TSH (as well as GH), and administration of antiserum to rats increases basal serum TSH concentrations and the serum TSH responses to both cold stress and TRH (ARIMURA and SCHALLY 1976; FERLAND et al. 1976). In humans, SS administration reduces the elevated serum TSH concentrations in patients with primary hypothyroidism, reduces the serum TSH response to TRH, abolishes the nocturnal elevation in TSH secretion, and prevents TSH release after administration of dopamine antagonist drugs. SS-14 and -28 exert equipotent effects on TSH release (RODRIGUEZ-ARNAO et al. 1981). Furthermore, GH administration in humans decreases basal and TRH-stimulated TSH secretion (LIPPE et al. 1975), probably because of direct stimulatory effects of GH on hypothalamic SS release (BERELOWITZ et al. 1981). In patients with pituitary disease, TSH secretory status correlates inversely with GH secretory status (COBB et al. 1981). Despite these potent acute inhibitory effects of SS on TSH secretion in humans, long-term treatment with SS or the long-acting analogue, octreotide, does not cause hypothyroidism (PAGE et al. 1990), presumably because the great sensitivity of the thyrotrophs to any decrease in serum thyroid hormone concentrations overrides the inhibitory effect of SS in the long term.

SS binds to at least five distinct types of specific, high-affinity receptors (SSTR 1 to 5) in the anterior pituitary, brain and other tissues (GONZALES et al. 1989; KIMURA 1989). The receptor subtypes differ in binding specifities, molecular weight and linkage to adenylate cyclase. The pituitary SS receptors (predominantly SSTR 2 and SSTR 5) are negatively coupled to adenylate cyclase through the inhibitory subunit of the guanine nucleotide regulatory protein, conventionally termed Ni, a mechanism that mediates at least some of the inhibitory actions of this neuropeptide. However, SS also acts independently of cAMP by reducing calcium influx and inducing hyperpolarization of membranes through conventional G protein linkage to calcium and potassium channels, respectively (Nilsson et al. 1989) (Fig. 2).

E. Actions of Neurotransmitters

An extensive network of neurotransmitter neurons terminates on the cells bodies of the hypophysiotropic neurons, and within the interstitial spaces of the median eminence, where they regulate neuropeptide release into hypophyseal portal blood. In addition, dopamine (and possibly other neurotransmitters) is released directly into hypophyseal portal blood and exerts direct actions on anterior pituitary cells, particularly as the major physiological inhibitor of prolactin release, but to a lesser extent as a physiological inhibitor of TSH release.

As a consequence of the specialised anatomical arrangements within the hypothalamus, each of the hypophysiotropic neuronal systems that regulate TSH secretion (TRH, SS and dopamine) are, in turn, influenced by networks of other neurons that project from several brain regions. Without these projections, basal TSH secretion (in rats and presumably in humans) and feedback regulation by thyroid hormones is relatively normal, suggesting that basal TRH secretion is regulated by intrinsic hypothalamic function interacting with pituitary and thyroid hormones. In contrast, circadian rhythms of TSH and pituitary-thyroid changes in response to stress and cold exposure (in lower animals) are mediated by nerve pathways that project to the medial basal hypothalamus (Fukuda and Greer 1975).

The principal systems that influence tuberoinfundibular neurons contain a bioamine neurotransmitter (dopamine, serotonin, histamine or adrenaline), although several other neuropeptides and amino acid neurotransmitters may play a role. Virtually all the dopaminergic, noradrenergic and serotoninergic pathways that project to the hypothalamus arise from groups of nuclei located in the midbrain. Two dopaminergic systems exist within the hypothalamus: one, entirely intrinsic to the hypothalamus, arises in the arcuate nuclei, and the other projects from the midbrain. Histaminergic pathways are intrinsic to the hypothalamus, whereas adrenergic pathways arise from cell groups in the midbrain, although an intrinsic hypothalamic noradrenergic system also may exist. Opioid and γ-aminobutyric acid systems are mainly intrinsic to the hypothalamus. Cholinergic systems appear to play little part in the neuroregulation of TSH secretion (Morley 1981).

In view of the complexity of these interacting neuronal networks, it is hardly surprising that neuropharmacological attempts to dissect the relative contributions of different neurotransmitter systems to the neuroregulation of TSH secretion have proved difficult. Furthermore, certain pathways have been studied extensively in rats yet hardly at all in humans, and the lack of availability of specific neuropeptide antagonists has limited study of the direct physiological relevance of many of these molecules. Despite these problems consensus views have developed concerning the roles of several neurotransmitter pathways.

Studies using central neurotransmiter agonist and antagonist drugs have indicated the existence of stimulatory α-noradrenergic and inhibitory dopaminergic pathways in the control of TSH secretion in rats. α-Adrenergic agonists injected systemically or into the third ventricle stimulate TSH release, and α-adrenergic antagonists or catecholamine-depleting drugs block TSH responses to cold (MORLEY 1981). More precisely, it appears that α_2 pathways are stimulatory, whereas α_1 pathways are inhibitory (KRULICH 1982). It has been assumed from such in vivo studies that these neurotransmitter effects are mediated by the appropriate modulation of the release of TRH, SS or both, into hypophyseal-portal blood. A clear example of this is that the acute TSH release that follows cold stress in rats can be abolished by pretreatment with either anti-TRH antibodies or α-adrenergic antagonists, suggesting that adrenergically stimulated TRH release mediates this effect (JACKSON 1982).

The results of in vitro studies using rat hypothalamic tissue, however, are not in keeping with this attactive and simple hypothesis. For example, dopamine and dopamine-agonist drugs stimulate both TRH and SS release from rat hypothalamus, acting through the DA_2 class of dopamine receptors (LEWIS et al. 1987, 1989). This may reflect a general action of DA_2 receptors to mediate enhanced neuropeptide release at the level of the median eminence, in contrast to the usual inhibitory action of DA_2 agonists at the level of the anterior pituitary.

Although little precise knowledge exists regarding central mechanisms, it is clear that dopamine and adrenaline exert opposing actions on TSH release directly at the anterior pituitary level. Furthermore, both these molecules are present in rat hypophyseal portal blood at higher concentrations than in peripheral blood and at concentrations that could exert physiological actions on the thyrotrophs (BEN-JONATHAN et al. 1977; JOHNSTON et al. 1983). Dopamine inhibits TSH release from rat (FOORD et al. 1980) and bovine (COOPER et al. 1983) anterior pituitary cells in a dose-related, stereospecific way, and there is striking parallelism between the inhibition of TSH and prolactin by dopamine and dopamine-agonist drugs (FOORD et al. 1983). As with prolactin, this inhibitory action on TSH release is mediated by DA_2 receptors (FOORD et al. 1983) that are negatively coupled to adenylate cyclase. TSH release by thyrotroph cells from hypothyroid animals is more sensitive to the inhibitory effects of dopamine, which may reflect increased DA_2 receptor number rather than affinity (FOORD et al. 1984). In contrast, the sensitivity of prolactin to the inhibitory effects of dopamine is reduced in lactotroph cells from hypothyroid animals (FOORD et al. 1984, 1986), a phenomenon that may contribute to the hyperprolactinaemia that occurs in some patients with primary hypothyroidism.

Evidence from in vitro studies using rat anterior pituitary cells suggests that TSH may specifically regulate its own release through the induction of DA_2 receptors on the thyrotroph cells (FOORD et al. 1985), perifused cells showing little dopaminergic sensitivity due to rapid dispersion of locally released TSH. These data indicate a mechanism for the ultrashort-loop feedback control of TSH secretion that is dependent on the functional integrity of the hypothalamo-pituitary axis and consequent catecholamine supply (Fig. 2).

In addition to its acute inhibitory effects on TSH secretion in vitro, dopamine also decreases the levels of α-subunit and TSH-β-subunit mRNAs and gene transcription by up to 75% in cultured anterior pituitary cells from hypothyroid rats. These effects occur within a few minutes and can be reversed by activation of adenylate cyclase with forskolin (SHUPNIK et al. 1986). Similar actions of dopamine have been described in relation to prolactin gene expression.

In contrast to dopamine, adrenergic activation stimulates TSH release by cultured rat and bovine anterior pituitary cells in a dose-related stereospecific fashion. This effect is mediated by high-affinity, α_1-adrenoreceptors (PETERS et al. 1983a; KLIBANSKI et al. 1983; DIEGUEZ et al. 1984), and both α_1-adrenoreceptors and α_1-receptor-mediated TSH release are reduced in cells from hypothyroid animals (DIEGUEZ et al. 1985). Quantitatively, the adrenergic release of TSH is almost equivalent to that induced by TRH (DIEGUEZ et al. 1984). Together, at maximal dosage, these two agents have additive effects on TSH release, indicating activation of separate intracellular pathways. It is likely that dopamine and adrenaline exert their direct actions on the thyrotrophs by opposing actions on cAMP generation, with DA_2 receptors being negatively linked to adenylate cyclase and α_1-adrenoreceptors being positively linked (Fig. 2).

In humans, it is well established that dopamine has a physiological inhibitory role in the control of TSH release, and some data suggest a stimulatory α-adrenergic pathway. In contrast to the situation in animals, evidence for direct effects of dopaminergic and adrenergic manipulation on TSH release by normal human pituitary cells is lacking. Data from the use of dopamine, dopamine agonists and specific dopamine-receptor antagonist drugs such as domperidone, which does not penetrate the blood-brain barrier to any appreciable extent, suggest that dopamine-induced decreases in TSH secretion are a direct pituitary or median eminence action mediated by the DA_2 class of dopamine receptor (BURROW et al. 1977; SCANLON et al. 1977, 1979).

The dopaminergic inhibition of TSH release varies according to sex, thyroid status, time of day and prolactin secretory status. TSH release after endogenous dopamine disinhibition with dopamine-receptor-blocking drugs, such as metoclopramide and domperidone, is greater in women than in men (SCANLON et al. 1979). It is assumed that oestrogens determine this effect, but the mechanism of action is unknown. The dopaminergic inhibition of TSH release, like the stimulation of TSH release by TRH, is also greater in patients with mild or subclinical hypothyroidism than in normal subjects or severely hypothyroid patients (SCANLON et al. 1980a). The mechanisms that underlie this biphasic relationship between the dopaminergic inhibition of TSH release and thyroid status are not known, but data from in vitro studies of anterior pituitary cells from hypothyroid rats suggest an increase in dopamine-receptor capacity rather than affinity (FOORD et al. 1984). Also, the concentration of dopamine in hypophyseal portal blood of thyroidectomised rats is greater than that of sham-operated rat. This is due to increased activity of tyrosine hydroxylase in the median eminence, an effect that can be reversed by thyroid hormone replacement (REYMOND et al. 1987; WANG et al. 1989). In addition to its effects on the release of TSH, dopamine also inhibits the release of α-subunit and TSH-β-subunit, the greatest effect occurring in patients with primary hypothyroidism (SCANLON et al. 1981; PETERS et al. 1983b).

Only limited data are available on the adrenergic control of TSH release in humans. α-Adrenergic blockade with phentolamine, which does not readily cross the blood-brain barrier, or with thymoxamine, which does, inhibits the serum TSH response to TRH (ZGLICZYNSKI and KANIEWSKI 1980) and reduces but does not abolish the nocturnal rise in TSH secretion (VALCAVI et al. 1987). Overall, these data suggest a small stimulatory role for endogenous adrenergic pathways in TSH control in humans. The catecholaminergic control of TSH secretion appears to act as a fine-tuning mechanism rather than being of primary importance. This is not to say that the effects of catecholamines are so small as to be without consequence. For example, acute dopaminergic blockade in humans releases enough TSH to elicit subsequent release of thyroid hormones. As with SS-agonist analogues, however, chronic administration of catecholaminergic drugs does not lead to long-term alterations in thyroid status, reflecting the action of compensatory mechanisms to maintain TSH secretion and euthyroidism.

The role of the serotoninergic system in the control of TSH release in animals and humans is unclear, both stimulatory and inhibitory actions having been described (MORLEY 1981; SMYTHE et al. 1982). Opioid pathways appear to play an important role in the inhibitory control of TSH secretion in rats because opioid peptides decrease basal TSH secretion. Their action can be blocked by the specific antagonist naloxone (SHARP et al. 1981), which also blocks the stress-induced fall in TSH secretion (JUDD and HEDGE 1982). In humans, however, endogenous opioids may have a stimulatory effect on TSH secretion, especially during the nocturnal TSH surge (SAMUELS et al. 1994). A variety of other neuropeptides including neurotensin, vasoactive intestinal polypeptide, bombesin, vasopressin, oxytocin, substance P and cholecystokinin can produce small alterations in TSH secretion both in vitro and in vivo in animals, but the lack of suitable specific antagonist drugs has not allowed adequate physiological studies to be undertaken. These molecules should be added to the list of agents that can affect TSH secretion, but their relevance is uncertain.

F. Actions of Cytokines and Inflammatory Mediators

Tumour necrosis factor (TNF; cachectin) is a peptide produced by macrophages that acts as an inflammatory mediator and can cause many of the clinical phenomena that accompany severe systemic illness. Interleukin-1 (IL-1) is a cytokine produced by many cells, including monocytes, that stimulates B- and T-lymphocytes to produce a range of other cytokines and lymphokines. Both TNF and IL-1β inhibit TSH secretion in rats and mice (DUBUIS et al. 1988; OZAWA et al. 1988; PANG et al. 1989), while IL-1β causes a relative and inappropriate reduction in TRH gene expression in the paraventricular nucleus in the face of low thyroid hormone concentrations (KAKUCSKA et al. 1994). These molecules each produce a biochemical pattern similar to that which occurs in patients with acute non-thyroidal illness (HERMUS et al. 1992; PANG et al. 1993) and they also activate the hypothalamo-pituitary-adrenal axis (WOLOSKI et al. 1985; BESODOVSKY et al. 1986; BERNTON et al. 1987) probably via stimulation of the release of hypothalamic corticotrophin-releasing hormone (SAPOLSKY et al. 1987). This family of molecules plays a crucial role in mediating and coordinating the thyroidal and adrenal responses to non-thyroidal illness. IL-1β is produced by rat anterior pituitary cells, and its release from them can be stimulated by bacterial lipopolysaccharide. It colocalises with TSH in thyrotroph cells (KOENIG et al. 1990). Presumably IL-1β subserves an important autocrine or paracrine role in anterior pituitary control, as has also been suggested for the IL-1-dependent cytokine IL-6, which is also produced by rat anterior pituitary cells (SPANGELO et al. 1990), particularly folliculo-stellate cells (VANKELECOM et al. 1989).

G. Physiological and Secondary TSH Changes

Alterations in TSH secretion occur in relation to both the pattern and degree of change in basal TSH secretion or in the pattern and degree of serum TSH responses to TRH or dopamine-receptor blockade. A clear circadian variation is evident in serum TSH concentrations. In most humans, serum TSH concentrations begin to rise several hours before the onset of sleep, reaching maximal concentrations between 2300 and 0400 hours and declining gradually thereafter, with the lowest concentrations occurring at about 1100 hours. The concentrations during the nocturnal surge are sometimes slightly above the normal range reported by most clinical laboratories. Sleep itself modulates TSH secretion, by reducing pulse amplitude rather than frequency (PARKER et al. 1987; BRABANT et al. 1990), but the underlying mechanisms are not clear. Furthermore, a seasonal variation in TSH secretion has been described in patients with primary hypothyroidism receiving T_4 therapy; some of these patients have higher basal serum TSH concentrations in the winter than in the summer (KONNO and MORIKAWA 1982). This may be a consequence of temperature effects on the peripheral metabolism of thyroid hormones, but such a difference was not found in euthyroid subjects (BRABANT et al. 1989). Although there is some evidence that oestrogens can enhance and androgens reduce serum TSH responses to TRH, no sex-related difference in amplitude or frequency of circadian TSH changes has been found (Brabant et al. 1989).

TSH is secreted in a pulsatile manner with increases in pulse amplitude and frequency at night (Rossmanith et al. 1988; Brabant et al. 1990). Patients with severe primary hypothyroidism have increased pulse amplitude throughout the day but loss of the usual nocturnal increase in pulse amplitude. The pulses of TSH-α and the gonadotrophins are concordant, consistent with the operation of a common hypothalamic pulse generator (Samuels et al. 1990).

The circadian and pulsatile changes in TSH secretion are not secondary to peripheral factors, such as changes in serum T_4 and T_3 concentrations, haemoconcentration, or changes in cortisol secretion (Salvador et al. 1988), although the latter may modulate TSH rhythms. Furthermore, circadian changes in serum TSH concentrations can be detected in some patients with mild thyrotoxicosis (Evans et al. 1986), suggesting that central mechanisms can to some extent override the powerful negative-feedback effects of thyroid hormones at the pituitary level.

Basal serum TSH concentrations rise slightly after serum cortisol concentrations are lowered by 11β-hydroxylase inhibition with metyrapone (Re et al. 1976), suggesting that cortisol exerts a small inhibitory influence on TSH secretion. Furthermore, pharmacological doses of glucocorticoids acutely inhibit basal TSH secretion and abolish the circadian variation in serum TSH concentrations (Brabant et al. 1989). This mechanism may well explain the reduction in basal and TRH-stimulated serum TSH concentrations and in circadian TSH changes that occurs in patients with depression (Souetre et al. 1988; Bartalena et al. 1990a), after major surgery (Bartalena et al. 1990b) and in non-thyroidal illness. Total abolition of the circadian rhythm of cortisol with metyrapone, however, did not cause disruption of overall circadian TSH changes, although a small but significant decrease did occur in the acrophase and amplitude of the TSH profile (Salvador et al. 1985).

The central mechanisms that underlie TSH pulsatility and rhythmicity are unknown. Pulsatile TRH release does not appear to be involved in TSH pulse frequency although it may influence amplitude (Samuels et al. 1993). Pulsatility is probably mediated in part by signals from the suprachiasmatic nuclei of the hypothalamus. These nuclei are paired structures situated just above the optic chiasm that initiate intrinsic circadian rhythmicity, the timing of which can be influenced by non-visual nerve impulses arising in the retina (Moore 1983). Although both dopamine and dopamine agonists acutely abolish the circadian change in TSH secretion (Sowers et al. 1982; Brabant et al. 1989), endogenous dopaminergic pathways probably do not play a role in determining the circadian changes in TSH secretion. The nocturnal increase in TSH secretion is not due to a decline in dopaminergic inhibition because dopaminergic inhibition of TSH release is greater at night than during the day (Scanlon et al. 1980b; Rossmanith et al. 1988). Dopamine is, however, a determinant of TSH pulse amplitude (but not frequency) (Rossmanith et al.

1988). It appears that dopamine acts as a fine-tuning control to dampen TSH pulsatility, presumably to maintain basal TSH concentrations and hence thyroid function in as steady a state as possible. Why the serum TSH response to dopamine blockade is greater at night than during the day is not known. It is unlikely to be due to increased central dopaminergic activity, since the serum prolactin response to dopamine blockade is the same during the day and night (Salvador et al. 1988).

Similarly, α-adrenergic pathways do not play a primary role in determining TSH circadian rhythmicity, since α-adrenergic blockade with thymoxamine, which penetrates the blood-brain barrier, did not affect the circadian pattern of TSH secretion, although serum TSH concentrations decreased slightly throughout the entire period of study (Valcavi et al. 1987). Serotonin, although present in high concentrations in the suprachiasmatic nucleus, does not play any major role in circadian TSH secretion in humans (O'Malley et al. 1984), nor does the pineal hormone melatonin (Strassman et al. 1988), which in animals exerts an inhibitory effect on hypothalamo-pituitary-thyroid function (Gordon et al. 1980). TSH may regulate its own secretion through an increase in dopamine receptors at the level of the thyrotrophs (Foord et al. 1985), a finding that could explain the higher serum TSH and unaltered serum prolactin responses to dopamine blockade at the time of greatest TSH secretion (Salvador et al. 1988). A further possible contributor to the changes in circadian TSH secretion in rats is the diurnal variation in the activity of anterior pituitary T_4-5′-deiodinase in this species (Murakami et al. 1988).

Cold exposure in rats causes an acute rise in serum TSH concentrations that is accompanied by an increase in hypothalamic TRH gene expression and increased TRH release (Zoeller et al. 1990; Rage et al. 1994). A similar phenomenon occurs in human neonates, but is unusual in adults; when it does occur the increase is very small. The cold-induced effect in rats can be abolished by either passive immunisation with anti-TRH antibodies or α-adrenergic blockade, indicating that adrenergic release of hypothalamic TRH mediates the phenomenon (Jackson 1982; Morley 1981; Scanlon et al. 1980). Lesions that affect the temperature-regulating centre of the preoptic nucleus of the hypothalamus abolish the serum TSH response to cold stres but do not cause hypothyroidism (Morley 1981).

Aging itself causes a slight decrease in TSH secretion. Thyroid secretion, however, changes little, due to a resetting of the threshold of TSH inhibition by thyroid hormones as a result of increased pituitary conversion of T_4 to T_3, increased T_4 uptake by thyrotrophs (Lewis et al. 1991) or decreased T_4 and T_3 clearance. In one study of healthy elderly subjects 5% had low basal serum TSH concentrations and those same subjects had a reduced serum TSH response to TRH (Finucane et al. 1989). In addition, TSH pulse amplitude was reduced, with preservation of the frequency of pulsatility and the overall pattern of circadian change (Van Coeverden et al. 1989). These data should introduce caution into the use of TSH assays alone in the assessment of thyroid function in the elderly. The underlying mechanism is unclear, but the change in TSH secretion may reflect an adaptive mechanism to the reduced need for thyroid hormones in the elderly (VAN COEVERDEN et al. 1989).

Calorie restriction causes a small decrease in basal and TRH-stimulated serum TSH concentrations despite a decline in serum T_3 concentrations (BORST et al. 1983). In rats this is associated with reduced hypothalamic TRH gene expression (BLAKE et al. 1991; SHI et al. 1993). The components of the decrease in TSH secretion in humans are a reduction in the daytime serum TSH concentration and in the nocturnal increase in TSH secretion, with an overall decrease in TSH pulse amplitude (ROMIJN et al. 1990). Passive immunisation with SS antiserum abolishes the starvation-induced decline in TSH secretion in rats (HUGUES et al. 1986), indicating a mediating role of hypothalamic SSergic pathways secondary to unknown metabolic signals. There is no evidence of increased dopaminergic inhibition of TSH secretion during caloric restriction (MORA et al. 1980; RODJMARK 1983), and TRH administration does not reverse the acute decline in serum TSH concentrations during fasting (SPENCER et al. 1983).

In rats stress causes an acute decline in serum TSH concentrations. In humans, surgical stress causes transient acute lowering of serum TSH (BARTALENA et al. 1990b). This occurs despite a fall in serum free T_3 concentrations, whereas serum free T_4 concentrations do not change (WARTOFSKY and BURMAN 1982; BARTALENA et al. 1990b). In animals, both opioids and dopamine may play a role in this stress phenomenon, whereas in humans glucocorticoids and dopamine have been implicated (JUDD and HEDGE 1982; WARTOFSKY and BURMAN 1982; ZALAGA et al. 1985). As with the effects of caloric restriction, these stress phenomena bear some resemblance to the altered neuroregulation of TSH that can occur in non-thyroidal illness and in certain neuropsychiatric disorders. Although basal serum TSH concentrations are usually normal in patients with both acute and chronic non-thyroidal illness, they may be either low or slightly raised. In addition to the frequent use of pharmacological agents such as glucocorticoids and dopamine that acutely inhibit TSH secretion (WEHMAN et al. 1985; HAMBLIN et al. 1986), intrinsic central suppression of thyrotroph function is common, as illustrated by the abolition of the nocturnal increase in serum TSH concentrations in up to 60% of acutely ill patients in the presence of low serum free T_3 concentrations (ROMIJN et al. 1990). However, true central hypothyroidism is rare in these patients, who usually, although not always, have normal serum free T_4 concentrations (FABER et al. 1987; ROMIJN et al. 1990).

Abnormalities in TSH secretion also occur in patients with anorexia nervosa and endogenous depression. A common abnormality is a reduced serum TSH response to TRH (MORA et al. 1980; LOOSEN 1988). Even more common is loss of the nocturnal increase in TSH secretion (BARTALENA et al. 1990a), which together with the low serum free thyroid hormone, ferritin, and sex hormone-binding globulin concentrations may indicate central hypothyroidism. Once again, the mechanisms are unclear. Dopamine is not involved in central TSH suppression in anorexia nervosa (MORA et al. 1980), but increased serum cortisol concentrations may contribute; both serum cortisol and body temperature changes have been implicated in depression (SOUETRE et al. 1988; BARTALENA et al. 1990a).

It seems clear that, in addition to peripheral alterations in thyroid hormone economy usually manifest as low serum free T_3, high reverse T_3 and normal free T_4 concentrations, there is central suppression of thyrotroph function in patients with severe non-thyroidal illness, for example, with heart failure, infection, diabetes mellitus (KABADI 1984; SMALL et al. 1986) or chronic renal failure (POKRAY et al. 1974). The precise initiating signals and underlying mechanisms are unknown, although alterations in opioidergic, dopaminergic and somatostatinergic activity may each contribute. In addition, peripheral, glucocorticoid-mediated inhibitory feedback probably plays an important role, particularly in acutely ill patients (DELITALA et al. 1987). Finally, activation of the cytokine pathways involving tumor necrosis factor-α and IL-β, each of which inhibit TSH and stimulate ACTH release in animals (DUBUIS et al. 1988; OZAWA et al. 1988), may be a crucial mediating event in the coordination of the thyroidal and adrenal responses to stress and non-thyroidal illness.

References

Arimura A, Schally AV (1976) Increase in basal and thyrotropin-releasing hormone stimulated secretion of thyrotropin by passive immunisation with antiserum to somatostatin. Endocrinology 98:1069–1072

Bartalena L, Placidi GF, Martino E et al (1990a) Nocturnal serum thyrotropin (TSH) surge and the TSH response to TSH-releasing hormone: dissociated behaviour in untreated depressives. J Clin Endocrinol Metab 71:650–655

Bartalena L, Martino E, Brandi LS, Falcone M, Pacchiarotti A, Ricci C, Bogazzi F, Grasso L, Mammoli C, Pinchera A (1990b) Lack of nocturnal serum thyrotropin surge after surgery. J Clin Endocrinol Metab 70:293–296

Ben-Jonathan N, Oliver C, Weiner HJ, Mical RS, Porter JC (1977) Dopamine in hypophyseal portal plasma of the rat during the estrous cycle and throughout pregnancy. Endocrinology 100:452–458

Berelowitz M, Firestone SL, Frohman LA (1981) Effects of growth hormone excess and deficiency on hypothalamic somatostatin content and release and on tissue somatostatin distribution. Endocrinology 109:714–719

Bernton EW, Beach JE, Holaday, Smallridge RC, Fein HG (1987) Release of multiple hormones by a direct action of interleukin-1 on pituitary cells. Science 238:519–521

Besedovsky H, Del Rey A, Sorkin E, Dinarello CA (1986) Immuno-regulatory feedback between interleukin-1 and glucocorticoid hormones. Science 233:652–654

Blake NG, Eckland DJ, Foster OJ, Lightman SL (1991) Inhibition of hypothalamic thyrotropin-releasing hormone messenger ribonucleic acid during food deprivation. Endocrinology 129:2714–2718

Borst GC, Osburne RC, O'Brian JT, Georges LP, Burman KD (1983) Fasting decreases thyrotropin responsiveness to thyrotropin-releasing hormone: a potential cause of misinterpretation of thyroid function tests in the critically ill. J Clin Endocrinol Metab 57:380–383

Brabant G, Ocran K, Ranft U, von zur Muhlen A, Hesch RD (1989) Physiological regulation of thyrotropin. Biochimie 71:293–301

Brabant G, Frank K, Ranft U et al (1990) Physiological regulation of circadian and pulsatile thyrotropin secretion in normal man and woman. J Clin Endocrinol Metab 70:403–409
Bruhn TO, Rondeel JM, Bolduc TG, Jackson IM (1994) Thyrotropin-releasing hormone (TRH) gene expression in the anterior pituitary. I. Presence of pro-TRH messenger ribonucleic acid and pro-TRH-derived peptide in a sub-population of somatotrophs. Endocrinology 134:815–820
Burrow GN, May PB, Spaulding SW, Donabedian RK (1977) TRH and dopamine interactions affecting pituitary hormone secretion. J Clin Endocrinol Metab 45:65–72
Carr FE, Galloway RJ, Reid AH, Kaseem LL, Dhillon G, Fein HG, Smallridge RC (1991) Thyrotropin-releasing hormone regulation of thyrotropin beta-subunit gene expression involves intracellular calcium and protein kinase C. Biochemistry 30:3721–3728
Carr FE, Fein HG, Fisher CU, Wessendorf MW, Smallridge RC (1992) A cryptic peptide (160–169) of thyrotropin-releasing hormone prohormone demonstrates biological activity in vivo and in vitro. Endocrinology 131:2653–2658
Carr FE, Reid AH, Wessendorf MW (1993) A cryptic peptide from the preprothyrotropin-releasing hormone precursor stimulates thyrotropin gene expression. Endocrinology 133:809–814
Cobb WE, Reichlin S, Jackson IMD (1981) Growth hormone secretory status is a determinant of the thyrotropin response to thyrotropin-releasing hormone in euthyroid patients with hypothalamic pituitary disease. J Clin Endocrinol Metab 52:324–329
Cooper DS, Klibanski A, Ridgway EC (1983) Dopaminergic modulation of TSH and its subunits: in vivo and in vitro studies. Clin Endocrinol (Oxf) 18:265–276
Croissandeau G, Grouselle D, Li JY, Roche M, Peillon F, Le Dafniet M (1994) Hypothyroidism increases TRH and TRH precursor levels in rat anterior pituitary. Biochem Biophys Res Commun 201:1248–1254
Delitala G, Tomasi P, Virdis R (1987) Prolactin, growth hormone and thyrotropin-thyroid hormone secretion during stress states in man. Baillieres Clin Endocrinol Metab 1:391–414
Dieguez C, Foord SM, Peters JR, Hall R, Scanlon MF (1984) Interactions among epinephrine, thyrotropin (TSH)-releasing hormone, dopamine and somatostatin in the control of TSH secretion in vitro. Endocrinology 114:957–961
Dieguez C, Foord SM, Peters JR, Hall R, Scanlon MF (1985) α_1-Adrenoreceptors and α_1-adrenoreceptor-mediated thyrotropin release in cultures of euthyroid and hypothyroid rat anterior pituitary cells. Endocrinology 117:624–630
Dubuis JM, Dayer JM, Siegrist-Kaiser CA, Burger AG (1988) Human recombinant interleukin-1β decreases plasma thyroid hormone and thyroid stimulating hormone levels in rats. Endocrinology 123:2175–2181
Evans RM (1988) The steroid and thyroid hormone receptor super family. Science 240:889–895
Evans PJ, Weeks I, Jones MK, Woodhead JS, Scanlon MF (1986) The circadian variation of thyrotropin in patients with primary thyroidal disease. Clin Endocrinol (Oxf) 24:343–348
Faber K, Kirkegaard C, Rasmussen B, Westh H, Busch-Sorensen M, Jensen IW (1987) Pituitary-thyroid axis in critical illness. J Clin Endocrinol Metab 65:315–320
Ferland L, Labrie F, Jobin M et al (1976) Physiological role of somatostatin in the control of growth hormone and thyro-tropin secretion. Biochem Biophys Res Commun 68:149–156
Finucane P, Rudra T, Church H, Hsu R, Newcombe R, Pathy MSJ, Scanlon MF, Woodhead JS (1989) Thyroid function tests in elderly patients with and without an acute illness. Age Ageing 18:398–402
Foord SM, Peters JR, Scanlon MF, Rees Smith B, Hall R (1980) Dopaminergic control of TSH secretion in isolated rat pituitary cells. FEBS Lett 121:257–259

Foord SM, Peters JR, Dieguez C, Scanlon MF, Hall R (1983) Dopamine receptors on intact anterior pituitary cells in culture: functional association with the inhibition of prolactin and thyrotropin. Endocrinology 112:1567–1577
Foord SM, Peters JR, Dieguez C, Jasani B, Hall R, Scanlon MF (1984) Hypothyroid pituitary cells in culture: an analysis of TSH and PRL responses to dopamine and dopamine receptor binding. Endocrinology 115:407–415
Foord SM, Peters JR, Dieguez C, Shewring AG, Hall R, Scanlon MF (1985) TSH regulates thyrotroph responsiveness to dopamine in vitro. Endocrinology 118:1319–1326
Foord SM, Peters JR, Dieguez C, Lewis MD, Lewis BM, Hall R, Scanlon MF (1986) Thyroid stimulating hormone. In: Lightman S, Everitt B (eds) Neuroendocrinology. Blackwell Scientific, London, pp 450–471
Fukuda H, Green MA (1975) The effect of basal hypothalamic deafferentiation in the nictohemeralAQ17 rhythm of plasma TSH. Endocrinology 97:749–754
Gesundheit N, Petrick PA, Nissim M, Dahlberg PA, Doppman JL, Emerson CH, Braverman LE, Oldfield EH, Weintraub BD (1989) Thyrotropin-secreting pituitary adnenomas: clinical and biochemical heterogeneity. Ann Intern Med 111:827–835
Gonzalez BJ, Leroux P, Bodenant C, Laquerriere A, Coy DH, Vaudry H (1989) Ontogeny of somatostatin receptors in the rat brain: biochemical and autoradiographic study. Neuroscience 29:629–644
Goodman RH, Aron DC, Roos BA (1983) Rat-preprosomatostatin: structure and processing by microsomal membranes. J Biol Chem 258:5570–5573
Gordon J, Morley JE, Hershman JM (1980) Melatonin and the thyroid. Horm Metab Res 12:71–73
Greer MA, Sato N, Wang X, Greer SE, McAdams S (1993) Evidence that the major physiological role of TRH in the hypothalamic paraventricular nuclei may be to regulate the set-point for thyroid hormone negative feedback on the pituitary thyrotroph. Neuroendocrinology 57:569–575
Haisenleder DJ, Yasin M, Yasin A, Marshall JC (1993) Regulation of prolactin, thyrotropin subunit, and gonadotropin subunit gene expression by pulsatile or continuous calcium signals. Endocrinology 133:2055–2061
Halasz B (1986) A view of the hypothalamic control of the anterior pituitary. In: Muller EE, MacLeod RM (eds) Neuroendocrine perspectives, vol 5,1. Elsevier, Amsterdam
Hamblin PS, Dyer SA, Mohr VS, Le Grand BA, Lim CF, Tuxen DV, Topliss DJ, Stockigt JR (1986) Relationship between thyrotropin and thyroxine changes during recovery from severe hypothyroxinaemia of critical illness. J Clin Endocrinol Metab 62:717–722
Hermus RM, Sweep CG, van der Meer MJ, Ross HA, Smals AG, Benraad TJ, Kloppenborg PW (1992) Continuous infusion of interleukin-1 beta induces a nonthyroidal illness syndrome in the rat. Endocrinology 131:2139–2146
Hinkle PM, Perrone MH, Schonbrunn A (1981) Mechanism of thyroid hormone inhibition of thyrotropin-releasing hormone action. Endocrinology 108:199–205
Hugues JN, Enjalbert A, Moyse E, Shu C, Voirol MJ, Sebaoun J, Epelbaum J (1986) Differential effects of passive immunization with somatostatin antiserum on adenohypophysial hormone secretions in starved rats. J Endocrinol 109:169–174
Jackson IMD (1982) Thyrotropin releasing hormone. N Engl J Med 306:145–155
Jackson IMD (1989) Controversies in TRH biosynthesis and strategies towards the identification of a TRH precursor. Ann N Y Acad Sci 553:7–10
Jackson IMD, Wu P, Lechan RM (1985) Immunohistochemical localisation in the rat brain of the precursor for thyrotropin-releasing hormone. Science 229:1097–1099
Johnston CA, Gibbs DM, Negro-Vilar A (1983) High concentrations of epinephrine derived from a central source and of 5-hydroxyindole-3-acetic acid in hypophysial portal plasma. Endocrinology 113:819–821

Jones KE, Chin WW (1991) Differential regulation of thyroid hormone receptor messenger ribonucleic acid levels by thyrotropin-releasing hormone. Endocrinology 128:1763–1768

Judd AM, Hedge GA (1982) The role of opioid peptides in controlling thyroid stimulating hormone release. Life Sci 31:2529–2536

Kabadi UM (1984) Impaired pituitary thyrotroph function in uncontrolled type II diabetes mellitus: normalisation on recovery. J Clin Endocrinol Metab 59:521–525

Kaji H, Hinkle PM (1987) Regulation of thyroid hormone receptors and responses by thyrotropin-releasing hormone in GH4C1 cells. Endocrinology 121:1697–1704

Kakucska I, Rand W, Lechan RM (1992) Thyrotropin-releasing hormone gene expression in the hypothalamic paraventricular nucleus is dependent upon feedback regulation by both triiodothyronine and thyroxine. Endocrinology 130:2845–2850

Kakucska I, Romero LI, Clark BD, Rondeel JM, Qi Y, Alex S, Emerson CH, Lechan RM (1994) Suppression of thyrotropin-releasing hormone gene expression by interleukin-1-beta in the rat: implications for nonthyroidal illness. Neuroendocrinology 59:129–137

Kim DS, Ahn SK, Yoon JH, Hong SH, Kim KE, Maurer RA, Park SD (1994) Involvement of a cAMP-responsive DNA element in mediating TRH responsiveness of the human thyrotropin alpha-subunit gene. Mol Endocrinol 8:528–536

Kimura N (1989) Developmental change and molecular properties of somatostatin receptors in the rat cerebral cortex. Biochem Biophys Res Commun 160:72–78

Klibanski A, Milbury PE, Chin WW, Ridgway EC (1983) Direct adrenergic stimulation of the release of thyrotropin and its subunits from the thyrotrope in vitro. Endocrinology 113:1244–1249

Koenig JI, Snow K, Clark BD, Toni R, Cannon JG, Shaw AR, Dinarelio CA, Reichlin S, Lee SL, Lechan RM (1990) Intrinsic pituitary interleukin-1 beta is induced by bacterial lipopolysaccharide. Endocrinology 126:3053–3058

Konno N, Morikawa K (1982) Seasonal variation of serum thyrotropin concentration and thyrotropin response to thyrotropin-releasing hormone in patients with primary hypothyroidism on constant replacement dosage of thyroxine. J Clin Endocrinol Metab 54:1118–1124

Krulich L (1982) Neurotransmitter control of thyrotropin secretion. Neuroendocrinology 35:139–144

Lechan RM, Wu P, Jackson IMD et al (1986) Thyrotropin releasing hormone precursor: characterisation in rat brain. Science 231:159–161

Lewis BM, Dieguez C, Lewis MD, Scanlon MF (1987) Dopamine stimulates release of thyrotrophin-releasing hormone from perfused intact rat hypothalamus via hypothalamic D_2 receptors. J Endocrinol 115:419–424

Lewis BM, Dieguez C, Ham J, Page MD, Creagh FM, Peters JR, Scanlon MF (1989) Effects of glucose on TRH, GHRH, somatostatin and LHRH release from rat hypothalamus in vitro. J Neuroendocrinol 1:437–441

Lewis GF, Alessi CA, Imperial JG, Refetoff S (1991) Low serum free thyroxine index in ambulating elderly is due to a resetting of the threshold of thyrotropin feedback suppression. J Clin Endocrinol Metab 73:843–849

Lippe BM, Van Herle AJ, La Franchi SH et al (1975) Reversible hypothyroidism in growth hormone deficient children treated with growth hormone. J Clin Endocrinol Metab 40:612–618

Loosen PT (1988) Thyroid function in affective disorders and alcholism. Endocrinol Metab Clin North Am 17:55–82

Magner JA (1990) Thyroid-stimulating hormone: biosynthesis, cell biology and bioactivity. Endocr Rev 11:354–385

Mason ME, Friend KE, Copper J, Shupnik MA (1993) Pit-1/GHF-1 binds to TRH-sensitive regions of the rat thyrotropin beta gene. Biochemistry 32:8932–8938

Millar RP, Sheward RJ, Wegener I, Fink G (1983) Somatostatin 28 is a hormonally active peptide secreted into hypophysial portal vessel blood. Brin Res 260:334–337

Miura Y, Perkel VS, Papenberg KA, Johnson MJ, Magner JA (1989) Concanavalin-A, lentil and ricin affinity binding characteristics of human thyrotropin: differences in the sialylation of thyrotropin in sera of euthyroid, primary, and central hypothyroid patients. J Clin Endocrinol Metab 69:985–995

Montminy MR, Goodman RH, Horovitch SJ, Habener JF (1984) Primary structure of the gene encoding rat pre-prosomatostatin. Proc Natl Acad Sci USA 81:3337–3340

Moore RY (1983) Organisation and function of a nervous system circadian oscillator. Fed Proc 42:2783–2789

Mora B, Hassanyeh F, Schapira K et al (1980) Calorie restriction, thyroid status and inhibitory dopaminergic control of thyrotrophin secretion in man. In: Stockigt JR, Nagataki S (eds) Proceedings of Australian Academy of Science. Thyroid research VIII. Proceedings of the VIIIth international thyroid congress, pp 59–61

Morley JE (1981) Neuroendocrine control of thyrotropin secretion. Endocr Rev 2:396–436

Murakami M, Tanaka K, Greer MA (1988) There is a nyctohemeral rhythm of type II iodothyronine 5′-deiodinase activity in rat anterior pituitary. Endocrinology 123:1631–1635

Nilsson T, Arkhammar P, Rorsman P, Berggren P-O (1989) Suppression of insulin release by galanin and somatostatin is mediated by a G-protein. An effect involving repolarisation and reduction in cytoplasmic free Ca^{2+} concentration. J Biol Chem 264:973–980

O'Malley BP, Jennings PE, Cook N, Barnette DB, Rosenthal FD (1984) The role of serotonin in the control of TSH and prolactin release in euthyroid subjects as assessed by the administration of ketanserin (5-HT_2 antagonist) and zimelidine (5-HT re-uptake inhibitor). Psychoneuroendocrinology 9:13–19

Ozawa M, Sato K, Han DC, Kawakami M, Tsushima T, Shizume K (1988) Effects of tumor necrosis factor-α/cachectin on thyroid hormone metabolism in mice. Endocrinology 123:1461–1467

Page MD, Millward ME, Hourihan M, Hall R, Scanlon MF (1990) Long-term treatment of acromegaly with a long-acting analogue of somatostatin, octreotide. J Med 74:189–201

Pang XP, Hershman JM, Mirell CJ, Pekary AE (1989) Impairment of hypothalamic-pituitary-thyroid function in rats treated with human recombinant tumour necrosis factor-a (cachectin). Endocrinology 125:76–84

Pang XP, Yoshimura M, Hershman JM (1993) Suppression of rat thyrotroph and thyroid cell function by tumor necrosis factor-alpha. Thyroid 3:325–330

Parker DC, Rossman LG, Pekary AE, Hershman JM (1987) Effect of 64-hour sleep deprivation on the circadian waveform of thyrotropin (TSH): further evidence of sleep-related inhibition of TSH release. J Clin Endocrinol Metab 64:157–161

Peters JR, Foord SM, Dieguez C, Scanlon MF, Hall R (1983a) α_1-Adrenoreceptors on intact rat anterior pituitary cells: correlation with thyrotropin release. Endocrinology 37:269–274

Peters JR, Foord SM, Dieguez C, Scanlon MF (1983b) TSH neuroregulation and alterations in disease states. Clin Endocrinol Metab 12:669–694

Pokroy N, Epstein S, Hendricks S, Pimstone B (1974) Thyrotropin response to intravenous thyrotropin releasing hormone in patients with hepatic and renal disease. Horm Metab Res 6:132–136

Rage F, Lazaro JB, Benyassi A, Arancibia S, Tapia-Arancibia L (1994) Rapid changes in somatostatin and TRH mRNA in whole rat hypothalamus in response to acute cold exposure. J Neuroendocrinol 6:19–23

Re RN, Kourides IA, Ridgway EC, Weintraub BD, Maloof F (1976) The effect of glucocorticoid administration on human pituitary secretion of thyrotropin and prolactin. J Clin Endocrinol Metab 43:338–346

Reymond MJ, Benotto W, Lemarchand-Beraud T (1987) The secretory activity of the tuberoinfundibular dopaminergic neurons is modulated by the thyroid status in the adult rat: consequence of prolactin secretion. Neuroendocrinology 46:62–68

Rodriguez-Arnao MD, Gomez-Pan A, Rainbow SJ et al (1981) Effects of prosomatostatin on growth hormone and prolactin response to arginine in man. Comparison with somatostatin. Lancet 1:353–356
Rojdmark S (1983) Are fasting-induced effects on thyrotropin and prolactin secretion mediated by dopamine? J Clin Endocrinol Metab 56:1266–1270
Romijn JA, Adriaanse R, Brabant G, Prank K, Endert E, Wiersinga WM (1990) Pulsatile secretion of thyrotropin during fasting: a decrease of thyrotropin pulse amplitude. J Clin Endocrinol Metab 70:1631–1636
Rossmanith WG, Mortola JF, Laughin GA, Yen SS (1988) Dopaminergic control of circadian and pulsatile pituitary thyrotropin release in women. J Clin Endocrinol Metab 67:560–564
Salvador J, Wilson DW, Harris PE, Peters JR, Edwards C, Foord SM, Dieguez C, Hall R, Scanlon MF (1985) Relationships between the circadian rhythms of TSH, prolactin and cortisol in surgically treated microprolactinoma patients. Clin Endocrinol (Oxf) 22:265–272
Salvador J, Dieguez C, Scanlon MF (1988) The circadian rhythms of thyrotropin and prolactin secretion. Chronobiol Int 5:85–93
Samuels MH, Veldhuis JD, Henry P, Ridgway EC (1990) Pathophysiology of pulsatile and copulsatile release of thyroid-stimulating hormone, luteinising hormone, follicle-stimulating hormone and α-subunit. J Clin Endocrinol Metab 71:425–432
Samuels MH, Henry P, Luther M, Ridgway EC (1993) Pulsatile TSH secretion during 48-hour continuous TRH infusions. Thyroid 3:201–206
Samuels MH, Kramer P, Wilson D, Sexton G (1994) Effects of naloxone infusions on pulsatile thyrotropin secretion. J Clin Endocrinol Metab 78:1249–1252
Sapolsky R, Rivier C, Yamamoto G et al (1987) Interleukin-1 stimulates the secretion of hypothalamic corticotropin-releasing factor. Science 238:522–524
Scanlon MF, Toft AD (1995) Regulation of thyrotropin secretion. In: Braverman LE, Utiger RD (eds) The thyroid. Lippincott, New York
Scanlon MF, Mora B, Shale DJ, Weightman DR, Heath M, Snow MH, Hall R (1977) Evidence for dopaminergic control of thyrotropin secretion in man. Lancet 2:421–423
Scanlon MF, Weightman DR, Shale DJ, Mora B, Heath M, Snow M, Lewis M, Hall R (1979) Dopamine is a physiological regulator of thyrotropin (TSH) secretion in normal man. Clin Endocrinol (Oxf) 10:7–15
Scanlon MF, Lewis M, Weightman DR, Chan V, Hall R (1980a) The neuroregulation of human thyrotropin secretion. In: Martini L, Ganong WF (eds) Frontiers in neuroendocrinology. Raven, New York, p 333
Scanlon MF, Weetman AP, Lewis M, Pourmand M, Rodriguez-Arnao MD, Weightman DR, Hall R (1980b) Dopaminergic modulation of circadian thyrotropin rhythms and thyroid hormone levels in euthyroid subjects. J Clin Endocrinol Metab 51:1251–1256
Scanlon MF, Chan V, Heath M, Pourmand M, Rodriguez-Arnao MD, Lewis M, Weightman DR, Hall R (1981) Dopaminergic control of thyrotropin, alpha-subunit and prolactin in euthyroidism and hypothyroidism: dissociated responses to dopamine receptor blockade with metoclopramide in hypothyroid subjects. J Clin Endocrinol Metab 53:360–365
Sharp B, Morley JE, Carlson HE et al (1981) The role of opiates and endogenous opioid peptides in their regulation of rat TSH secretion. Brain Res 219:335–344
Shen L-P, Pictet RL, Rutter WJ (1982) Human somatostatin. I. Sequence of the cDNA. Proc Natl Acad Sci USA 79:4575–4579
Sheward WJ, Harmar AJ, Fraser HM, Fink G (1983) TRH in rat pituitary stalk blood and hypothalamus. Studies with high performance liquid chromatography. Endocrinology 113:1865–1869
Shi ZX, Levy A, Lightman SL (1993) The effect of dietary protein on thyrotropin-releasing hormone and thyrotropin gene expression. Brain Res 606:1–4

Shupnik MA, Greenspan SL, Ridgway EC (1986) Transcriptional regulation of thyrotropin subunit genes by thyrotropin-releasing hormone and dopamine in pituitary cell culture. J Biol Chem 261:12675–12679
Shupnik MA, Rosenzweig BA, Friend KE, Mason ME (1992) Thyrotropin (TSH)-releasing hormone-responsive elements in the rat TSH beta gene have distinct biological and nuclear protein-binding properties. Mol Endocrinol 6:43–52
Siaud P, Tapia-Arancibia L, Szafarczyk A, Alonso G (1987) Increase of thyrotropin-releasing hormone immunoreactivity in the nucleus of the solitary tract following bilateral lesions of the hypothalamic paraventricular nuclei. Neurosci Lett 79:47–52
Silva JE, Larsen PR (1978) Contributions of plasma triiodothyronine and local thyroxine monodeiodination to nuclear triiodothyronine receptor saturation in pituitary, liver and kidney of hypothyroid rats. J Clin Invest 61:1247–1259
Silva JE, Dick TE, Larsen PR (1978) The contribution of local tissue thyroxine monodeiodination to the nuclear 3,5,3-triiodothyronine in pituitary, liver and kidney of euthyroid rats. Endocrinology 103:1196–1207
Small M, Cohen HN, McLean JA, Beastall GH, MacCuish AC (1986) Impaired thyrotropin secretion following the administration of thyrotropin-releasing hormone in type II diabetes mellitus. Postgrad Med J 62:445–448
Smythe GA, Bradshaw JE, Cat WI, Symons RG (1982) Hypothalamic serotoninergic stimulation of thyrotropin secretion and related brain-hormone and drug interactions in the rat. Endocrinology 111:1181–1191
Souetre E, Salvati E, Wehr TA, Sack DA, Krebs B, Darcourt G (1988) Twenty-four hour profiles of body temperature and plasma TSH in bipolar patients during depression and during remission and in normal control subjects. Am J Psychiatry 145:1133–1137
Sowers JR, Catania RA, Hershman JM (1982) Evidence for dopaminergic control of circadian variations in thyrotropin secretion. J Clin Endocrinol Metab 54:673–675
Spangelo BL, MacLeod RM, Isaacson PC (1990) Production of interleukin-6 by anterior pituitary cells in vitro. Endocrinology 126:582–586
Spencer CA, Lun SMC, Wilbur JF, Kaptein EM, Nicoloff JT (1983) Dynamics of serum thyrotropin and thyroid hormone changes during fasting. J Clin Endocrinol Metab 56:883–888
Steinfelder HJ, Radovick S, Wondisford FE (1992) Hormonal regulation of the pituitary-specific transcription factor Pit-1. Proc Natl Acad Sci USA 89:5492–5495
Strassman RJ, Peake GT, Qualls CR, Lisansky EJ (1988) Lack of an acute modulatory effect of melatonin on human nocturnal thyrotropin and cortisol secretion. Neuroendocrinology 48:387–393
Taylor T, Wondisford FE, Blaine T, Weintraub BD (1990) The paraventricular nucleus of the hypothalamus has a major role in thyroid hormone feedback regulation of thyrotropin synthesis and secretion. Endocrinology 126:317–323
Valcavi R, Dieguez C, Azzarito C, Artioli C, Portioli I, Scanlon MF (1987) Alpha-adrenoreceptor blockade with thymoxamine reduces basal thyrotrophin levels but does not influence circadian thyrotrophin changes in man. J Endocrinol 115:187–191
Vale W, Brazeau P, Rivier C et al (1975) Somatostatin. Rec Prog Horm Res 31:365–397
Van Coeverden A, Laurent E, Decoster C, Kerkhofs M, Neve F, van Cauter E, Mockel J (1989) Decreased basal and stimulated thyrotropin secretion in healthy elderly men. J Clin Endocrinol Metab 69:177–185
Vankelecom H, Carmeliet P, Van Damme J, Billian A, Denef C (1989) Production of interleukin-6 by folliculo-stellate cells of the anterior pituitary gland in a histiotype cell aggregate culture system. Neuroendocrinology 49:102–106
Wang PS, Gonzalez HA, Reymond MJ, Porter JC (1989) Mass and in situ molar activity of tyrosine hydroxylase in the median eminence. Neuroendocrinology 49:659–663

Wartofsky L, Burman KD (1982) Alterations in thyroid function in patients with systemic illness: the "euthyroid sick syndrome". Endocr Rev 3:164–217
Wehman RE, Gregerman RI, Burns WH, Saral R, Santos GW (1985) Suppression of thyrotropin in the low-thyroxine state of severe nonthyroidal illness. N Engl J Med 312:546–552
Woloski BM, Smith EM, Meyer WJ III, Fuller GM, Blalock JE (1985) Corticotropin-releasing activity of monokines. Science 230:1035–1037
Yamada M, Monden T, Satoh T, Iizuka M, Murakami M, Iriuchijima T, Mori M (1992) Differential regulation of thyrotropin-releasing hormone receptor mRNA levels by thyroid hormone in vivo and in vitro (GH3 cells). Biochem Biophys Res Commun 184:367–372
Zaloga GP, Chernow B, Smallridge RC, Zajtchuk R, Hall-Boyer K, Hargraves R, Lake CR, Burman KD (1985) A longitudinal evaluation of thyroid function in critically ill surgical patients. Ann Surg 201:456–464
Zgliczynski S, Kaniewski M (1980) Evidence for a-adrenergic receptor mediated TSH release in men. Acta Endocrinol (Oxf) 95:172–176
Zoeller RT, Kabeer N, Albers HE (1990) Cold exposure elevates cellular levels of messenger ribonucleic acid encoding thyrotropin-releasing hormone in paraventricular nucleus despite elevated levels of thyroid hormones. Endocrinology 127:2955–2962

CHAPTER 3

The TSH Receptor

M. MISRAHI and E. MILGROM

A. Introduction

The thyroid-stimulating hormone (TSH) receptor (TSHR) plays a key role in the control of thyroid growth and function. This G-protein-coupled receptor essentially activates adenylate cyclase and to a lesser extent phospholipase C. The role of the cAMP cascade in the production of thyroid hormones and in the mitogenic effect of TSH has been thoroughly studied (reviewed in DUMONT et al. 1989).

Interest in this receptor also stemmed from its implication in autoimmune diseases (reviewed in REES SMITH et al. 1988; WEETMAN and MCGREGOR 1994). Autoantibodies directed against the TSHR which are able to mimic TSH function are found in Graves' disease patients: this leads to hyperthyroidism. The frequency of this organ-specific autoimmune disease is unique among endocrine diseases (reviewed in WILKIN 1990). Understanding of the specificity of the TSHR among glycoprotein hormone receptors, and more generally among G-protein-coupled receptors, has offered a challenge to many researchers. The establishment of the structure of the TSHR in thyroid tissue, as well as the identification of the epitopes recognised by the autoantibodies, were obvious first steps for the elucidation of the pathophysiology of the disease.

Due to the fragility of the receptor and its scarcity in thyroid tissue, the cloning of the TSHR lagged behing other G-protein-coupled receptors. The classical approach through immunopurification and monoclonal antibodies production failed, and indeed several reported monoclonal antibodies were later demonstrated to be directed against unrelated proteins (KOHN et al. 1984). The use of autoantibodies from patients was also deceptive as the heterogeneity of these autoantibodies led to the identification of other thyroid autoantigens (LEEDMAN et al. 1993).

The structure of TSHR was a matter of considerable debate prior to its cloning, with a reported molecular mass varying from 90 to 500 kDa and the number of subunits ranging from one to three. Unexpectedly, controversy as to the structure of the TSHR still remains after its cloning. Different molecular masses between 46 and 210 kDa are still proposed for various receptor species with either one or two subunits. A ganglioside has also been reported to be an integral component of the purified TSHR (KIELCZYNSKI et al. 1991). It must, however, be stressed that very few of these recent studies have been performed with human thyroid tissue using completely characterised antibodies.

B. TSH Receptor Cloning

Cloning relied on the presupposed homologies between the TSHR and other related glycoprotein hormone receptors and/or other G-protein-coupled receptors. The LH/CG receptor was the first member of the glycoprotein hormone receptor family to be cloned (LOOSFELT et al. 1989; MCFARLAND et al. 1989): it was subsequently used as a probe in cross-hybridisation experiments to clone the TSHR from human thyroid tissue (MISRAHI et al. 1990). A parallel approach was the use of low stringency polymerase chain reaction (PCR) based on conserved regions of the transmembrane domain of more distant G-protein-coupled receptors (LIBERT et al. 1989). NAGAYAMA et al. (1989) also reported the cloning of the human TSHR.

The mature protein deduced from the cDNA sequence is 743 residues long and has a calculated MW of ~85 kDa. It comprises a seven transmembrane domain of 266 amino acids, characteristic of G-protein-coupled receptors, and a large extracellular domain of 394 amino acids which corresponds to the hormone-binding domain. This domain contains six potential glycosylation sites; it is formed by the juxtaposition of repetitive leucine-rich sequences. Such motifs have been previously described in a family of proteins able to interact with other proteins implicated in cell adhesion. The crystallographic structure of one member of this familly, the ribonuclease inhibitor, has recently been described (review in KOBE and DEISENHOFER 1994). Leucine-rich repeats correspond to β-α structural units comprising a short β-strand and an α-helix approximately parallel to each other. The structural units are arranged so that all the β-strands and the helices are parallel to a common axis. The protein has a non-globular horseshoe-shaped structure with a curved parallel β-sheet lining the inner circumference of the horseshoe and α-helices flanking its outer circumference. Strong protein-protein interactions very probably occur in the concave surface. Modelling of the three-dimensional structure of the TSHR was subsequently performed on the basis of these findings (KAJAVA et al. 1995).

Two clusters of cysteines are found at both extremities of the extracellular domain of the TSHR. They may be implicated in the formation of disulphide bridges. The extracellular domain can be divided into regions according to their homology to luteinising hormone (LH) and follicle-stimulating hormone (FSH) receptors. The conservation of the limits of these regions in all three receptors is quite striking and this suggests a similar arrangement of their functional domains (Fig. 1).

The seven transmembrane domain of the TSHR is the transduction domain. It is highly conserved (~70%) among glycoprotein hormone receptors (Fig. 1) but has very poor sequence homology with other G-protein-coupled

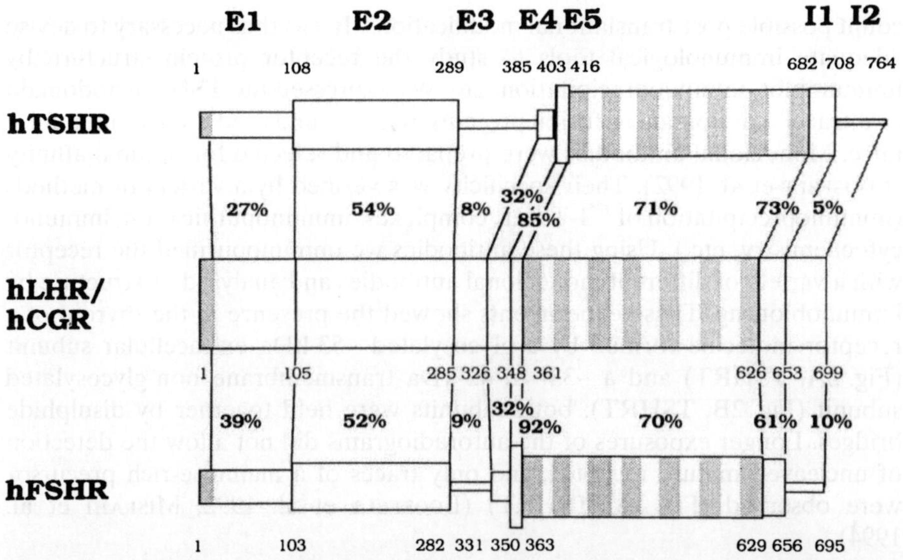

Fig. 1. Comparison of the structure of human LH/CG (MINEGISH et al. 1990), human FSH (MINEGISH et al. 1991) and human TSH (MISRAHI et al. 1990) receptors. Receptors are divided into regions according to the extent of homology (indicated by *thickness of the figure representing the FSH and TSH receptors*). *Dashed regions* represent the putative signal peptide and the seven membrane spans. *E1-5* are the putative extracellular and *I1, I2* the intracellular domains. Amino acid numbering is shown *above and below the figure*. (From MISRAHI et al. 1993)

receptors. However, certain amino acids are remarkably conserved between TSHR, gonadotrophin receptors and other G-protein-coupled receptors. This suggests that there may be similarities in the mechanisms of ligand binding and signal transmission. A computer search also showed the existence within the third cytoplasmic loop of a motif found in non-receptor-type tyrosine kinases (MISRAHI et al. 1990); this motif is absent in the corresponding viral oncogenes, but its function within the TSHR is currently unknown.

The intracellular domain of the TSHR is 83 amino acids long. It can be divided into two regions according to its homology with gonadotrophin receptors. The initial (amino-terminal) part of the domain is highly conserved while the remaining part is divergent. This domain contains several serines and threonines which are potential substrates for phosphorylation. A target protein kinase C sequence is found, but whether and how the TSHR is phosphorylated remains unknown.

C. Structure of the TSHR in the Human Thyroid Gland

Cloning the cDNA encoding the TSHR allowed its sequencing and thus the deduction of its amino acid sequence. However, this does not take into account possible post-translational modifications. It was thus necessary to devise adequate immunological tools to study the receptor protein structure by immunoblot, immunoprecipitation, etc. We expressed the TSHR ectodomain or intracellular domain as fusion proteins in *E. coli* and used them to immunise mice. Monoclonal antibodies were prepared and selected for optimal affinity (LOOSFELT et al. 1992). Their specificity was verified by a variety of methods (immunoprecipitation of ^{125}I-TSHR complexes, immunopurification, immunocytochemistry, etc.). Using these antibodies we immunopurified the receptor with a variety of different monoclonal antibodies and analysed its structure by immunoblotting. These experiments showed the presence in the thyroid of a receptor molecule formed by a glycosylated ~53-kDa extracellular subunit (Fig. 2A, TSHRT) and a ~33- to 42-kDa transmembrane non-glycosylated subunit (Fig. 2B, TSHRT): both subunits were held together by disulphide bridges. Longer exposures of the autoradiograms did not allow the detection of uncleaved mature receptor, and only traces of a mannose-rich precursor were observed (Fig. 2A, TSHRT) (LOOSFELT et al. 1992; MISRAHI et al. 1994).

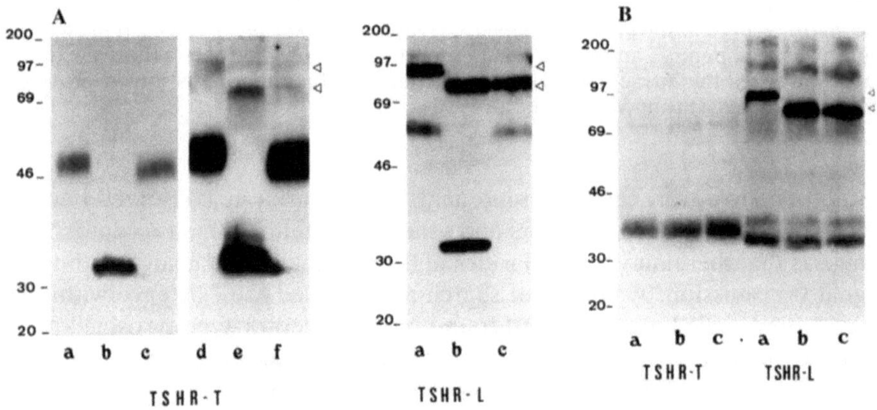

Fig. 2A,B. Comparison of the TSHR species present in human thyroid glands and in permanently transfected L cells. The immunopurified receptor preparations were resolved by SDS/PAGE under reducing conditions and detected by immunoblot. **A** Immunoblot with T5-51 (monoclonal antibody raised against the extracellular domain of the TSHR). **B** Immunoblot with T3-365 (monoclonal antibody raised against the intracellular domain of the TSHR). *TSHR-T,* receptor from human thyroid gland; *TSHR-L,* receptor expressed in L cells. *Lanes a, d,* untreated receptors; *lanes b, e,* receptors treated with peptide *N*-glycanase F (note the deglycosylated form of the TSHR is more strongly labelled by the T5-51 monoclonal antibody); *lanes c, f,* receptors treated with endoglycosidase H. *Lanes a, b, c,* 2 days autoradiography of the immunoblots; *lanes d, e, f,* overexposure (15 days) of the immunoblot of extracts of human thyroid. *Arrows* designate the endoglycosidase-H-sensitive 95-kDa monomer which accumulates in L cells and is present in trace amounts in the thyroid. Size of the molecular mass markers is indicated *on the left in kilodaltons.* (From MISRAHI et al. 1994)

This structure is similar to that suggested previously by Rees Smith (review in Rees Smith et al. 1988), but diverges from several other reports. Pötter et al. (1994) observed two main bands at ~150 kDa and ~90 kDa in non-reducing conditions, while after reduction these were replaced by a diffuse band at 50–55 kDa (thus similar to the α-subunit we have observed). Costagliola et al. (1991) detected a unique ~93-kDa species whereas Marion et al. (1992) described receptor species of 46–48 kDa and 86–88 kDa and Grossman et al. (1995) described receptor species of ~230, 180 and 95 kDa.

D. Structure of the TSHR in Transfected Cells

We also used these tools to analyse the TSHR in stably transfected L cells. In these cells we observed a complex pattern of three receptor species (Misrahi et al. 1994) (Fig. 2A, B TSHRL):

1. An α-β dimer held together by disulphide bonds, similar to that observed in the thyroid. Glycosylation of the α-subunit was more extensive in L cells yielding a protein with an apparent molecular weight of ~60 kDa. However, deglycosylation by N glycanase F of human thyroid and L-cell α-subunits yielded the same polypeptide core of ~35 kDa (Fig. 2A, TSHRL). Two individualised sharp β-subunits are observed in L cells instead of the broad band present in the thyroid. This may be due to differences in the post-translational modifications of the β-subunits in thyroid and L cells or to the existence of alternative cleavage (Fig. 2B, TSHRL).
2. A small amount of uncleaved mature receptor of ~120 kDa. The carbohydrates of this receptor can be digested by N glycanase F but not endoglycosidase H. The amount of the mature ~120 kDa species was variable and seemed to be related to cell growth conditions and cell confluence.
3. A large amount of a mannose-rich precursor of molecular weight ~95 kDa. The carbohydrates of the latter can be digested by both N glycanase F and endoglycosidase H. It should be noted that glycosylation of N-linked oligosaccharides occurs in two steps. The protein first undergoes glycosylation of the high-mannose type in the endoplasmic reticulum. The mannose residues are then trimmed and complex oligosaccharides are added within the Golgi apparatus. The two types of glycosylated proteins can be differentiated by the use of endoglycosidase H. This enzyme removes only the mannose-rich carbohydrates while both types of glycosylated residues are removed by N glycanase F.

Pulse-chase experiments performed in L cells confirmed the nature of these precursors. They showed the successive appearance in L cells of the ~95-kDa high-mannose precursor glycoprotein followed by a ~120-kDa species containing mature oligosaccharides. This latter precursor was then processed into the mature α- and β-subunits. In primary cultures of human thyrocytes, precursors of similar size could be detected (Misrahi et al. 1994).

Finally, immunoelectron microscopy studies were performed with the same monoclonal antibodies. They demonstrated the distribution of the different forms of the TSHR in thyroid and transfected cells. In human thyrocytes most of the receptor was present on the cell surface. In L cells the receptors were likewise detected on the cell surface but a large proportion of receptor was also found inside the cell (in the endoplasmic reticulum and in the Golgi apparatus). The latter pool of receptor probably corresponds to the high mannose-rich precursor. This accumulation is probably due to the overexpression of the receptor and to the insufficiency of the cellular machinery required for the processing of the receptor in these transfected cells (Misrahi et al. 1994).

A great number of other experiments have been performed on transfected cells with diverging results. The group of Rapoport initially reported a monomeric ~100-kDa protein in CHO cells. They also observed a ~54-kDa species the proportion of which varied in different experiments and which they considered to be a product of artefactual proteolysis (Russo et al. 1991a). However, they recently reported that variation in the concentration of the ~54-kDa species was due to incomplete reduction of disulphide bridges, and thus seems to suggest that this receptor form is not a proteolysis artefact (Chazenbalk and Rapoport 1994).

The group of Kohn (Ban et al. 1992) has transfected TSHR in Cos-7 cells and observed receptor species of 230, 180, 95–100 kDa as well as minor bands of 54 and 48 kDa. Their assumption was that the 230- and 180-kDa species corresponded to precursor forms whereas the 54-kDa and 48-kDa bands corresponded to degradation products. It is, however, difficult to understand how a receptor with a polypeptide core deduced from its cDNA sequence of 84.5 kDa can have precursors of 230 and 180 kDa molecular weight. A monomeric 104-kDa receptor has also been observed in CHO cells (Endo et al. 1992), while Harfst et al. (1994) describe in the same cells receptor species of 180 kDa (attributed to an artefact of aggregation), 55 kDa (thought to be a proteolytic artefact) and ~100 kDa.

E. Controversies on Receptor Structure

As described above, there has been an extraordinary variety of receptor forms observed by various authors. In our experience this is for several reasons.

Immunoblot experiments with glycoprotein hormone receptors (LH/CGR, FSHR, TSHR) are difficult to interpret due to the fact that these heterogeneous proteins yield wide bands. Thus, the specific signal is "diluted" and can be difficult to distinguish from non-specific bands. Furthermore, there is a strong tendency for these proteins to aggregate and to interact with other proteins. If precautions are not taken the majority of the receptor may remain on the top of the gel. For these reasons it has proved very difficult for us to obtain meaningful results in Western blots of whole membrane extracts: only prior enrichment of receptor (for instance immunoprecipitation or immunopurification) allowed us to get rid of the majority of the non-specific bands. Of course, high-affinity antibodies with well controlled specificity are a prerequisite.

Finally, in transfected cells the mannose-rich precursor has often been mistaken for a mature full-length receptor. N glycanase F and endoglycosidase H treatments are necessary to clearly identify the bands which are observed.

The possibility has been frequently raised that the cleavage of receptor does not occur in vivo but is an artefact of tissue (or cell) homogenisation and of receptor handling. There is now a wealth of evidence disproving this possibility. First, in human thyroid we never found even a trace of mature uncleaved receptor, suggesting that the "artefactual" phenomenon should have been improbably complete in every single experiment. In addition, the use of a variety of protease inhibitors during tissue homogenisation and handling was without effect.

Furthermore, in both human thyroid cells and in transfected cells the cleavage reaction occurs in vivo as shown by the spontaneous shedding of the receptor ectodomain (Couet et al. 1996a). In the same transfected L cells, the related LH/CG (Vu Hai et al. 1992) and FSH (Vannier et al. 1996) receptors do not undergo cleavage whereas the TSHR does. This cleavage is specifically inhibited in vivo by the incubation of cells with the specific matrix metalloprotease inhibitor BB 2116 (Couet et al. 1996a and see below).

F. Expression of the TSH Receptor in the Baculovirus System

Various groups have used the baculovirus system to produce high levels of receptor proteins. *Spodoptera frugiperda* insect cells (Sf9 and Sf21) infected with a recombinant baculovirus encoding the complete human TSHR synthesise a monomeric protein of ~90kDa (Misrahi et al. 1994). It has been shown in these cells that many proteins are expressed as incompletely processed forms. Comparison of this receptor with the product of in vitro transcription-translation (~85kDa) suggested that some incomplete glycosylation did occur, probably of the high-mannose type. The insolubility of this receptor precluded characterisation by the use of endoglycosidases. Immunoelectron microscopy showed that nearly all the receptor molecules expressed in insect cells were trapped in the endoplasmic reticulum. Thus, the baculovirus system cannot be used to obtain large amounts of intact functional receptor.

Expression of the extracellular domain of the TSHR in Sf9 cells has also been reported. The receptor produced is either non-functional (Huang et al. 1993; Harfst et al. 1992) or only very partially able to bind hormone (Seetharamaiah et al. 1994; Chazenbalk and Rapoport 1995).

G. Shedding of TSH Receptor Ectodomain in Thyroid and Transfected Cells

Quantification of TSHR subunits in human thyroid membranes demonstrated an unexpected 2.5- to 3-fold excess of β- over α-subunits (LOOSFELT et al. 1992). This observation led to the hypothesis that the α-subunit might be shed from cell membranes and released into the extracellular space or bloodstream. Such a phenomenon could be relevant in the context of autoimmune diseases. Indeed, using a quantitative immunoradiometric assay, performed with two monoclonal antibodies directed against the extracellular domain of the TSHR, we have detected a spontaneous shedding of the ectodomain of the TSHR in the culture medium of L cells and CHO cells stably transfected with the TSHR, as well as in primary cultures of human thyrocytes (COUET et al. 1996a). Accumulation of this soluble receptor was time dependent and reached ~25% of the total cellular receptor by 48h. This soluble TSHR (sTSHR) specifically bound TSH. Immunopurification of sTSHR from the L-cell line conditioned media and deglycosylation experiments demonstrated that its polypeptide core corresponds to the α-subunit (~35kDa) of the receptor.

The presence of sTSHR in normal human serum was also detected using the same assay. Our assumption is that this sTSHR is generated by shedding. TSHR-related peptide-like immunoreactivity (MURAKAMI et al. 1992) and TSH-binding protein (HUNT et al. 1992) have been previously detected in human serum. Alternatively, spliced TSHR mRNAs have been cloned from normal and Graves' disease thyroids (TAKESHITA et al. 1992; GRAVES et al. 1992; HUNT et al. 1995). Further experiments should allow us to determine what is the main source for the sTSHR found in human serum, differentiating between post-transcriptional or post-translational mechanisms. More experiments are also needed to ascertain whether there is a correlation between the serum sTSHR and specific pathological conditions such as autoimmune diseases or thyroid cancers.

Various cell surface receptors are shed into the extracellular milieu (reviewed in EHLERS and RIORDAN 1991; TEDDER 1991). In several cases receptor shedding is increased by ligand binding or by protein kinase C activation. TSH induced a significant but limited (25%–30%) increase in the shedding of the sTSHR. Phorbol esters and calcium ionophores mimicked the effect of TSH, while agents acting on the cAMP pathway had no effect.

Lowering serum concentrations from 10% to 1% greatly enhanced TSHR shedding by an unknown mechanism. There was no relationship between the inhibitory effect of serum and cell growth. When cell division was stimulated by insulin and other growth factors there was no inhibition of TSHR shedding.

The use of various inhibitors of intracellular trafficking of the receptor led to the conclusion that receptor modifications involved in the shedding occur at (or close to) the cell membrane. The subtilisin family of serine proteases corresponds to the best-known convertases involved in the maturation of precursor proteins (SEIDAH and CHRETIEN 1992). One member of this family, furin, is involved in the maturation of the insulin proreceptor (BRAVO et al. 1994). This maturation occurs in the late Golgi compartment. However, previous pulse chase experiments indicated that the cleavage mechanisms are nonidentical for TSH and insulin receptors (MISRAHI et al. 1994).

While most protease inhibitors were ineffective in modulating sTSHR production, BB2116, a synthetic hydroxamic acid acting as a specific inhibitor of zinc-dependent matrix metalloproteases, which has been shown to inhibit the maturation of tumour necrosis factor α (GEARING et al. 1994), totally suppressed sTSHR accumulation in culture medium. This effect was secondary to a strong inhibition of TSHR cleavage into α/β-heterodimers (COUET et al. 1996a).

BB2116 inhibits the activity of several matrix metalloprotease in vitro: collagenases, stromelysins, gelatinases and PUMP I. These enzymes are secreted by the cells and are implicated in the physiological remodelling of connective tissue in destructive inflammatory pathologic processes and in tumour invasion (reviewed in WOESSNER 1991; STETLER-STEVENSON et al. 1993). The cleavage sites cannot be predicted as matrix metalloproteases exhibit broad substrate and sequence specificities. Cross-linking of radiolabelled TSH to intact cells expressing mutant TSHR localised the proteolytic cleavage site between residues 261 and 418 (RUSSO et al. 1992). Immunopurification of receptor subunits followed by protein sequencing should allow us to establish the precise cleavage site.

The shedding of the TSHR is a two-step process: cleavage of the receptor followed by disulphide bond(s) reduction (Fig. 3). The membrane impermeant sulphhydryl reagent DTNB was used to determine whether disulphide bonds of the receptor are reduced at the cell surface. This compound markedly

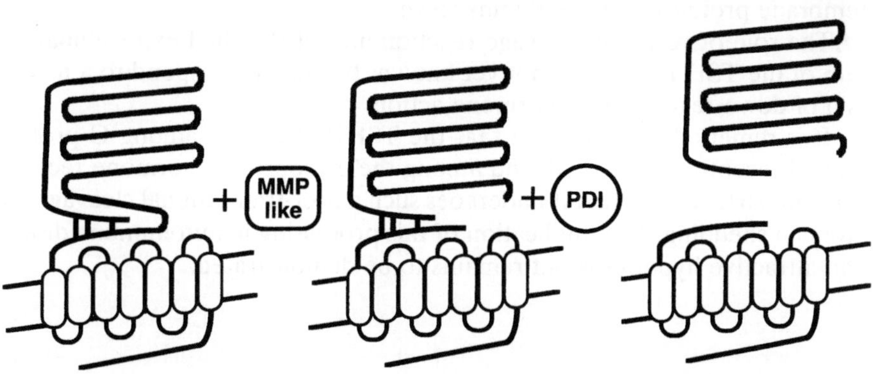

Fig. 3. Schematic representation of the two steps involved in sTSHR shedding. The first step corresponds to a cleavage of the ~120-kDa precursor by a matrix metalloprotease-like enzyme (*MMP*-like) leading to the formation of a heterodimeric receptor (COUET et al. 1996a). The second step corresponds to the reduction of the disulphide bonds holding the two subunits of the receptor by protein disulfide isomerase (PDI), (COUET et al. 1996b)

inhibited receptor shedding, confirming that thiol-disulphide exchange reactions are involved at the cell membrane. Furthermore, the antibiotic bacitracin also elicited a marked inhibition of TSH receptor shedding both from transfected cells and from primary cultures of human thyrocytes. This inhibition was not due to a decreased cleavage of the TSH receptor, as shown by western blots. Three enzymes are known to catalyze disulphide oxidoreduction reactions in mammalian cells: protein disulphide isomerase, thioredoxin and glutaredoxin.

Bacitracin is known to be an inhibitor of PDI (ROTH et a. 1981; MANDEL et al. 1993). Monoclonal antibodies raised against PDI were used to confirm that the latter enzyme is involved in receptor shedding. Three of these antibodies have been shown to be inhibitory of its activity (KAETZEL et al. 1987). These three inhibitory antibodies markedly inhibited the shedding of TSH receptor ectodomain when compared to a control-unrelated antibody (COUET et al. 1996b). PDI is a major intracellular protein and a multifunctional enzyme. Most of PDI is localized in the endoplasmic reticulum, where it catalyzes disulphide bridge formation, isomerization, and reduction (FREEDMAN et al. 1994). These reactions are necessary for the correct folding of newly synthesized proteins. PDI has recently been detected at the surface of mammaliam cells. It has been implicated in the reduction of disulphide bonds occurring during endocytosis of exogenous macromolecules (FEENER et al. 1990) or necessary for the action of diphtheria toxin (MANDEL et al. 1993) or the infection of human lymphoid cells by membrane-bound human immunodeficiency virus (RYSER et al. 1994).

Shedding of extracellular domains has been described for a variety of membrane proteins. PDI involvement in the shedding of other endogenous membrane proteins is currently unknown.

The role of receptor cleavage reaction and of the shed extracellular domain of the TSH receptor is not yet known. It might correspond to a mechanism of down regulation of hormone action.

It is remarkable to observe that the TSHR is unique among G-protein-coupled receptors in general, and among the glycoprotein hormone receptor family in particular, in that it undergoes such a post-translational cleavage and ectomain shedding. The implication of this processing in autoimmune disease is an attractive hypothesis but remains to be demonstrated.

H. Cellular Expression of the TSH Receptor

I. Polarised Expression in the Thyroid

The use of monoclonal antibodies raised against the human TSHR, and more generally against the porcine and human LH/CG and human FSH receptors, has allowed the study of the cellular expression of these receptors. Immunocytochemistry has shown that the TSHR is expressed only at the basolateral surface of thyroid follicular cells (LOOSFELT et al. 1992). The same polarised distribution is observed for the FSH receptor in Sertoli cells (VANNIER et al. 1996). On the contrary, the LH/CG receptor is spread over the whole surface of thecal, granulosa and luteal cells in the ovary, and of Leydig cells in the testes (MEDURI et al. 1992 and unpublished results).

Such differences in cellular distribution might be due either to differences in the structure of the receptor or simply to the fact that thyroid and Sertoli cells are polarised whereas LH/CG receptor expressing cells are not. The use of a polarised cellular system has allowed to answer this question. (see I I)

II. Expression in Other Cell Types

The expression of TSHR mRNAs has been detected in peripheral lymphocytes by PCR (FRANCIS et al. 1991). The TSHR cDNA has been cloned from rat adipose tissue (ENDO et al. 1995). TSHR mRNAs have also been detected in retro-orbital tissues but this is still controversial (review in PASCHKE et al. 1995). It has been suggested that the extrathyroidal localisations of the TSHR might play a role in the pathogenesis of extrathyroidal manifestations of Graves' disease. However, while PCR may detect rare transcripts of mRNAs the expression of the receptor protein in these tissues has not been demonstrated.

TSH stimulates mitogen-activated protein kinase (MAP kinase) in rat astrocytes (TOURNIER et al. 1995). Further experiments are needed to know whether a functional TSHR is found in the central nervous system.

I. Intracellular Trafficking of the Receptor

Little is known about the cellular trafficking of G-protein-coupled receptors in general and of this subgroup of receptors in particular. Ultrastructural immunocytochemistry has revealed LH/CGR-driven hormone transcytosis through endothelial cells of testicular vessels (GHINEA et al. 1994). Thus, the same receptor found in Leydig cells of the testes is also found in the testicular microvasculature and is involved in the transport and concentration of the hormone in the subendothelial space, in close contact with target cells. Preliminary experiments have shown the existence of the TSHR in the microvasculature of the thyroid (Ghinea and Milgrom, unpublished results). Thus, a similar mechanism may possibly be involved in the transendothelial transport of TSH toward thyroid cells.

I. Polarized Expression in MDCK Cells

Madin-Darby canine kidney (MDCK) cell lines expressing the TSH, FSH and LH receptors were established to study the polarized expression of TSH and gonadotropin receptors (Beau et al. 1997; see Sect. H.I). MDCK cells are the best known system for studying the polarization of proteins.

The physiological basolateral localization of TSH and FSH receptors, observed in thyrocytes and Sertoli cells, respectively, was reproduced in the heterologous MDCK cells (Fig. 4). This suggested that the corresponding targetting signals are included in the proteins themselves and are functional in heterologous polarized cells. Furthermore, the LH receptor, which is not physiologically polarized, has basolateral polarized expression in MDCK cells (MEDURI et al. 1992, 1996). This suggested that the LH receptor also possesses a basolateral targetting signal, as the other members of this receptor subgroup. In vitro mutagenesis will allow identification of the signal involved in all three receptors.

A basolateral localization has previously been observed for two other G-protein-coupled receptors: the α_{2A}-adrenergic receptor in MDCK cells (KEEFER and LIMBIRD 1993) and the parathormone receptor in epithelial kidney cells (SHLATZ et al. 1975; MOHR and HESCH 1980; ZHOU et al. 1990). Conversely, the adenosine A_1 receptor is localized essentially on the apical

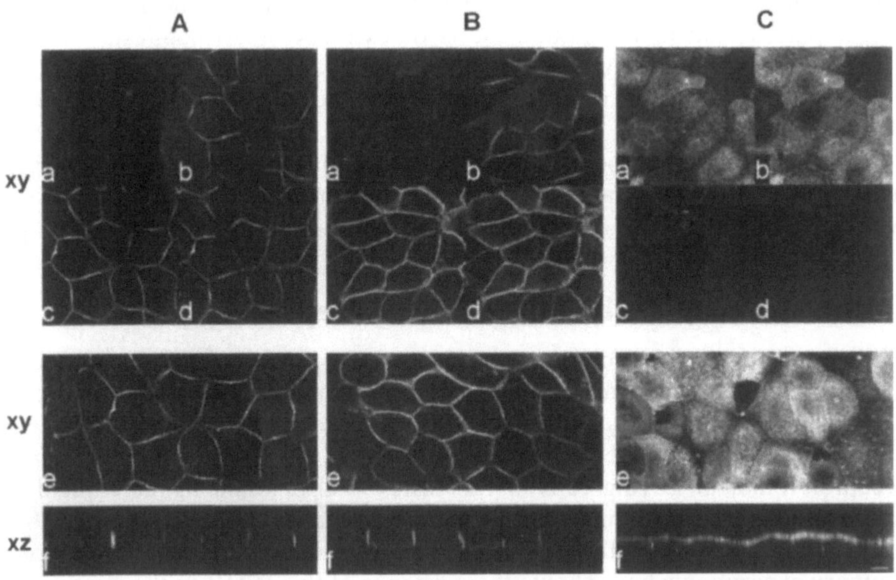

Fig. 4A–C. Confocal microscopic examination of the distribution of TSH and gonadotropin receptors in polarized MDCK cells (BEAU et al. 1997). Polarized monolayers of cells transfected with the TSH, LH or FSH receptor cDNA were grown to confluence on coverslips and treated with EGTA to open the tight junction. They were then processed for indirect immunofluorescence microscopy. Primary antibodies corresponded to control monoclonal antibodies BC11 (**A**) and BB18 (**C**), recognizing, respectively, a basolateral and an apical endogenous antigen of MDCK cells. Monoclonal antibodies directed against the TSH, FSH or LH receptors were also used to study the corresponding cell line. xy horizontal focal sections (parallel through MDCK cells) were performed from the apical (*a*) to the basal level (*d*) of the cells. The same polarized expression was observed for the three receptors. This experiment shows the example of the LH receptor. *Below*, an xy section (*e*) of a selected area of cells and the corresponding zy sections (*f*) taken in 0.1-μm steps through the cells at 90° to the xy sections. The apical region of the cells is oriented topmost. *Bar*, 10 μm surface of MDCK cells (SAUNDERS et al. 1996). The basolateral targetting of proteins in epithelial cells may occur via any of various mechanisms. Indeed, different mechanisms may even be used for closely related proteins: the α_{2A}- and α_{2C}-adrenergic receptors are delivered directly to the basolateral surface of MDCK cells, whereas the α_{2B}-adrenergic receptor is inserted randomly into both cell surface domains but is retained preferentially on the basolateral surface (its half-life being shorter on the apical surface; WOZNIAK and LIMBIRD 1996). In the case of FSH receptor both time course studies of receptor appearance on the cell surface and protease-digestion experiments show a direct basolateral targetting.

A small proportion (10%–15%) of the gonadotropin FSH and LH receptors are localized on the apical surface of MDCK cells. In fact, these receptors are initially delivered to the basolateral surface and secondarily undergo transcytosis to the apical surface (BEAU et al. 1997). In MDCK cells previous studies involving a number of protiens have shown that apical localization in most cases results from direct targeting (SIMONS and WANDINGER-NESS 1990). This is not the case for gonadotropin receptors.

Brefeldin A inhibits the basolateral localization of low-density lipoprotein receptor (MATTER et al. 1993) and of the polymeric immunoglobulin receptor (APODACA et al. 1993) but has no effect on the polarization of various other proteins (LOW et al. 1991, 1992) including the FSH receptor. Two hypotheses have been proposed to explain these differneces: either different carrier vesicles are used to reach the same compartment, or brefeldin A acts by selectively altering only some of them.

Monomeric G proteins, especially those of the rab and ARF families, are involved in practically all of the steps of vesicular trafficking (GOUD and MCCAFFREY 1991; NUOFFER and BALCH 1994). The role of the heterotrimeric G proteins in this respect has only recently been shown (STOW and DE ALMEIDA 1993; STOW et al. 1991). PIMPLIKAR and SIMARS (1993) established that the apical and basolateral targeting of surface proteins is regulared in the trans-golgi compartment by heterotrimeric G proteins. These authors proposed a general mechanism by which Gi inhibits basolateral transport while Gs stimulates apical trransport. Gs has also been implicated in the transcytosis of the polymeric immunoglobulin receptor (BOMSEL and MOSTOV 193). The FSH receptor does not follow the model proposed by PIMPLIKAR and SIMONS (1993) since inhibition of Gi is without effect on receptor distribution whereas stimulation of Gs does not increase direct receptor apical transport but markedly enhances receptor transcytosis. This may be due to a rerouting of internalized receptor from the degradative lysozymal pathway toward the transcytotic pathway.

The compartmentalization and surface targeting of the LH receptor closely resembles those of the FSH receptor in MDCK cells. For both receptors a minimal transcytosis of receptor and hormone is observed, which is increased by the activation of Gs. This phenomenon, which is very limited in MDCK cells, may be more important in other cell types. Receptor-mediated transcytosis of hormone has been described in endothelial cells of testicular vessels (GHINEA et al. 1994).

The TSH receptor also displays a basolateral localization in MDCK cells, but no transcytosis is observed, and there is no apparent effect of Gs activation. These differences between gonatropin and TSH receptors may be related to a possible interaction of the TSH receptor with a cellular or an extracellular component of MDCK cells. Interaction of Na^+/K^+ ATPase with the cytoskeleton has been shown to stabilize the protein at the basolateral surface (HAMMERTON et al. 1991). The possibility remains, however, that in other cell types (endothelial cells) transcytosis may occur.

II. Receptor Downregulation

Following exposure of target cells to the agonist, a diminished response upon reexposure is observed: this process is called desensitisation and is a stepwise phenomenon. The fastest mechanism seems to be the diminution or downregulation of hormone-binding sites secondary to internalisation of hormone-receptor complexes. This mechanism may itself be secondary to post-translational modifications of the receptor, such as phosphorylation, as described for β-adrenergic receptor (review in STROSBERG 1991). Other mechanisms may involve functional uncoupling of the receptor from the G protein as also proposed for the adrenergic receptors, together with the decrease in cellular responses. A second phase of agonist-induced downregulation is dependent on the reduction of receptor mRNA levels (see Sect. K).

Desensitisation has also been described in thyroid cells (RAPOPORT and ADAMS 1976). However, as permanent stimulation of TSHR is observed in Graves' disease patients, this mechanism seems to be less important in vivo in the case of the TSHR as compared to the LH/CGR. The existence of a desensitisation mechanism in transfected cells expressing the human TSHR is under debate.The group of Rapoport did not observe TSH-induced desensitisation using CHO cells which express the full-length TSHR. They concluded that desensitisation was dependent on a thyroid cell-specific factor (CHAZENBALK et al. 1990a). However, this conclusion is not supported by other studies which describe densitisation of the TSHR in stably transfected CHO cells (TEZELMAN et al. 1994; HARAGUCHI et al. 1993) or in other transfected cells (HELDIN et al. 1994; NAGAYAMA et al. 1994).

Phosphorylation on serines or threonines of the intracellular domain is involved in the downregulation of G-protein-coupled receptors. Internalisation sequences of several membrane receptors have been shown to include a tyrosine residue located next to the transmembrane domain. However, deletion mutants have demonstrated that the carboxy-terminal part of the cytoplasmic tail of the TSHR, up to residues 726 (HARAGUCHI et al. 1994) or even 708 (SHI et al. 1993), which includes serines and threonine residues, is not involved in these processes. Serine 694 and tyrosine 706 located next to the membrane also do not participate in receptor downregulation (SHI et al. 1993).

Deletion of 56 amino acids from the C terminus of the cytoplasmic tail *enhances* TSHR internalisation as compared to the wild-type receptor (SHI et al. 1995). Enhancement of internalisation resulting from deletions of the cytoplasmic tail is also observed for the rat LH/CG and avian β-adrenergic receptors (HERTEL et al. 1990; RODRIGUEZ et al. 1992). This suggests that the cytoplasmic tail may exert a negative control on receptor internalisation either by the existence of inhibitory sequences within this tail or by the occlusion of an internalisation sequence within a secondary structure in basal conditions.

A sequence resembling the NPXY sequences corresponding to internalisation sequences found in insulin, insulin-like growth factor-I and low-density lipoprotein receptors is found within the seventh transmembrane helix of TSHR. Mutation of Tyr 678, which is included in this NPXXY sequence, completely abolishes the adenylate cyclase transduction pathway without impairing high-affinity hormone binding and significantly reduces TSHR internalisation in CHO cells (SHI et al. 1995). The NPXXY sequence of TM7 is highly conserved in G-protein-coupled receptors. Mutation of the tyrosine residue within this motif in the β_2-adrenergic receptor completely abolishes agonist-mediated receptor sequestration without affecting the ability of the receptor to undergo rapid desensitisation and downregulation in response to the agonist (BARAK et al. 1994). Further experiments will determine whether other internalisation sequences are also used in the TSHR.

J. Structure-Function Relationships

I. Transduction Pathways of the TSH Receptor

Although many effects of TSH on thyroid cell growth and function can be mimicked by cAMP agonists, the existence of other transduction pathways has been raised by different groups. TSH stimulates two different transduction pathways in human thyroid, mainly the adenylate cyclase pathway but also the phospholipase C pathway (reviewed in VASSART and DUMONT 1992). Higher concentrations of TSH are needed (1–10 mU/ml) to stimulate the latter. It has been shown that the same recombinant TSHR is coupled to both cascades (VAN SANDE et al. 1990). Two different G proteins are involved: Gs and Gq/11. Both are activated by TSH in human thyroid membranes (ALLGEIER et al. 1994). It has been suggested that the difference in the doses of TSH necessary to activate the two classes of G protein might be due to differences in the efficiency of coupling of the G proteins with their respective effectors.

In FRTL5 cells TSH stimulates phospholipase A_2 activity and it has been shown that TSH-induced hydrogen peroxide production is mediated by the cascade of Ca^{2+}-dependent phospholipase A_2/arachidonate cascade (KIMURA et al. 1995). TSH can also activate phospholipase D in these cells as a consequence of prior protein kinase C activation (GUPTA et al. 1995).

Very recently it has also been shown that activation of theTSHR by TSH led to increased incorporation of a GTP analogue into immunoprecipitated α-subunits of all G proteins detected in thyroid cells (Gs, Gi, Go, Gq, G11, G12, G13; LAUGWITZ et al. 1996). To prove the specificity of the observed effect, a blocking antiserum from a patient with autoimmune hypothyroidism was used which suppressed the effect of TSH. The TSHR would then appear as a general G-protein-activating receptor.

Some effects of TSH on thyroid cell growth might not be mediated by cAMP. It has been shown in WRT cells that the full mitogenic response to TSH requires the adenylate cyclase and a *Ras*-dependent pathway. Microinjection of a dominant interfering *Ras* protein reduces TSH-stimulated DNA synthesis in these cells. This *Ras*-dependent pathway is, however, unusual in that it is *Raf1* and *MEK* independent as shown by microinjection of *Raf*1 antibodies and dominant interfering *MEK* proteins (AL-ALAWI et al. 1995). The effector of *Ras* in TSH mediating signalling in these cells is unknown at the present. The cooperation of PKA and *Ras*-dependent pathways in thyroid growth is also supported by the fact that activating mutations in both *Gs* and *Ras* are frequently found in thyroid tumours.

In human thyroid membranes it has been shown that TSH stimulates the mitogen activated (MAP) kinase cascade through a cAMP-independent pathway. This effect was suppressed by immunoprecipitation of hormone by a monoclonal anti-TSH antibody, which suggests that it is not an artefact due to factors contaminating the hormone used (SAUNIER et al. 1995).

II. Mutagenesis of Transmembrane and Intracellular Domains of the TSH Receptor

Mutagenesis of the transmembrane and intracellular domains of the TSHR has provided insight into some important regions in signal transduction.

The group of Rapoport has shown that the first cytoplasmic loop, the carboxy-terminal region of the second cytoplasmic loop and the carboxy-terminal region of the third cytoplasmic loop, are important in the ability of the TSHR to mediate an increase in cAMP production in stably transfected CHO cell lines (CHAZENBALK et al. 1990b). The second cytoplasmic loop has been shown by another group also to be important for agonist-induced phosphoinositide signalling (KOSUGI et al. 1994a). Even if a single loop is involved in the interaction with two different G proteins, the regions within this second loop critical for each signalling pathway could be discriminated.

Controversy exists for the first and third cytoplasmic loops. Using transient transfection in Cos-7 cells of receptor mutants, KOSUGI and MORI (1994a) reported that the first cytoplasmic loop is important for phosphoinositide signalling but not for agonist-induced adenylate cyclase activation. KOSUGI et al. (1993a) reproduced a mutation in the carboxy terminus of the third cytoplasmic loop identical to the one performed by CHAZENBALK et al. (1990b) with opposite results. Transfection of the mutant TSHR in Cos 7 cells revealed that it retained the TSH-induced cAMP response but displayed no TSH-induced inositol phosphate response. They concluded that the third loop is less important for agonist-induced Gs-interactions.

Concerning the contradictions described in the literature with receptor mutants, some specific points need to be stressed: The exact limits of a region which is mutated need to be considered. Indeed, multiple amino acid residues may function as a group and individual mutations may not reproduce the mutation of a whole region (CHAZENBALK et al. 1991). Moreover, the type of substitution performed may alter the secondary structure of a whole region of the TSHR or even of the whole receptor. Therefore, the alteration of TSHR function may be due to a repercussion of the mutation at a distance. This is exemplified by alterations of TSH binding in some receptors with intracellular mutations. Furthermore, TSHRs of different species may differ in their functional topology.

These observations might explain why mutation of alanine 623 in the third cytoplasmic loop to lysine or glutamic acid impairs TSH-mediated phosphoinositide formation but not cAMP production (KOSUGI et al. 1992a), while the same residue mutated to other amino acids yields a constitutive receptor spontaneously coupled to Gs (PARMA et al. 1993 and see below). Other engineered mutations of neighbouring amino acids (residues 617–620) also yielded constitutive receptors which produced elevated basal cAMP levels as well as small increases in basal inositol phosphatate production (KOSUGI et al. 1993a).

The role of the cytoplasmic tail in signal transduction was also examined. Deletion of the entire cytoplasmic tail of the TSHR markedly reduced TSH binding, which did not allow for the investigation of the role of this region in signal transduction. Removal of the two thirds of the carboxy-terminal end of the cytoplasmic tail of the TSHR, a region not conserved with gonadotrophin receptors, did not impair TSHR function (CHAZENBALK et al. 1990b). Substitution of the amino-terminal part of the cytoplasmic tail (residues 684–692) with α_1- or β_2-adrenergic receptor sequences impaired agonist-induced phosphoinositide signalling but not adenylate cyclase activation (KOSUGI and MORI 1994b). Also receptor mutants truncated between residues 700 and 722 showed a decreased or suppressed inositol phosphate response to TSH without alteration of the cAMP response. Thus the amino-terminal half of the cytoplasmic tail, up to residue 721, seems to be essential for full TSHR function (KOSUGI and MORI 1994c).

The extracellular loops also have a critical conformational role for the whole TSHR transmembrane domain and thus for TSHR function. Mutations of two cysteines (494 and 569) located respectively in the first and second extracellular loops of the TSHR impair TSH function. These cysteines are potentially involved in a disulphide bond by analogy with other G-protein-coupled receptors. A single mutation impaired the hormone-binding ability of the receptor, while a double mutant retained the ligand-binding capacity but lost most of the cAMP response (GUSTAVSSON et al. 1994). Receptor mutants in which the length or sequence of the first and second extracellular loops has been changed display no TSH-binding ability. Substitution of the third extracellular loop alters the TSH-stimulated cAMP response (KOSUGI and MORI 1994d).

III. Mutagenesis of the Extracellular Domain of the TSH Receptor

Alteration in hormone binding of receptor mutants may result from different causes: The mutation may have disrupted a specific high-affinity TSH-binding site within the extracellular domain of the receptor, but it may also have altered receptor stability, intracellular trafficking or membrane insertion. No definitive conclusions can be drawn from mutagenesis experiments if the expression of the receptor at the cell surface is not demonstrated (for example, by immunocytochemical experiments). The lack of immunological tools has often prevented such experiments being done. Again, this might explain some discrepancies in the conclusions derived from different studies.

The regions involved in TSH binding have been studied through different approaches. As the conformation of the extracellular domain is an important element in the hormone-binding ability of the receptor, one interesting approach was the use of chimeric TSH-LH/CG receptors. Replacement of the entire extracellular domain of the TSHR with the corresponding region of the LH/CGR resulted in high-affinity hCG binding and complete loss of TSH binding. The symmetrical substitution yielded a chimeric receptor able to bind TSH with high affinity and to stimulate adenylate cyclase (NAGAYAMA et al. 1991a). Thus, there is no doubt that the extracellular domain of receptors of this class are involved in high-affinity hormone binding. However, hormonal activation of an N terminally truncated LHR lacking most of the extracellular domain had been obtained (JI and JI 1991). This led to the hypothesis that hCG could also interact directly with the transmembrane segments, albeit with low affinity. The construction of similar TSHR mutants did not show any TSH-induced increase in cAMP in transfected cells (PASCHKE et al. 1994a). These results suggested that activation of the TSHR does not implicate direct interaction of TSH with the transmembrane domain, or that the latter has to undergo previous conformational changes triggered by TSH binding to its extracellular domain.

The use of a series of TSHR-LH/CGR chimeras led to the conclusion that the TSH-binding regions are likely to span the entire extracellular domain with multiple discontinuous contact sites (NAGAYAMA et al. 1991a). This conclusion is also supported by the modelling of the TSHR ectodomain (KAJAVA et al. 1995). The middle region (residues 171–260) is, however, especially important for TSH binding (NAGAYAMA et al. 1990). Construction of other chimeric receptors indicates that Lys 201 to Lys 211 and Gly 222 to Leu 230 are also involved in TSH binding (NAGAYAMA et al. 1991b). In contrast, residues 303 to 382 of the rat TSHR can be deleted without loss of TSH function (KOSUGI et al. 1991a). This region is flanked by possible TSH-binding sites at residues 295–306 and around tyrosine 385. Mutation of the downstream cysteine 390 markedly impairs TSH binding (Kosugi et al. 1991b). However, in these experiments an alteration of cell surface expression of the TSHR has not been excluded.

Both extremities of the extracellular domain of TSH and gonadotrophin receptors contain several cysteine residues. They might be implicated in the formation of disulphide bonds. Mutations of several cysteines 41 (Wadsworth et al. 1992), 301 (Akamizu et al. 1994) and 390 (Kosugi et al. 1991b) resulted in a loss of TSH binding. However, this may be due to disruption of disulphide bonds, to alteration of receptor tertiary structure or to modification of its insertion in the cell membrane.

There is controversy as to a possible role of the extracellular domain of the TSHR in signal transduction. The use of partial chimeric receptors suggested that the middle region and carboxyl half of the extracellular domain of the TSHR are involved in signal transduction. Indeed, their substitution with the corresponding regions of the LH/CGR did not abolish TSH binding but impaired signal transduction. Within the carboxy-terminal half of the extracellular domain of the human TSHR, two short regions corresponding to amino acids 270–278 and 287–297 were particularly important in signal transduction (Nagayama and Rapoport 1992a). However, these results were not confirmed by another group. Using chimeric TSH-LH/CG receptors, Akamizu et al. (1993) reported that substitution of residues 268–304 of the TSHR with homologous residues from the LH/CGR markedly decreased high-affinity TSH binding but there was minimal change in TSH-stimulated adenylate cyclase activity. Within this region, cysteine 301 was shown to play an important role in TSH binding (Akamizu et al. 1994).

The role of the glycosylation of the receptor in TSHR function has also been studied by site-directed mutagenesis. The TSHR has six potential N-linked glycosylation sites within the extracellular domain. Substitution of asparagine 77 and 113 suppressed or greatly impaired TSH binding and signal transduction. Substitution of the four other potential glycosylation sites had no deleterious effects on TSHR function (Russo et al. 1991b). This suggested that either those sites are not glycosylated or that glycosylation at these residues does not play a major role in TSHR trafficking and expression at the cell surface.

To identify regions involved in high-affinity hormone binding, another approach was to use synthetic peptides (reviewed in Endo and Onaya 1993). These studies were focused on specific regions in the extracellular domain of the TSHR. The TSHR has two unique insertions in its extracellular domain that are not found in the LH/CG or FSH receptors (Fig. 1). Thus, these two regions were investigated initially for their hormone-binding ability. Study of direct binding of TSH to synthetic peptides led to the conclusion that peptides 2–30 and 324–344 contain specific binding regions for TSH (Atassi et al. 1991). Preincubation of bovine TSH with peptide 35–50 resulted in a dose-dependent decrease in cAMP accumulation induced by TSH (Ohmori et al. 1991). The use of competition experiments led to identification of residues 256–275 as TSH-binding sites. Within this region nine specific amino acids were especially important (BRYANT et al. 1994).

This methodology, however, does not take into account the whole conformation of the extracellular domain of the receptor: different regions may be necessary to create a hormone-binding pocket. The peptides are used at concentrations usually orders of magnitude higher than hormone or receptor concentrations. It should be emphasised that this approach yielded contradictory results in the study of the sites of interaction of Graves' disease IgG with the TSHR (see below).

K. Gene Structure and Regulation

I. Gene Organisation

The structure of the human TSHR gene has been determined. This gene spans 60 kbp and is split into 10 exons (Fig. 5) (GROSS et al. 1991). All the introns are located in the 5′ region of the gene corresponding to the extracellular part of the receptor. This domain is thus encoded by the entire nine first exons and the beginning of the tenth exon. The limits of exons correspond to the limits of leucine-rich repeats. The transmembrane and intracellular domains of the receptor are encoded by the last exon. This organisation is similar to that of

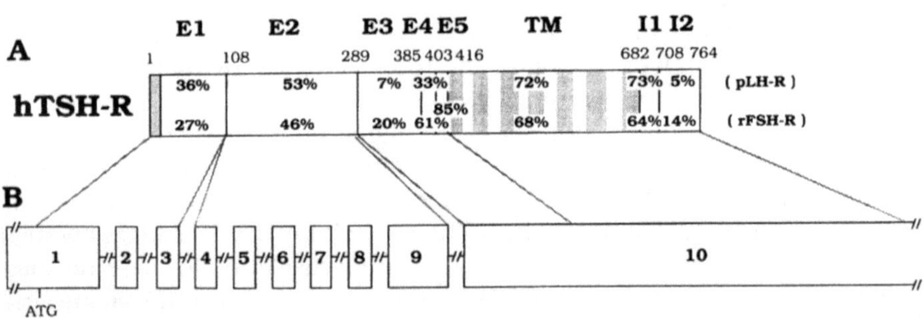

Fig. 5. Organisation of the human TSH-R gene. *A* Structure of the human TSHR, comparison with LH and FSH receptors. The human TSHR (*hTSH-R*) has been divided into domain according to the extent of homology with the porcine LH receptor (*pLH-R*) and the rat FSH receptor (*rFSH-R*). The extracellular part is divided into E1-5. *TM* is the transmembrane domain with its seven dashed membrane spans. The intracellular part of the receptor is divided into I1 and I2. *In the boxes,* percentages of homology of hTSH-R with pLH-R are *written on top,* percentages with rFSH-R *below.* For E5, the homology of 85% is identical for both receptors. The signal peptide is shown by *a dashed box.* Amino acid numbering is shown *above the figure. B* Exon/intron organisation of the hTSH-R gene. Exons, *represented by boxes, are numbered from 1 to 10.* Introns *are represented by interrupted thin lines.* Position of the translation initiation (ATG) codon is indicated. The limits of the exons are compared to the limits of the domains of hTSH-R. (From GROSS et al. 1991)

related genes encoding the LH/CG or the FSH receptors. The human LH/CGR gene displays 11 exons (ATGER et al. 1995) and the human FSHR gene 10 exons (AITTOMAKI et al. 1995).

The existence of a single large exon encoding a short part of the extracellular domain and the whole transmembrane domain of this class of receptors recalls the structure of adrenergic and muscarinic receptor genes which are also devoid of introns. Thus, an evolutionary relationship of the TSH and gonadotrophin receptor genes to other G-protein-coupled receptors has been hypothesised (GROSS et al. 1991). This class of genes would have arisen from the fusion of a gene encoding a leucine-rich glycoprotein and a gene for a protoreceptor similar to the β-adrenergic-type receptor.

II. Chromosomal Localisation and Genetic Mapping

The LH/CG and FSH receptors have been assigned to the same chromosomal location: 2p21 (ROUSSEAU-MERCK et al. 1990a, 1993). This is a supplementary argument for their evolutionary relationship, as they might have evolved by gene duplication from a common ancestor. However, the TSHR gene, which is closely related to the previous genes, has been localised on chromosome 14q31 (ROUSSEAU-MERCK et al. 1990b). It is thus possible that recombination events caused the scattering of this receptor gene during evolution.

Three polymorphic markers localised within introns 2 and 7 of the TSHR gene have been described recently. They have allowed us to map precisely the TSHR gene on chromosome 14q31 between D14S287 and D14S68 (DE ROUX et al. 1996a). Furthermore, the establishment of the structure of intron/exon junctions has allowed for the definition of the optimal conditions for PCR amplification and direct genomic sequencing of the ten exons of the TSHR gene. All these tools will be useful in all pathological situations where mutations of the TSHR may be present.

1. Structure and Function of TSHR Promoter and 5′ Flanking Region

The promoter of the human TSHR gene is very G + C rich and displays no typical TATA or CAAT boxes: three initiation sites are found. The main site is located 157 bp upstream from the site of translation (GROSS et al. 1991). The TSHR mRNA is essentially regulated by TSH, cyclic AMP and growth factors. Putative *cis*-acting elements regulated by cyclic AMP are found in the 5′ flanking region of the human TSHR gene: a cyclic AMP-responsive element (CRE) is present at position –132, and several AP2 consensus sequences are also found (GROSS et al. 1991).

The 5′ flanking regions of the rat thyrotrophin receptor gene have also been characterised. Deletion analyses demonstrated a minimal region exhibiting promoter activity, tissue specificity and negative regulation by TSH between –195 and –39 bp (IKUMAYA et al. 1992). This region is highly conserved in rat and human TSHR genes. It comprises a cAMP-responsive element

(CRE) which has been shown to be functional. However, this element is not thyroid specific. By analogy with the promoters of two other main thyroid differentiation markers, thyroperoxidase and thyroglobulin, it has been suggested that thyroid transcription factor 1 (TTF-1), a thyroid-specific homeodomain-containing transcription factor, binds to the TSHR gene promoter. Indeed, a TTF-1-binding site is found at position –189 to –175 and is involved in thyroid-specific gene transcription (Civitareale et al. 1993; Shimura et al. 1994a). The activity of the TTF-1-binding element requires a functioning CRE and a cooperative effect between the two factors has been described (Saiardi et al. 1995).

The functioning of the TTF-1-binding element in the TSHR gene differs from that of the one found in thyroglobulin and thyroperoxidase genes. In these latter genes TTF-1 interacts with *Pax 8*, a paired domain containing protein, whose binding site overlaps the recognition site of TTF-1 (review in Damante and di Lauro 1994). In the TSHR gene no such interactions have been shown. In addition, the TTF-1 site in the minimal promoter of the TSHR gene is associated with both upregulation and downregulation of the TSHR gene by cAMP. However, the mechanisms involved are different in each case. Positive regulation has been linked to TSH-induced phosphorylation of TTF-1 via the cAMP pathway; downregulation of TSHR gene expression is associated with a TSH-induced decrease in TTF-1 RNA levels by the cAMP pathway.

Other transcription factors are also involved in the regulation of the TSHR gene. A single-strand DNA-binding protein which has an adjacent binding site to TTF-1 acts with the latter in an additive way on constitutive TSHR expression, and also on the negative regulation of TSHR by cAMP (Shimura et al. 1995). An upstream TTF-1-binding site (position –881 to –866 bp) has also been detected in the thyrotrophin promoter which functions as a thyroid-specific enhancer but requires the presence of the downstream TTF-1 site (Ohmori et al. 1995).

Insulin and insulin-like growth factor-1 (IGF-1) are required for thryrotrophin (TSH) regulation of thyroid cell growth and function. An insulin-responsive element has been identified in the rat thyrotrophin receptor promoter immediately upstream of the proximal TTF-1-binding site. Both sites seem to cooperate at least partially in the response to insulin (Shimura et al. 1994b). Thus, it seems that the thyroid-specific activity of the TSHR promoter relies on the coordinated action of many transcription factors.

Prolonged incubation of cells with TSH reduces the cAMP response to a subsequent hormonal stimulation. This long-term homologous desensitisation of the TSHR involves downregulation at the transcriptional level. Recently, it has been shown that TSH induces a transcriptional repressor in the rat thyroid gland and in the FRTL5 cell line. This repressor has been identified as the inducible cAMP early repressor isoform (ICER) of the CRE modulator gene (CREM). ICER binds to a CRE-like sequence in the TSHR promoter and represses its expression (LALLI and SASSONE-CORSI 1995). Thus, CREM as well as TTF-1 is involved in the negative regulation of the TSHR promoter.

L. The TSH Receptor and Pathology

I. Autoimmunity

1. The TSHR and the Genetics of Graves' Disease

Several pieces of evidence implicate genetic factors in the aetiology of Graves' disease. Ten percent of cases of Graves' disease are clustered in affected families (BARTELS 1941). There is a higher concordance of Graves' disease between homozygous twins (50% probability of the other twin developing the disease) than for heterozygotic twins (only 7% probability) (VOLPE et al. 1972). These observations have led to speculation that Graves' disease is a polygenic disease with concomitant involvement of environmental factors in its pathogenesis.

Various genes have been examined for their implication in the genetic pathology of Graves' disease, particularly genes of the immune system (reviewed in WEETMAN and MCGREGOR 1994). A genetic linkage has been established recently between the HLA-DR3 loci and Graves' disease. This study concluded that whereas HLA-DR3 may increase susceptibility to autoimmune thyroid disease, the major genetic influence is probably at a different locus (SHIELDS et al. 1994).

Concerning one of the major thyroid autoantigens, the TSHR, two possibilities have been raised by different authors: an anomaly of the structure of the TSHR might render the receptor more "immunogenic", or an alteration of its regulation might be involved in the pathogenesis of Graves' disease (for review see DEGROOT and QUINTANS 1989; MIZUKAMI et al. 1994). A polymorphism was recently described at codon 52 of the TSHR, changing a proline into a threonine (BOHR et al. 1993; SUNTHORNTHEPVARAKUL et al. 1994); preliminary studies have shown this polymorphism is associated with severe cases of Graves' disease, and it was suggested that this mutant form may have unique immunogenic properties (BAHN et al. 1994). This variant was also claimed to display enhanced coupling to adenylate cyclase (LOOS et al. 1995). However, no association was found between this polymorphism and Graves' disease in another study (WATSON et al. 1995), while a further investigation concluded that the polymorphism was associated with autoimmune thyroid diseases in a female population (CUDDIHY et al. 1995a). The variant was shown to have a normal function in vivo (CUDDIHY et al. 1995b). A somatic polymorphism of codon 36 (Asp, His) has also been described in association with Graves' disease (HELDIN et al. 1991). Functional analysis of the variant revealed no abnormality (GUSTAVSSON et al. 1995).

To study the role of the TSHR in the genetic pathogenesis of Graves' disease, a linkage study was performed in 14 large multiplex and strongly informative families (SHIELDS et al. 1994). Several microsatellites, particularly informative with regard to the introns of the gene, were used for the study. A variety of disease models and statistical methods were used which all gave the same result. No linkage could be observed between the TSHR gene and the occurrence of Graves' disease. Furthermore there was no linkage disequilibrium between a marker allele of the TSHR and the disease (DE ROUX et al. 1996b). These results are incompatible with the existence of a specific more "immunogenic" structural variant of the TSHR, and they thus contradict the previous report (CUDDIHY et al. 1995a) proposing the existence of an association between Graves' disease and a polymorphism of codon 52 of the receptor in a region considered especially immunogenic (KOSUGI et al. 1993b). They also contradict the suggestion of an abnormal regulation of the TSHR gene expression in Graves' disease which has been raised by several authors (DEGROOT and QUINTANS 1989; GOODNOW et al. 1990; MIZUKAMI et al. 1994). However, a minor role of the TSHR locus in the genetic susceptibility to Graves' disease cannot be excluded, although such a role might only be detected by an association study involving a large cohort of subjects using the allele-sharing methodology (LANDER and SCHORK 1994). A possible role of the TSHR gene in the pathogenesis of Graves' disease in other ethnic groups also cannot be entirely eliminated.

2. Epitopes of the TSH Receptor Recognised by the Auto-antibodies

The direct study of autoantibodies found in patients is hampered by the heterogeneity of these antibodies, their possible low concentration in serum and the difficulty in finding an efficient expression system to obtain large amounts of native TSHR. Expression of the receptor in *E. coli* yielded large amounts of receptor but in a non-native state. The expression of the complete TSHR or of its extracellular domain in the baculovirus system yielded a protein which is processed into a non-functional species (see Sect. F). Thus many different groups have performed studies on the possible interaction between TSHR and the autoantibodies with either a denatured or improperly processed receptor or synthetic peptides. Varied and even contradictory results have been published (review in MORI et al. 1994; NAGAYAMA 1995). These approaches might have produced negative results if conformational epitopes are recognised by autoantibodies, as suggested by several groups (LIBERT et al. 1991; GRAVES et al. 1995), or if folding or glycosylation were also important parameters for antibody recognition.

Mutagenesis experiments have also been used to localise the epitopes recognised by the autoantibodies. While most studies conclude that the extracellular domain of the TSHR contains epitopes for TSHR autoantibodies, the involvement of the extracellular loops of the transmembrane domain has not been excluded. It appears that binding sites for stimulating (TSAbs) or blocking antibodies (TSBAbs) and for TSH are dispersed within the extracellular domain of the TSHR and are different while sometimes overlapping (TAHARA et al. 1991; NAGAYAMA and RAPOPORT 1992b; KOSUGI et al. 1992b, 1993b, c).

The use of chimeric LH/CG-TSHRs led to the conclusion that regions 1–260 (NAGAYAMA et al. 1991c) or 8–89 (TAHARA et al. 1991) were important for functional response to TSAb. Mutagenesis experiments showed that the binding sites for the autoantibodies were located in specific regions of the TSHR which are not homologous with gonadotrophin receptors. Thyroid-stimulating autoantibodies recognised N-terminal epitopes at residues 34–37, 40, 42–45 and 52–56 while thyroid-stimulating blocking autoantibodies recognised epitopes located mainly in the middle portion of the ectodomain of the TSHR at residues 295–306, 387–395 and tyrosine 385 (KOSUGI et al. 1992b, 1993b,c).

The mechanism of action of the autoantibodies found in Graves' disease is still unknown. They might produce a conformational change of the extracellular domain of the TSHR in a way very similar to the action of TSH. The latter structural change may then be transmitted to the transmembrane domain by unknown mechanism(s). The existence of constitutive mutations of TSHR has led to the hypothesis that the receptor might exist in two different forms, active and inactive, in constant equilibrium (see below). The activating autoantibodies might also act in a manner reminiscent of catalytic antibodies (TRAMONTANO et al. 1986): they might displace the receptor steady-state towards the active (or reactive) conformational state by favouring its stabilisation.

II. Mutations of the TSH Receptor in Pathology

1. TSH Receptor and Tumorigenesis

The pioneering study on $\alpha_1\beta$-adrenergic receptors showed that activating mutations of G-protein-coupled receptors could lead to transformation in NIH3T3 cells or tumorigenesis in nude mice (review in DHANASEKARAN et al. 1995). In the thyroid, cAMP activates a mitogenic cascade. Thus, a similar situation might be expected for chronic stimulation of the cAMP cascade in the thyroid. Indeed, the Gs-coupled A_2 adenosine receptor targeted into thyroid cells in transgenic mice provokes thyroid hyperplasia (LEDENT et al. 1992). Somatic activating mutations of Gs proteins in patients with the McCune Albright syndrome may also lead to thyroid nodules and hyperthyroidism (WEINSTEIN et al. 1991). Mutations of Gsα (gsp mutations) have been found in ~30% of the hyperfunctioning thyroid adenomas (SUAREZ et al. 1991; YOSHIMOTO et al. 1993). Furthermore, thyroid-targeted expression of constitutive Gsα-subunit in transgenic mice yields hyperfunctioning thyroid adenomas (MICHIELS et al. 1994). All these examples supported the possibility of finding TSHR mutations activating the cAMP cascade in thyroid tumours (VAN SANDE et al. 1995). Indeed, somatic mutations of the TSHR have been found in autonomously hyperfunctioning adenomas (PARMA et al. 1993, 1995;

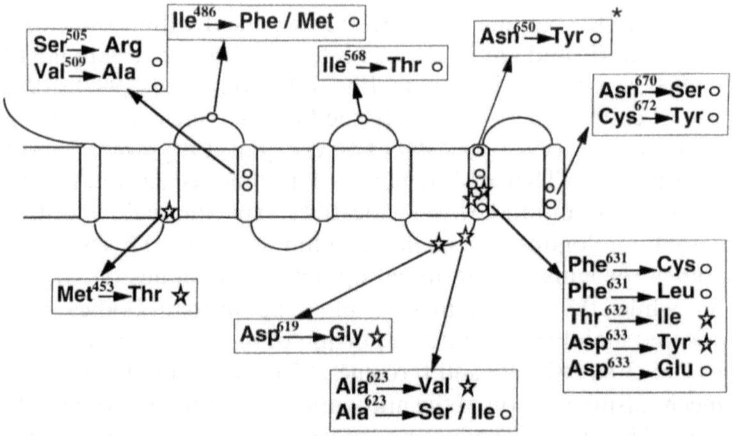

Fig. 6. Constitutive mutations of the TSHR. *Open circle,* mutation found only in TSHR; *star,* mutation found in TSHR and LH/CGR. *Asterisk* indicates a residue which is specific for the TSHR. *Numbering* corresponds to the sequence of hTSHR (Asp^{619}/gly, Ala^{623}/Ile, PARMA et al. 1993; Ala^{623}/Val, PASCHKE et al. 1994b; Ala^{623}/Ser, RUSSO et al. 1995; Asp^{633}/Glu, PORCELLINI et al. 1994; Phe^{631}/Cys, PORCELLINI et al. 1994, KOSUGI et al. 1994b; Phe^{631}/Leu, KOPP et al. 1995; Val^{509}/Ala, Cys^{672}/Tyr, DUPREZ et al. 1994; Thr^{632}/Ile, PASCHKE et al. 1994, KOSUGI et al. 1994b, PORCELLINI et al. 1995; Ile^{486}/Phe or Met, Ile^{568}/Thr, PARMA et al. 1995; Asp^{633}/Tyr or Glu, KOSUGI et al. 1994; Ser^{505}/Arg, Asn ^{670}/Ser, TONACCHERA et al. 1996; Asn^{650}/Tyr, TONACCHERA et al. 1996 and our unpublished results; Met^{453}/Thr, DE ROUX et al. 1996c)

PORCELLINI et al. 1994, 1995; PASCHKE et al. 1994b; KOSUGI et al. 1994b; RUSSO et al. 1995a) (Fig. 6). In one study 7 out of 11 (73%) of such tumours exhibited heterozygous constitutive activations of the TSHR confined to the tumour (PORCELLINI et al. 1994). All these mutations were shown to yield a spontaneously activated receptor able to stimulate the adenylate cyclase pathway in the absence of hormone.

A constitutive somatic mutation of the TSHR identical to a mutation previously detected in autonomously hyperfunctioning adenomas has also been detected in thyroid cancers (RUSSO et al. 1995b). However, it is not known at which step of the development of the cancer this mutation occurred. Thus the question is raised as to whether one of the molecular events leading to neoplasia might correspond to activating neomutations of the TSHR.

2. TSHR and Non-immune Hyperthyroidism

Germline constitutive mutations of the TSHR have been detected in familial non-immune hyperthyroidism (DUPREZ et al. 1994; TONACCHERA et al. 1996). Neomutations of the TSHR have also been detected in two cases of neonatal hyperthyroidism (KOPP et al. 1995; DE ROUX et al. 1996c) (Fig. 6). The phenotype of the disease is very similar and is independent of the localisation of the mutation; it consists in an isolated severe hyperthyroidism resistant to treatment with (initially) no or moderate thyroid enlargement and no ocular signs, the latter being considered to be pathognomonic of autoimmune disease. However, in one case of neonatal non-immune hyperthyroidism due to a neomutation of the TSHR the infant presented ocular signs. Proptosis was confirmed on CT scanning. The mutation which was detected had an unusual location in the second transmembrane segment of the receptor (Fig. 6). The pathogenesis of bilateral exophthalmos in thyroid disease is still debated. This observation may explain previous observations of "Graves' disease" with exophthalmos but without evidence of an immune mechanism (HOLLINGSWORTH and MABRY 1976). In these cases an autosomal dominant pattern of inheritance was observed, compatible with hypothetical TSHR mutations.

The highly variable age of onset of the disease (from 18 months to adulthood) in members of a family harbouring the same mutation is not understood (DUPREZ et al. 1994). However, the evolution of the disease is always severe, with the hyperthyroidism being resistant to medical treatment, and surgery is needed to achieve euthyroidism.

III. Constitutive Mutations and Model of Receptor Activation

Constitutive mutations of G-protein-coupled receptors implicated in human diseases were first described for rhodopsin. Engineered constitutive mutations of adrenergic receptors were subsequently established. A constitutive variant of the MSH receptor has also been described in mice (review in COUGHLIN 1994).

Mutations in the TSH and gonadotrophin receptors were sought and subsequently detected initially within or close to regions which had been implicated in direct interaction with G proteins such as the third intracellular loop. Other mutations were later detected within transmembrane segments and thus in regions which could not a priori establish direct contact with G proteins. This led to the hypothesis of the existence of a modification of the whole tridimensional structure of the transmembrane domain in the mutated receptor.

Previous studies on engineered mutants of adrenergic receptors suggested a model of receptor activation. These receptors would exist in an equilibrium between an inactive (R) and an active (R*) conformation. Hormone-binding drives the inactive constrained receptor into the activated "relaxed" form in which a portion of the molecule becomes available for G-protein activation (SAMAMA et al. 1993). This agonist-mediated allosteric modification of the receptor is mimicked by the unliganded mutated constitutive receptors. This configuration would allow a spontaneous functional coupling of the receptor with the G protein.

Until now constitutive mutations of the TSHR have been detected in the third intracellular loop, in the second, third, sixth and seventh transmembrane segments of the TSHR and in the first and second extracellular loops (Fig. 6). The same residues (Phe 631 and Ala 623) were found mutated in non-immune hyperthyroidism (germline mutations) and in hyperfunctioning adenomas (somatic mutations; Fig. 6). This suggests that a similar mechanism is involved in these two different pathologies.

Most of the mutations described in the TSHR activate only the adenylate cyclase pathway. However, mutations in the first and second extracellular loops, found in hyperfunctioning adenomas, activate both pathways (PARMA et al. 1995). This suggests that the active configuration adopted by the different mutants may differ. The ability of the constitutive mutants to be stimulated by TSH varies greatly. The identification of novel mutations yielding to constitutive activation of the TSHR and other gonadotrophin receptors will allow a better understanding of the mechanism of receptor activation. Each mutated residue might have a crucial role in maintaining the receptor in a locked inactive state.

The mutated amino acids found in constitutive receptors have to be distinguished in that some of them are highly conserved in all G-protein-coupled receptors. The mutated residue Ala 623 in TSHR corresponds to Ala 293 of the $\alpha_1\beta$-adrenergic receptor (reviewed in COUGHLIN 1994). This confirms the hypothesis that basic mechanisms implicated in the activation of G-protein-coupled receptors are highly conserved. Other mutated residues (the majority of them) are, on the contrary, strictly conserved in the restricted subgroup of glycoprotein hormone receptors (TSHR, LHR and FSHR) and may play a similar role in this subgroup of receptors (Fig. 6). This suggests that the mechanisms of TSH-R and LH/CG-R activation share important similarities. Finally, mutated residues may also be specific for a single receptor. Only two such cases have been described. Asn 650, specific for the TSHR, was mutated in a family of non-immune hyperthyroidism (TONACCHERA et al. 1996 and our unpublished results) (Fig. 6) while Ile 542 (which is replaced by a valine in the homologous position of the TSHR) was found mutated in a male patient with precocious puberty (LAUE et al. 1995). This suggests that some specificity in receptor activation may also exist within members of this subgroup of receptors.

Some antagonists named "inverse agonists" display the property of inhibiting the ability of the β_2-adrenergic receptor to adopt an active configuration (SAMAMA et al. 1994). Similar antagonists could be developed for other G-protein-coupled receptors and be useful and novel therapeutic agents.

IV. Loss of Function Mutations

1. Animal Model

In *hyt/hyt* hypothyroid mice a change of Pro to Leu in the fourth transmembrane segment of the TSHR has been found (STEIN et al. 1994) (Fig. 7). This proline is highly conserved in members of the G-protein-coupled receptor family and the mutation yielded a receptor expressed on the cell surface of transfected cells but unable to bind the hormone (GU et al. 1995). The impor-

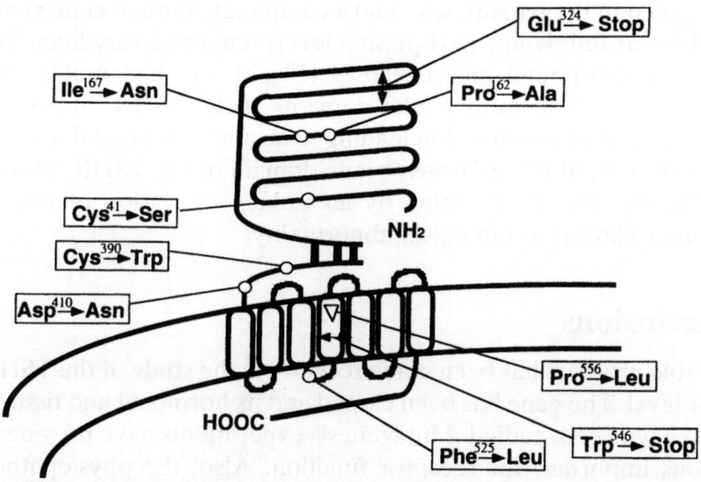

Fig. 7. Loss-of-function mutations of the TSHR. *Open circle,* mutations found in human (Ile^{167}/Asn and Pro^{162}/Ala are from SUNTHORNTHEPVARAKUL et al. 1995; Glu^{324}/stop, Cys^{41}/Ser, Cys^{390}/Trp, Asp^{410}/Asn, Phe^{525}/Leu, Trp^{546}/stop are from DE ROUX et al. 1996d). *Triangle,* mutation found in the *hyt/hyt* mouse: Pro^{556}/Leu (STEIN et al. 1994). As the exact localisation of the cleavage site of the TSHR is presently unknown, it has been positioned arbitrarily at the end (C-terminal region) of the extracellular domain of the TSHR

tance of this proline in the fourth transmembrane segment of G-protein-coupled receptors was initially demonstrated by the fact that its mutation in rhodopsin causes retinis pigmentosa. In the muscarinic M_3 receptor, mutation of the homologous proline greatly reduces the affinity for the ligand. Molecular modelling suggests that this proline resides on the outside surface of the α-helix, facing the lipid bilayer (HULME et al. 1991), and might play an important conformational role.

2. Thyroid Resistance to TSH Due to TSHR Mutations

Loss of function mutations of the TSHR have been described in three siblings who were euthyroid and had normal concentrations of thyroid hormones but high concentrations of thryrotrophin (SUNTHORNTHEPVARAKUL et al. 1995). The thyroid gland was normal on radioiodide scanning. Germline mutations of both alleles of the gene for the thryrotrophin receptor made the patients compound heterozygotes. Both mutations were located in the extracellular domain of the receptor (Fig. 7). The parents who were heterozygous for each mutation had slightly increased serum TSH concentrations.

We also detected mutations within the TSHR gene in three similar cases (DE ROUX et al. 1996d). The patients were detected at birth by the high levels of blood TSH which were confirmed by plasma assays. Serum T_3 and T_4 concentrations were in the normal range. The radioiodide scan showed eutopic thyroids of subnormal size or slightly enlarged. In one case no treatment was given to the patient, who had a completely normal clinical evolution during a 10-year follow-up. TSH plasma levels remained very high. The three patients were compound heterozygotes (Fig. 7) and had mutations in the extracellular and/or the intracellular domains of the TSHR. In two cases the mutation introduced a stop codon leading to an amputation of the whole, or of an important part, of the transmembrane domain of the TSHR. Mutations of the TSHR may thus be revealed by an isolated elevation of plasma TSH without other clinical or biological abnormality.

M. Conclusions

Considerable progress has been made recently in the study of the TSHR at the molecular level. The gene has been cloned and its hormonal and tissue specific regulation have been studied. Mutagenesis experiments have provided insight into regions important for receptor function. Also, the physiopathology of some thyroid disease (non-immune hyperthyroidism, hyperfunctioning adenomas, resistance to TSH) has been elucidated in certain cases through the finding of TSHR mutations. Constitutive mutants will also lead to a better understanding of the mechanism of TSHR activation.

However, unexpectedly, and in contrast to these developments at the molecular level, the structure of the TSHR protein itself is still a matter of debate and very little is known about its cellular expression and intracellular trafficking. This is mainly due to the lack of development of adequate immunological tools to perform such studies. However, a consensus has been slowly emerging from the literature in favour of a heterodimeric structure of the TSHR. Some questions are still unanswered: what is the role of cleavage in TSHR function, what is the role of the shed α-subunit, and is the latter implicated in the development of Graves' disease or other thyroid disease?

Six years after the cloning of the TSHR nothing certain is known regarding the pathogenesis of Graves' disease. Genetic studies do not favour a major role for the TSHR in the ontogeny of Graves' disease. The epitopes recognised by the autoantibodies have not been clearly mapped up to now, and their mechanism of action is still unknown. The possibility of developing an in vitro test for the direct detection and for the study of these autoantibodies requires the purification of large amounts of native receptor. These developments will probably be a major issue in the next few years.

References

Aittomäki K, Lucena Jld, Pakarinen P, Sistonen P, Tapanainen J, Gromoll J, Kaskikari R, Sankila EM, Lehväslaiho H, Engel AR, Nieschlag E, Huhtaniemi I, De La Chapelle A (1995) Mutation in the follicle-stimulating hormone receptor gene causes hereditary hypergonadotropic ovarian failure. Cell 82:959–968

Akamizu T, Inoue D, Kosugi S, Ban T, Kohn LD, Imura H, Mori T (1993) Chimeric studies of the extracellular domain of the rat thyrotropin (TSH) receptor: amino acids (268–304) in the TSHR are involved in ligand high affinity binding, but not in TSHR-specific signal transduction. Endocr J 40:363–372

Akamizu T, Inoue D, Kosugi S, Kohn LD, Mori T (1994) Further studies of amino acids (268–304) in thyrotropin (TSH)-lutropin/chorionic gonadotropin (LH/CG) receptor chimeras: cysteine-301 is important in TSH binding and receptor tertiary structure. Thyroid 4:43–48

Al-Alawi N, Rose DW, Buckmaster C, Ahn N, Rapp U, Meinkoth J, Feramisco JR (1995) Thyrotropin-induced mitogenesis is ras dependent but appears to bypass the raf-dependent cytoplasmic kinase cascade. Mol Cell Biol 15:1162–1168

Allgeier A, Offermanns S, Van Sande J, Spicher K, Schultz G, Dumont JE (1994) The human thyrotropin receptor activates G-proteins Gs and Gq/11. J Biol Chem 269:13733–13735

Apodaca G, Aroeti B, Tang K, Mostov KE (1993) Brefeldin-A inhibits the delivery of the polymeric immunoglobulin receptor to the basolateral surface of MDCK cells. J Biol Chem 27:20380–20385

Atassi MZ, Manshouri T, Sakata S (1991) Localization and synthesis of the hormone-binding regions of the human thyrotropin receptor. Proc Natl Acad Sci USA 88:3613–3617

Atger M, Misrahi M, Sar S, Le Flem L, Dessen P, Milgrom E (1995) Structure of the human luteinizing hormone-choriogonadotropin receptor gene: unusual promoter and 5′ non-coding regions. Mol Cell Endocrinol 111:113–123

Bahn RS, Dutton CM, Heufelder AE, Sarkar G (1994) A genomic point mutation in the extracellular domain of the thyrotropin receptor in patients with Graves' ophthalmopathy. J Clin Endocrinol Metab 78:256–260

Ban T, Kosugi S, Kohn LD (1992) Specific antibody to the thyrotropin receptor identifies multiple receptor forms in membranes of cells transfected with wild-type receptor complementary deoxyribonucleic acid: characterization of their relevance to receptor synthesis, processing, structure, and function. Endocrinology 131:815–830

Barak LS, Tiberi M, Freedman NJ, Kwatra MM, Lefkowitz RJ, Caron MG (1994) A highly conserved tyrosine residue in G protein-coupled receptors is required for agonist-mediated β_2 adrenergic receptor sequestration. J Biol Chem 269:2790–2795

Bartels ED (1941) Heredity in Graves' disease. Munksgaard, Copenhagen

Beau I, Misrahi M, Vannier B, Loosfelt H, Vu Hai MT, Pichon C, Milgrom E (1997) Basolateral localization and transcytosis of gonadotropin and thyrostimulin receptors expressed in MDCK cells. J Biol Chem 272:5241–5248

Bohr URM, Behr M, Loos U (1993) A heritable point mutation in an extracellular domain of the TSHR involved in the interaction with Graves' immunoglobulins. Biochim Biophys Acta 1216:504–508

Bomsel M, Mostov KE (1993) Possible role of both the α and $\beta\gamma$ subunits of the heteotrimeric G protein, Gs, in transcytosis of the polymeric immunoglobulin receptor. J Biol Chem 268:25824–25825

Bravo DA, Gleason JB, Sanchez RL, Roth RA, Fuller RS (1994) Accurate and efficient cleavage of the human insulin proreceptor by the human proprotein-processing protease furin. J Biol Chem 269:2583–2587

Bryant WP, Bergert ER, Morris JC (1994) Delineation of amino acid residues within hTSHr 256–275 that participate in hormone binding. J Biol Chem 269:30935–30938

Chazenbalk GD, Rapoport B (1994) Cleavage of the thyrotropin receptor does not occur at a classical subtilisin-related proprotein convertase endoproteolytic site. J Biol Chem 269:32209–32213

Chazenbalk GD, Rapoport B (1995) Expression of the extracellular domain of the thyrotropin receptor in the baculovirus system using a promoter active earlier than the polyhedrin promoter. J Biol Chem 270:1543–1549

Chazenbalk GD, Nagayama Y, Kaufman KD, Rapoport B (1990a) The functional expression of recombinant human thyrotropin receptors in nonthyroidal eukary-

otic cells provides evidence that homologous desensitization to thyrotropin stimulation requires a cell-specific factor. Endocrinology 127:1240–1244
Chazenbalk GD, Nagayama Y, Russo D, Wadsworth HL, Rapoport B (1990b) Functional analysis of the cytoplasmic domains of the human thyrotropin receptor by site-directed mutagenesis. J Biol Chem 265:20970–20975
Chazenbalk GD, Nagayama Y, Wadsworth H, Russo D, Rapoport B (1991) Signal transduction by the human thyrotropin receptor: studies on the role of individual amino acid residues in the carboxyl terminal region of the third cytoplasmic loop. Mol Endocrinol 5:1523–1526
Civitareale D, Castelli MP, Falasca P, Saiardi A (1993) Thyroid transcription factor 1 activates the promoter of the thyrotropin receptor gene. Mol Endocrinol 7:1589–1595
Costagliola S, Ruf J, Durand-Gorde MJ, Carayon P (1991) Monoclonal antidiotypic antibodies interact with the 93 kilodalton thyrotropin receptor and exhibit heterogeneous biological activities. Endocrinology 128:1555–1562
Couet J, Sar S, Jolivet A, Vu Hai MT, Milgrom E, Misrahi M (1996a) Shedding of human thyrotropin receptor ectodomain. Involvement of a matrix metalloprotease. J Biol Chem 271:4545–4552
Couet J, Sar S, Jolivet A, Vu Hai MT, Milgrom E, Misrahi M (1996b) Shedding of human thyrotropin receptor ectodomain. Involvement of a matrix metalloprotease. J Biol Chem 271:4545–4552
Coughlin SR (1994) Expanding horizons for receptors coupled to G proteins: diversity and disease. Curr Opin Cell Biol 6:191–197
Cuddihy RM, Dutton CM, Hahn RS (1995a) A polymorphism in the extracellular domain of the thyrotropin receptor is highly associated with autoimmune thyroid disease in females. Thyroid 5:89–95
Cuddihy RM, Bryant WP, Bahn RS (1995b) Normal function in vivo of a homozygotic polymorphism in the human thyrotropin receptor. Thyroid 5:255–257
Damante G, di Lauro R (1994) Thyroid-specific gene expression. Biochim Biophys Acta 1218:255–266
DeGroot LJ, Quintans J (1989) The causes of autoimmune thyroid disease. Endocr Rev 10:537–562
de Roux N, Misrahi M, Chatelain N, Milgrom E (1996a) Three microsatellites localised within the human TSH receptor gene: characterization and genetic localisation. Mol Cell Endocrinol 117:253–256
de Roux N, Schields DC, Misrahi M, Ratanachaiyavong S, McGregor A, Milgrom E (1996b) Analysis of the Thyrotropin Recetor as a Candidate Gene in Familial Graves' Disease. J Clin Endocrinol Metab 81:3483–3486
de Roux N, Polak M, Couet J, Leger J, Czernichow P, Milgrom E, Misrahi M (1996c) Neomutation of the TSH receptor in a severe neonatal hyperthyroidism. J Clin Endocrinol Metab 81:2023–2026
de Roux N, Misrahi M, Brauner R, Houang M, Carel JC, Granier M, Le Bouc Y, Ghinea N, Boumedienne A, Toublanc JE, Milgrom E (1996d) J Clin Endocrinol Metab 81:4229–4235
Dhanasekaran N, Heasley LE, Johnson GL (1995) G protein-coupled receptor systems involved in cell growth and oncogenesis. Endocr Rev 16:259–270
Dumont JE, Jauniaux JC, Roger PP (1989) The cyclic AMP-mediated stimulation of cell proliferation. Trends Biochem Sci 14:67–71
Duprez L, Parma J, Van Sande J, Allgeier A, Leclere J, Schvartz C, Delisle MJ, Decoulx M, Orgiazzi J, Dumont J, Vassart G (1994) Germline mutations in the thyrotropin receptor gene cause non-autoimmune autosomal dominant hyperthyroidism. Nat Genet 7:396–401
Ehlers MRW, Riordan JF (1991) Membrane proteins with soluble counterparts: role of proteolysis in the release of transmembrane proteins. Biochemistry 30:10065–10073
Endo T, Onaya T (1993) Analysis of the interaction of thyrotropin receptor with the ligands by using its synthetic peptides. Endocr J 40:625–631

Endo T, Ikeda M, Ohmori M, Anzai E, Haraguchi K, Onaya T (1992) Single subunit structure of the human thyrotropin receptor. Biochem Biophys Res Commun 187:887–893

Endo T, Ohta K, Haraguchi K, Onaya T (1995) Cloning and functional expression of a thyrotropin receptor cDNA from rat fat cells. J Biol Chem 270:10833–10837

Feener EP, Shen WC, Ryser HJP (1990) Cleavage of disulfide bonds in endocytosed macromolucules. J Biol Chem 265:18780–18785

Francis T, Burch HB, Cai WY, Lukes Y, Peele M, Carr FE, Wartofsky L, Burman KD (1991) Lymphocytes express thyrotropin receptor-specific mRNA as detected by the PCR technique. Thyroid 1:223–228

Freedman RB, Hirst TR, Tuite MF (1994) Protein disulphide isomerase: building bridges in protein folding. Trends Biochem Sci 19:331–336

Gearing AJH, Beckett P, Christodoulou M, Churchill M, Clements J, Davidson AH, Drummond AH, Galloway WA, Gilbert R, Gordon JL, Leber TM, Mangan M, Miller K, Nayee P, Owen K, Patel S, Thomas W, Weils G, Wood LM, Wooley K (1994) Processing of tumour necrosis factor-α precursor by metalloproteinases. Nature 370:555–557

Ghinea N, Vu Hai MT, Groyer-Picard MT, Milgrom E (1994) How protein hormones reach their target cells. Receptor-mediated transcytosis of hCG through endothelial cells. J Cell Biol 125:87–97

Goodnow CC, Adelstein S, Basten A (1990) The need for central and peripheral tolerance in the B cell repertoire. Science 248:1373–1379

Goud B, McCaffrey M (1991) Small GTP-binding proteins and their role in trasport. Curr Opin Cell Bio 3:626–633

Graves PN, Tomer Y, Davies T (1992) Cloning and sequencing of a 1.3 kb variant of human thyrotropin receptor mRNA lacking the transmembrane domain. Biochem Biophys Res Commun 187:1135–1143

Graves PN, Vlase H, Davies TF (1995) Folding of the recombinant human thyrotropin (TSH) receptor extracellular domain: identification of folded monomeric and tetrameric complexes that bind TSH receptor autoantibodies. Endocrinology 136:521–527

Gross B, Misrahi M, Sar S, Milgrom E (1991) Composite structure of the human thyrotropin receptor gene. Biochem Biophys Res Commun 177:679–687

Grossman RF, Ban T, Duh QY, Tezelman S, Jossart G, Soh EY, Clark OH, Siperstein AE (1995) Immunoprecipitation isolates multiple TSH receptor forms from human thyroid tissue. Thyroid 5:101–105

Gu WX, Du GG, Kopp P, Rentoumis A, Albanese C, Kohn LD, Madison LD, Jameson JL (1995) The thyrotropin (TSH) receptor transmembrane domain mutation (Pro556-Leu) in the hypothyroid hyt/hyt mouse results in plasma membrane targeting but defective TSH binding. Endocrinology 136:3146–3153

Gupta S, Gomez-Munoz A, Matowe WC, Brindley DN, Ginsberg J (1995) Thyroid-stimulating hormone activates phospholipase D in FRTL-5 thyroid cells via stimulation of protein kinase C. Endocrinology 136:3794–3799

Gustavsson B, Westermark B, Heldin NE (1994) Point mutations of the thyrotropin receptor determining structural requirements for its ability to bind thyrotropin and to stimulate adenylate cyclase activity. Biochem Biophys Res Commun 199:612–618

Gustavsson B, Eklöf C, Westermark K, Westermark B, Heldin NE (1995) Functional analysis of a variant of the thyrotropin receptor gene in a family with Graves' disease. Mol Cell Endocrinol 111:167–173

Hammerton RW, Krzeminnski KA, Mays RW, Ryan TA, Wollner DA, Nelson WJ (1991) Mechanism for regulating cell surface distribution of Na^+, K^+-ATPase in polarized epithelial cells. Scienence 254:847–850

Haraguchi K, Peng X, Kaneshige M, Anzai E, Endo T, Onaya T (1993) Thyrotropin-dependent desensitization by Chinese hamster ovary cells that express the recombinant human thyrotropin receptor. J Endocrinol 139:425–429

Haraguchi K, Saito T, Kaneshige M, Endo T, Onaya T (1994) Desensitization and

internalization of a thyrotrophin receptor lacking the cytoplasmic carboxy-terminal region. J Mol Endocrinol 13:283–288
Harfst E, Johnstone AP, Gout I, Taylor AH, Waterfield MD, Nussey SS (1992) The use of the amplifiable high-expression vector pEE14 to study the interactions of autoantibodies with recombinant human thyrotropin receptor. Mol Cell Endocrinol 83:117–123
Harfst E, Ross MS, Nussey SS, Johnstone AP (1994) Production of antibodies to the human thyrotropin receptor and their use in characteristing eukaryotically expressed functional receptor. Mol Cell Endocrinol 102:77–84
Heldin NE, Gustavsson B, Westermark K, Westermark B (1991) A somatic point mutation in a putative ligand binding domain of the TSH receptor in a patient with autoimmune hyperthyroidism. J Clin Endocrinol Metab 73:1374–1376
Heldin NE, Gustavsson B, Hermansson A, Westermark B (1994) Thyrotropin (TSH)-induced receptor internalization in nonthyroidal cells transfected with a human TSH-receptor complementary deoxyribonucleic acid. Endocrinology 134:2032–2036
Hertel C, Nunnally MH, Wong SKF, Murphy EA, Ross EM, Perkins JP (1990) A truncation mutation in the avian beta adrenergic receptor causes agonist-induced internalization and GTP sensitive agonist binding characteristic of mammalian receptors. J Biol Chem 265:17988–17994
Hollingsworth DR, Mabry CC (1976) Congenital Graves' disease. Am J Dis Child 130:148–155
Huang GC, Page MJ, Nicholson LB, Collison KS, McGregor AM, Banga JP (1993) The thyrotropin hormone receptor of Graves' disease: overexpression of the extracellular domain in insect cells using recombinant baculovirus, immunoaffinity purification and analysis of autoantibody binding. J Mol Endocrinol 10:127–142
Hulme EC, Kurtenback E, Curtis CA (1991) Muscarinic acetylcholine receptors: structure and function. Biochem Soc Trans 19:133–138
Hunt N, Willey KP, Janher D, Ivell R, Northemann W, Castel MA, Leidenberger F (1992) Multiple forms of thyroid stimulating hormone receptor associated with Graves' disease. Exp Clin Endocrinol 100:22–27
Hunt N, Willey KP, Abend N, Balvers M, Jähner D, Northemann W, Ivell R (1995) Novel splicing variants of the human thyrotropin receptor encode truncated polypeptides without a membrane-spanning domain. Endocrine 3:233–240
Ikuyama S, Helmut Niller H, Shimura H, Akamizu T, Kohn LD (1992) Characterization of the 5′-flanking region of the rat thyrotropin receptor gene. Mol Endocrinol 6:793–804
Ji I, Ji TH (1991) Human choriogonadotropin binds to a lutropin receptor with essentially no N-terminal extension and stimulates cAMP synthesis. J Biol Chem 266:13076–13079
Kajava AV, Vassart G, Wodak SJ (1995) Modeling of the three-dimensional structure of proteins with the typical leucine-rich repeats. Structure 3:867–877
Kaetzel CS, Rao CK, Lamm ME (1987) Protein disulphide-isomerase from human placenta and rat liver. Biochem J 241:39–47
Keefer JR, Limbird LE (1993) The a_{2A}-adrengergic receptor is targeted directly to the basolateral membrane domain of Madin-Darby canine kidney cells independent of coupling to pertussis toxin-sensitive GTP-binding proteins. J Biol Chem 268:11340–11347
Kielczynski W, Harrison LC, Leedman PJ (1991) Direct evidence that ganglioside is an integral component of the thyrotropin receptor. Proc Natl Acad Sci USA 88:1991–1995
Kimura T, Okajima F, Sho K, Kobayashi I, Kondo Y (1995) Thyrotropin-induced hydrogen peroxide production in FRTL-5 thyroid cells is mediated not by adenosine 3′,5′-monophosphate, but by Ca^{2+} signalling followed by phospholipase-A2 activation and potentiated by an adenosine derivative. Endocrinology 136: 116–123

Kobe B, Deisenhofer J (1994) The leucine-rich repeat: a versatile binding motif. Trends Biochem Sci 19:415–421
Kohn LD, Valente wa, Laccetti P, Marcocci C, de Luca M, Ealey PA, Marshall NJ, Grollman EF (1984) Monoclonal antibodies as probes of thyrotropin receptor structure. In: Venter JC, Fraser CM, Lindström JM (eds) Monoclonal and anti-idiotypic antibodies: probes for receptor structure and function. Liss, New York, pp 85–116
Kopp P, van Sande J, Parma J, Duprez L, Gerber H, Joss E, Jameson JL, Dumont JE, Vassart G (1995) Brief report: congenital hyperthyroidism caused by a mutation in the thyrotropin-receptor gene. N Engl J Med 19:150–154
Kosugi S, Mori T (1994a) The first cytoplasmic loop of the thyrotropin receptor is important for phosphoinositide signaling but not for agonist-induced adenylate cyclase activation. FEBS Lett 341:162–166
Kosugi S, Mori T (1994b) The intracellular region adjacent to plasma membrane (residue 684–692) of the thyrotropin receptor is important for phosphoinositide signaling but not for agonist-induced adenylate cyclase activation. Biochem Biophys Res Commun 199:1497–1503
Kosugi S, Mori T (1994c) The amino-terminal half of the cytoplasmic tail of the thyrotropin receptor is essential for full activities of receptor function. Biochem Biophys Res Commun 200:401–407
Kosugi S, Mori T (1994d) The third exoplasmic loop of the thyrotropin receptor is partially involved in signal transduction. FEBS Lett 349:89–92
Kosugi S, Ban T, Akamizu T, Kohn LD (1991a) Site-directed mutagenesis of a portion of the extracellular domain of the rat thyrotropin receptor important in autoimmune thyroid disease and non homologous with gonadotropin receptors. J Biol Chem 266:19413–19418
Kosugi S, Ban T, Akamizu T, Kohn LD (1991b) Further characterization of a high affinity thyrotropin binding site on the rat thyrotropin receptor which is an epitope for blocking antibodies from idiopathic myxedema patients but not thyroid stimulating antibodies from Grave's patients. Biochem Biophys Res Commun 180:1118–1124
Kosugi S, Okajima F, Ban T, Hidaka A, Shenker A, Kohn LD (1992a) Mutation of Alanine 623 in the third cytoplasmic loop of the rat thyrotropin (TSH) receptor results in a loss in the phosphoinositide but not cAMP signal induced by TSH and receptor autoantibodies. J Biol Chem 267:24153–24156
Kosugi S, Ban T, Akamizu T, Kohn LD (1992b) Identification of separate determinants on the thyrotropin receptor reactive with Graves' thyroid-stimulating antibodies and with thyroid-stimulating blocking antibodies in idiopathic myxedema: these determinants have no homologous sequence on gonadotropin receptors. Mol Endocrinol 6:168–180
Kosugi S, Okajima F, Ban T, Hidaka A, Shenker A, Kohn LD (1993a) Substitutions of different regions of the third cytoplasmic loop of the thyrotropin (TSH) receptor have selective effects on constitutive, TSH-, and TSH receptor autoantibody-stimulated phosphoinositide and 3′,5′-cyclic adenosine monophosphate signal generation. Mol Endocrinol 7:1009–1020
Kosugi S, Ban T, Kohn LD (1993b) Identification of thyroid-stimulating antibody-specific interaction sites in the N-terminal region of the thyrotropin receptor. Mol Endocrinol 7:114–130
Kosugi S, Ban T, Akamizu T, Valente W, Kohn LD (1993c) Use of thyrotropin receptor (TSHR) mutants to detect stimulating TSHR antibodies in hypothyroid patients with idiopathic myxedema who have blocking TSHR antibodies. J Clin Endocrinol Metab 77:19–24
Kosugi S, Kohn LD, Akamizu T, Mori T (1994a) The middle portion in the second cytoplasmic loop of the thyrotropin receptor plays a crucial role in adenylate cyclase activation. Mol Endocrinol 8:498–509
Kosugi S, Shenker A, Mori T (1994b) Constitutive activation of cyclic AMP but not

phosphatidylinositol signaling caused by four mutations in the 6th transmembrane helix of the human thyrotropin receptor. FEBS Lett 356:291–294
Lalli E, Sassone-Corsi P (1995) Thyroid-stimulating hormone (TSH)-directed induction of the CREM gene in the thyroid gland participates in the long-term desensitization of the TSH receptor. Proc Natl Acad Sci USA 92:9633–9637
Lander ES, Schork JN (1994) Genetic dissection of complex traits. Science 265:2037–2048
Laue L, Chan WY, Hsueh AJW, Kudo M, Hsu SY, Wu SM, Blomberg L, Cutler GB Jr (1995) Genetic heterogeneity of constitutively activating mutations of the human luteinizing hormone receptor in familial male-limited precocious puberty. Proc Natl Acad Sci 92:1906–1910
Laugwitz KL, Allgeier A, Offermanns S, Spicher K, van Sande J, Dumont JE, Schultz G (1996) The human thyrotropin receptor: a heptahelical receptor capable of stimulating members of all four G protein families. Proc Natl Acad Sci USA 93:116–120
Ledent C, Dumont JE, Vassart G, Parmentier M (1992) Thyroid expression of an A_2 adenosine receptor transgene induces thyroid hyperplasia and hyperthyroidism. EMBO J 11:537–542
Leedman PJ, Harrison PJ, Harrison LC (1991) Immunoblotting for the detection of TSH receptor autoantibodies. J Autoimmun 4:529–542
Leedman PJ, Faulkner-Jones B, Cram DS, Harrison PJ, West J, O'Brien E, Simpson R, Coppel RL, Harrison LC (1993) Cloning from the thyroid of a protein related to actin binding protein that is recognised by Graves' disease immunoglobulins. Proc Natl Acad Sci USA 90:5994–5998
Libert F, Lefort A, Gerard C, Parmentier M, Perret J, Ludgate M, Dumont JE, Vassart G (1989) Cloning sequencing and expression of the human thyrotropin (TSH) receptor: evidence for binding of autoantibodies. Biochem Biophys Res Commun 165:1250–1255
Libert F, Ludgate M, Dinsart C, Vassart G (1991) Thyroperoxidase, but not the thyrotropin receptor, contains sequential epitopes recognised by autoantibodies in recombinant peptides expressed in the pUEX vector. J Endocrinol Clin Metab 13:857–860
Loos U, Hagner S, Bohr URM, Bogatkewitsch GS, Jakobs KH, van Koppen CJ (1995) Enhanced cAMP accumulation by the human thyrotropin receptor variant with the Pro52Thr substitution in the extracellular domain. Eur J Biochem 232:62–65
Loosfelt H, Misrahi M, Atger M, Salesse R, Vu Hai MT, Jolivet A, Guiochon-Mantel A, Sar S, Jallal B, Garnier J, Milgrom E (1989) Cloning and sequencing of Porcine LH/hCG receptor: variants lacking transmembrane domain. Science 245:525–528
Loosfelt H, Pichon C, Jolivet A, Misrahi M, Caillou B, Jamous M, Vannier B, Milgrom E (1992) Two-subunit structure of the human thyrotropin receptor. Proc Natl Acad Sci USA 89:3765–3769
Low SH, Wong SH, Tang BL, Tan P, Subramaniam VN, Hong W (1991) Inhibition by brefeldin A of protein secretion from the apical cell surface of Madin-Darby canine kidney cells. J Biol Chem 266:17729–17732
Low SH, Tang BL, Wong SH, Hong W (1992) Selective inhibition of protein targeting to the apical domain of MDCK cells by bredfeldin A. J Cell Biol 118:51–62
Mandel R, Ryser HJP, Ghani F, Wu M, Peak D (1993) Inhibition of a reductive function of the plasma membrane by bacitracin and antibodies against protein disulfide-isomerase. Proc Natl Acad Sci USA 90:4112–4116
Marion S, Ropars A, Ludgate M, Braun JM, Charreire J (1992) Characterization of monoclonal antibodies to the human thyrotropin receptor. Endocrinology 130: 967–975
McFarland KC, Sprengel R, Phillips H, Kohler M, Rosemblit N, Nokolics K, Segaloff D, Seeburg P (1989) Lutropin-choriogonadotropin receptor: an unusual member of the G protein-coupled receptor family. Science 245:494–499
Meduri G, Vu Hai MT, Jolivet A, Milgrom E (1992) New functional zonation in the

ovary as shown by immunohistochemistry of luteinizing hormone receptor. Endocrinology 131:366–373

Meduri G, Vu Hai MT, Jolivet A, Takemorei S, Kominami S, Driancourt MA, Milgrom E (1992) Comparison of cellular distribution of LH receptors and steroidogenic enzymes in the porcine ovary. J Endocrinol 148:435–446

Michiels FM, Caillou B, Talbot M, Dessarps-Freichey F, Maunoury MT, Schlumberger M, Mercken L, Monier R, Feunteun J (1994) Oncogenic potential of guanine nucleotide stimulatory factor α subunit in thyroid glands of transgenic mice. Proc Natl Acad Sci USA 91:10488–10492

Minegish T, Nakamura K, Takakura Y, Miyamoto K, Hasegawa Y, Ibuki Y, Igarashi M (1990) Cloning and sequencing of human LH/hCG receptor cDNA. Biochem Biophys Res Commun 172:1049–1054

Minegish T, Nakamura K, Takakura Y, Ibuki Y, Igarashi M (1991) Cloning and sequencing of human FSH receptor cDNA. Biochem Biophys Res Commun 175:1125–1130

Misrahi M, Loosfelt H, Atger M, Sar S, Guiochon-Mantel A, Milgrom E (1990) Cloning, sequencing and expression of human TSH receptor. Biochem Biophys Res Commun 166:394–403

Misrahi M, Vu Hai Mt, Ghinea N, Loosfelt H, Meduri G, Atger M, Jolivet A, Gross B, Savouret JF, Dessen P, Milgrom E (1993) Molecular and cellular biology of gonadotropin receptor. In: Adashi EY, Leung CK (eds) The ovary. Raven, New York, pp 57–92

Misrahi M, Ghinea N, Sar S, Saunier B, Jolivet A, Loosfelt H, Cerutti M, Devauchelle G, Milgrom E (1994) Processing of the precursors of the human thyroid-stimulating hormone receptor in various eukaryotic cells (human thyrocytes, transfected L cells and baculovirus-infected insect cells). Eur J Biochem 222:711–719

Mizukami Y, Hashimoto T, Nonomura A, Michigishi T, Nakamura S, Noguchi M, Matsukawa S (1994) Immunohistochemical demonstration of thyrotropin (TSH)-receptor in normal and diseased human thyroid tissues using monoclonal antibody against recombinant human TSH-receptor protein. J Clin Endocrinol Metab 79:616–619

Mohr H, Hesch RD (1980) Different handling of parathyrin by a basal-lateral and brush-border membranes of the bovine kidney cortex. Biochem J 188:649–656

Mori T, Akamizu T, Kosugi S, Sugawa H, Inoue D, Okuda J, Ueda Y (1994) Recent progress in TSH receptor studies with a new concept of "autoimmune TSH receptor disease". Endocr J 41:1–11

Murakami M, Miyashita K, Yamada M, Iriuchijima T, Mori M (1992) Characterization of human thyrotropin receptor-related peptide-like immunoreactivity in peripheral blood of Graves' disease. Biochem Biophys Res Commun 186:1074–1080

Nagayama Y (1995) Continuous versus discontinuous B-cell epitopes on thyroid-specific autoantigens: thyrotropin receptor and thyroid peroxidase. Eur J Endocrinol 132:9–11

Nagayama Y, Rapoport B (1992a) Role of the carboxyl-terminal half of the extracellular domain of the human thyrotropin receptor in signal transduction. Endocrinology 131:548–552

Nagayama Y, Rapoport B (1992b) Thyroid stimulatory autoantibodies in different patients with autoimmune thyroid disease do not all recognise the same components of the human thyrotropin receptor: selective role of receptor amino acids Ser_{25}-Glu_{30}. J Clin Endocrinol Metab 75:1425–1430

Nagayama U, Kaufman KD, Seto P, Rapoport B (1989) Molecular cloning, sequence and functional expression of the cDNA for the human thyrotropin receptor. Biochem Biophys Res Commun 165:1184–1190

Nagayama Y, Russo D, Chazenbalk GD, Wadsworth LH, Rapoport B (1990) Extracellular domain chimeras of the TSH and LH/CG receptors reveal the mid-region (amino acids 171–260) to play a vital role in high affinity TSH binding. Biochem Biophys Res Commun 173:1150–1156

Nagayama Y, Wadsworth HL, Chazenbalk GD, Russo D, Seto P, Rapoport B (1991a) Thyrotropin-luteinizing hormone/chorionic gonadotropin receptor extracellular domain chimeras as probes for thyrotropin receptor function. Proc Natl Acad Sci USA 88:902–905

Nagayama Y, Russo D, Wadsworth HL, Chazenbalk GD, Rapoport B (1991b) Eleven amino acids (Lys-201 to Lys-211) and 9 amino acids (Gly-222 to Leu-230) in the human thyrotropin receptor are involved in ligand binding. J Biol Chem 266:14926–14930

Nagayama Y, Wadsworth HL, Russo D, Chazenbalk GD, Rapoport B (1991c) Binding domains of stimulatory and inhibitory thyrotropin (TSH) receptor autoantibodies determined with chimeric TSH-lutropin/chorionic gonadotropin receptors. J Clin Invest 88:336–340

Nagayama Y, Chazenbalk GD, Takeshita A, Kimura H, Ashizawa K, Yokoyama N, Rapoport B (1994) Studies on homologous desensitization of the thyrotropin receptor in 293 human embryonal kidney cells. Endocrinology 135:1060–1065

Nuoffer C, Balch WE (1994) GTPases: multifunctional molecular switches regulating vesicular traffic. Annu Rev Biochem 63:949–990

Ohmori M, Endo T, Ikeda M, Onaya T (1991) Role of N-terminal region of the thyrotropin (TSH) receptor in signal transduction for TSH or thyroid stimulating antibody. Biochem Biophys Res Commun 178:733–738

Ohmori M, Shimura H, Shimura Y, Ikuyama S, Kohn LD (1995) Characterization of an upstream thyroid transcription factor-1-binding site in the thyrotropin receptor promoter. Endocrinology 136:269–282

Parma J, Duprez L, van Sande J, Cochaux P, Gervy C, Mockel J, Dumont J, Vassart G (1993) Somatic mutations in the thyrotropin receptor gene cause hyperfunctioning thyroid adenomas. Nature 365:649–651

Parma J, van Sande J, Swillens S, Tonacchera M, Dumont J, Vassart G (1995) Somatic mutations causing constitutive activity of the thyrotropin receptor are the major cause of hyperfunctioning thyroid adenomas: identification of additional mutations activating both the cyclic adenosine 3′,5′-monophosphate and inositol phosphate-Ca^{2+} cascades. Mol Endocrinol 9:725–733

Paschke R, Parmentier M, Vassart G (1994a) Importance of the extracellular domain of the human thyrotrophin receptor for activation of cyclic AMP production. J Mol Endocrinol 13:199–207

Paschke R, Tonacchere M, van Sande J, Parma J, Vassart G (1994b) Identification and functional characterization of two new somatic mutations causing constitutive activation of the thyrotropin receptor in hyperfunctioning autonomous adenomas of the thyroid. J Endocrinol Metab 79:1785–1789

Paschke R, Vassart G, Ludgate M (1995) Current evidence for and against the TSH receptor being the common antigen in Graves' disease and thyroid associated ophthalmopathy. Clin Endocrinol (Oxf) 42:565–569

Pimplikar SW, Simons K (1993) Regulation of apical transport in epithelial cells by a Gs class of heterotrimeric G protein. Nature 362:456–458

Porcellini A, Ciullo I, Laviola L, Amabile G, Fenzi G, Avvedimento VE (1994) Novel mutations of thyrotropin receptor gene in thyroid hyperfunctioning adenomas. J Clin Endocrinol Metab 79:657–661

Porcellini A, Ciullo I, Pannain S, Fenzi G, Avvedimento E (1995) Somatic mutations in the VI transmembrane segment of the thyroid hyperfunctioning adenomas. Oncogene 11:1089–1093

Pötter E, Horn R, Scheumann GFW, Dralle H, Costagliola S, Ludgate M, Vassart G, Dumont JE, Brabant G (1994) Western blot analysis of thyrotropin receptor expression in human thyroid tumours and correlation with TSH-binding. Biochem Biophys Res Commun 205:361–367

Rapoport B, Adams RJ (1976) Induction of refractoriness to thyrotropin stimulation in cultured thyroid cells. J Biol Chem 251:6653–6661

Rees Smith B, Melissa S, McLachlan SM, Furmaniak J (1988) Autoantibodies to the thyrotropin receptor. Endocr Rev 9:106–121

Rodriguez MC, Xie YB, Wang H, Collison K, Segaloff D (1992) Effects of truncations of the cytoplasmic tail of the luteinizing hormone/chorionic gonadotropin receptor on receptor-mediated hormone internalization. Mol Endocrinol 6:327–336

Roth RA (1981) Bacitracin: an inhibitor of the insulin degrading activity of glutathione-insulin transhydrogenase. Biochem Biophys Res Commun 98:431–438

Rousseau-Merck MF, Misrahi M, Loosfelt H, Atger M, Milgrom E, Berger R (1990a) Assignment of the human thyroid stimulating hormone receptor (TSHR) gene to chromosome 14q31. Genomics 8:233–236

Rousseau-Merck MF, Misrahi M, Atger M, Loosfelt H, Milgrom E (1990b) Localization of the human luteinizing hormone/choriogonadotropin receptor gene (LHCGR) to chromosome 2p21. Cytogenet Cell Genet 54:77–79

Rousseau-Merck MF, Atger M, Loosfelt H, Milgrom E, Berger R (1993) The chromosomal localization of the human follicle stimulating hormone receptor gene (FSHR) on 2p21p16 is similar to that of the luteinizing hormone receptor gene. Genomics 15:222–224

Russo D, Chazenbalk GD, Nagayama Y, Wadsworth HL, Seto P, Rapoport B (1991a) A new structural model for the thyrotropin (TSH) receptor, as determined by covalent cross-linking of TSH to the recombinant receptor in intact cells: evidence for a single polypeptide chain. Mol Endocrinol 5:1607–1612

Russo D, Chazenbalk GD, Nagayama Y, Wadsworth HL, Rapoport B (1991b) Site-directed mutagenesis of the human thyrotropin receptor: role of asparagine-linked oligosaccharides in the expression of a functional receptor. Mol Endocrinol 5:29–33

Russo D, Nagayama Y, Chazenbalk GD, Wadsworth HL, Rapoport B (1992) Role of amino acids 261–418 in proteolytic cleavage of the extracellular region of the human thyrotropin receptor. Endocrinology 130:2135–2138

Russo D, Arturi F, Wicker R, Chazenbalk GD, Schlumberger M, Dugas du Villard JA, Caillou B, Monier R, Rapoport B, Filetti S, Suarez HG (1995a) Genetic alteration in thyroid hyperfunctioning adenomas. J Clin Endocrinol Metab 80:1347–1351

Russo D, Arturi F, Schlumberger M, Caillou B, Monier R, Filetti S, Suarez HG (1995b) Activating mutations of the TSH receptor in differentiated thyroid carcinomas. Oncogene 11:1907–1911

Ryser JP, Levy EM, Manderl R, Disciullo GJ (1994) Inhibition of human immunodeficiency virus infection by agents that interfere with thiol disulfide interchange yupon virus-receptor interaction. Proc Natl Acad Sci USA 91:4559–4563

Saiardi A, Falasca P, Civitareale D (1995) Synergistic transcriptional activation of the thyrotropin receptor promoter by cyclic AMP-responsive-element-binding protein and thyroid transcription factor 1. Biochem J 310:491–496

Samama P, Cotecchia S, Costa T, Lefkowitz RJ (1993) A mutation-induced activated state of the β_2-adrenergic receptor. J Biol Chem 268:4625–4636

Samama P, Pei G, Costa T, Cotecchia S, Lefkowitz RJ (1994) Negative antagonists promote an inactive conformation of the β_2-adrenergic receptor. Mol Pharmacol 45:390–394

Saunders C, Keefer JR, Kennedy AP, Wells JN, Limbird E (1996) Receptors coupled to pertussis toxin-sensitive G-proteins traffic to opposite surfaces in Madin-Darby canine kidney cells. J Biol Chem 271:995–1002

Saunier B, Tournier C, Jacquemin C, Pierre M (1995) Stimulation of mitogen-activated protein kinase by thyrotropin in primary cultured human thyroid follicles. J Biol Chem 270:3693–3697

Seetharamaiah GS, Kurosky A, Desai RK, Dallas JS, Prabhakar BS (1994) A recombinant extracellular domain of the thyrotropin (TSH) receptor binds TSH in the absence of membranes. Endocrinology 134:549–554

Seidah NG, Chretien M (1992) Proprotein and prohormone convertases of the subtilisin family: recent developments and future perspectives. Trends Endocrinol Metab 3:133–140

Shi Y, Zou M, Ahring P, Farid NR (1993) Exhibition of TSH-induced desensitization in human TSH receptor transfected CHO cells: truncation of TSH receptor cytoplasmic tail does not affect homologous desensitization. Endocr J 1:157–162

Shi Y, Zou M, Ahring P, Al-Sedairy ST, Farid NR (1995) Thyrotropin internalization is directed by a highly conserved motif in the seventh transmembrane region of its receptor. Endocrine 3:409–414

Shields DC, Ratanachaiyavong B, McGregor AM, Collins A, Morton NE (1994) Combined segregation and linkage analysis of Grave's disease with a thyroid antoantibody diathesis. Am J Hum Genet 55:540–554

Shimura H, Okajima F, Ikuyama S, Shimura Y, Kimura S, Saji M, Kohn LD (1994a) Thyroid-specific expression and cyclic adenosine 3′,5′-monophosphate autoregulation of the thyrotropin receptor gene involves thyroid transcription factor-1. Mol Endocrinol 8:1049–1069

Shimura Y, Shimura H, Ohmori M, Ikuyama S, Kohn LD (1994b) Identification of a novel insulin-responsive element in the rat thyrotropin receptor promoter. J Biol Chem 269:31908–31914

Shimura H, Shimura Y, Ohmori M, Ikuyama S, Kohn LD (1995) Single strand DNA-binding proteins and thyroid transcription factor-1 conjointly regulate thyrotropin receptor gene expression. Mol Endocrinol 9:527–539

Shlatz LJ, Schwartz IL, Kinne-Saffran E, Kinne R (1975) Distribution of parathyroid hormone-stimulated adenylate cyclase in plasma membranes of cells of the kidney cortex. J Membr Biol 24:131–144

Simons K, Wandinger-Ness A (1990) Polarized sorting in epithelia. Cell 62:207–210

Stein SA, Oates EL, Hall CR, Grumbles RM, Fernandez LM, Taylor NA, Puett D, Jin S (1994) Identification of a point mutation in the thyrotropin receptor of the hyt/hyt hypothyroid mouse. Mol Endocrinol 8:129–138

Stetler-Stevenson WG, Liotta LA, Kleiner DE (1993) Extracellular matrix 6: role of matrix metalloproteinases in tumor invasion and metastasis. FASEB J 7:1434–1441

Stosberg AD (1991) Structure/function relationship of proteins belonging to the family of receptors coupled to GTP-binding proteins. Eur J Biochem 196:1–10

Stow JL, de Almeida JB, Narula N, Holtzman EJ, Ercolani L, Ausiello DA (1991) A heterotrimeric G protein, $G\alpha_{i\text{-}3}$, on golgi membranes regulates the secretion of a heparan sulfate proteoglycan in $LLC\text{-}PK_1$ epithelial cells. J Cell Biol 114:1113–1124

Suarez HG, du Villard JA, Caillou B, Schlumberger M, Parmentier C, Monier R (1991) gsp mutations in human thyroid tumors. Oncogene 6:677–679

Sunthornthepvarakul T, Hayashi Y, Refetoff S (1994) Polymorphism of a variant human thyrotropin receptor (hTSHR) gene. Thyroid 4:147–149

Sunthornthepvarakul T, Gottschalk ME, Hayashi Y, Refetoff S (1995) Brief report: resistance to thyrothropin caused by mutations in the thyrotropin-receptor gene. N Engl J Med 19:155–160

Tahara K, Ban T, Minegishi T, Kohn LD (1991) Immunoglobulins from Graves' disease patients interact with different sites on TSH receptor/LH-CG receptor chimeras than either TSH or immunoglobulins from idiopathic myxedema patients. Biochem Biophys Res Commun 179:70–77

Takeshita A, Nagayama Y, Fujiyama K, Yokoyama N, Namba H, Yamashita S, Izumi M, Nagataki S (1992) Molecular cloning and sequencing an alternatively spliced form of the human thyrotropin receptor transcript. Biochem Biophys Res Commun 188:1214–1219

Tedder FT (1991) Cell-surface receptor shedding: a means of regulating function. Am J Respir Cell Mol 5:305–306

Tezelman S, Shaver JK, Grossman RF, Liang W, Siperstein AE, Duh QY, Clark OH (1994) Desensitization of adenylate cyclase in Chinese hamster ovary cells transfected with human thyroid-stimulating hormone receptor. Endocrinology 134:1561–1569

Tonacchera M, van Sande J, Cetani F, Swillens S, Schvartz C, Winiszewski P, Portmann L, Dumont JE, Vassart G, Parma J (1996) Functional characteristics of three new

germline mutations of the thyrotropin receptor gene causing autosomal dominant toxic thyroid hyperplasia. J Clin Endocrinol Metab 81:547–554
Tournier C, Gavaret JM, Jacquemin C, Pierre M, Saunier B (1995) Stimulation of mitogen-activated protein kinase by thyrotropin in astrocytes. Eur J Biochem 228:16–22
Tramontanon A, Janda KK, Lerner RA (1986) Catalytic antibodies. Science 234:1566–1570
Van Sande J, Raspe E, Perret J, Lejeune C, Maenhaut C, Vassart G, Dumont JE (1990) Thyrotropin activates both the cyclic AMP and the PIP_2 cascades in CHO cells expressing the human cDNA of TSH receptor. Mol Cell Endocrinol 74:R1–R6
Van Sande J, Parma J, Tonacchera M, Swillens S, Dumont J, Vassart G (1995) Genetic basis of endocrine diseases. Somatic and germline mutations of the TSH receptor gene in thyroid diseases. J Clin Endocrinol Metab 80:2577–2585
Vannier B, Loosfelt H, Meduri G, Pichon C, Milgrom E (1996) Anti-human FSH receptor monoclonal antibodies: immunochemical and immunocytochemical characterization of the receptor. Biochemistry 35:1359–1366
Vassart G, Dumont JE (1992) The thyrotropin in receptor and the regulation of thyrocyte function and growth. Endocr Rev 13:596–611
Volpe R, Edmonds M, Lamki L, Clarke PV, Row VV (1972) The pathogenesis of Graves' disease. Mayo Clin Proc 47:824–834
Vu Hai MT, Misrahi M, Houllier A, Jolivet A, Milgrom E (1992) Variant forms of the pig lutropin/choriogonadotropin receptor. Biochemistry 31:8377–8383
Wadsworth HL, Russo D, Nagayama Y, Chazenbalk GD, Rapoport B (1992) Studies on the role of amino acids 38–45 in the expression of a functional thyrotropin receptor. Mol Endocrinol 6:394–398
Watson PF, French A, Pickerill AP, McIntosh RS, Weetman AP (1995) Lack of association between a polymorphism in the coding region of the thyrotropin receptor gene and Graves' disease. J Clin Endocrinol Metab 80:1032–1035
Weetman AP, McGregor AM (1994) Autoimmune thyroid disease: further developments in our understanding. Endocr Rev 15:788–830
Weinstein LS, Shenker A, Gejman PV, Merino MJ, Friedman E, Spiegel MA (1991) Activating mutations of the stimulatory G protein in the McCune-Albright syndrome. N Engl J Med 12:1688–1695
Wilkin TJ (1990) Receptor autoimmunity in endocrine disorders. N Engl J Med 8:1318–1324
Wozniak, Limbird LE (1996) The three α_2-adrenergic receptor subtypes achieve basolateral localization in Madin-Darby canine kidney II cells via different targeting mechanisms. J Biol Chem 271:5017–5024
Woessner FJ (1991) Matrix metalloproteinases and their inhibitors in connective tissue remodeling. FASEB J 5:2145–2154
Yoshimoto K, Iwahana H, Fukuda A, Sano T, Itakura M (1993) Rare mutations of the Gs alpha subunit gene in human endocrine tumors. Mutations detection by polymerase chain – reaction – primer – introduced restriction analysis. Cancer 72:1386–1393
Zhou J, Sims C, Chang CH, Berti-Mattera L, Hopfer U (1990) Proximal tubular epithelial cells possess a novel 42-kilodalton guanine nucleotide-binding regulatory protein. Proc Natl Acad Sci USA 87:7532–7535

CHAPTER 4

Thyroid Hormone Synthesis, Plasma Membrane Transport and Metabolism

G. HENNEMANN and T.J. VISSER

A. Thyroid Hormone Synthesis

The most important iodothyronine secreted by the thyroid gland is 3,5,3′,5′-tetraiodothyronine (thyroxine, T_4). Thyroxine has little, if any, biological activity, and is converted to the active hormone par excellence, i.e. 3,5,3′-triiodothyronine (T_3). In man about 80% of total plasma T_3 production is extrathyroidally converted to T_3 (see below), while 20% is secreted by the thyroid gland.

In the process of synthesis of thyroid hormone the following important steps will be discussed: iodide transport through the plasma membrane of the thyroid follicular cell, biosynthesis of T_4 and T_3, endocytosis of iodinated thyroglobulin from the colloid into the follicular cell (see also Chap. 7, this volume), and release of T_3 and T_4 into the bloodstream (Fig. 1).

I. Iodide Transport

Iodide is concentrated in the thyroid gland against a gradient by virtue of an energy-dependent, carrier-mediated transport mechanism in the plasma membrane of the thyroid cell. Usually, the concentration of iodide in the serum is around or less than 50 n*M*. However, large variations are possible, relative to iodine intake. The concentration gradient across the plasma membrane of the thyroid cell varies by a factor of 20–50 (DEGROOT et al. 1996). The iodide transporter is a Na^+/I^- symporter and the transport system requires O_2 and is inhibited in vitro by CN^- and dinitrophenol. Transport is dependent on plasma membrane Na^+/K^+-activated ATPase and is inhibited by ouabain, digitoxin and other cardiac glycosides in vitro. This inhibition is overcome by potassium (WOLFF 1960). The anion transport system is not specific for iodide and is competitively inhibited by the following monovalent anions: $TcO_4^- \geq ClO_4^- > ReO_4^- > BF_4^- > SCN^- > I^- > NO_3^- > Br^- > Cl^-$. Perchlorate ($ClO_4^-$) is clinically used in combination with thionamides to treat severe forms of hyperthyroidism and also to study discharge of previously administered radioactive iodine from the thyroid in cases of presumed organification defects. $^{99m}TcO_4^-$ (pertechnetate) is used as a radiolabel to visualize the thyroid and also to measure the activity of the "iodide pump". Following uptake, TcO_4^- is not covalently bound to proteins in the thyroid and therefore solely measures the

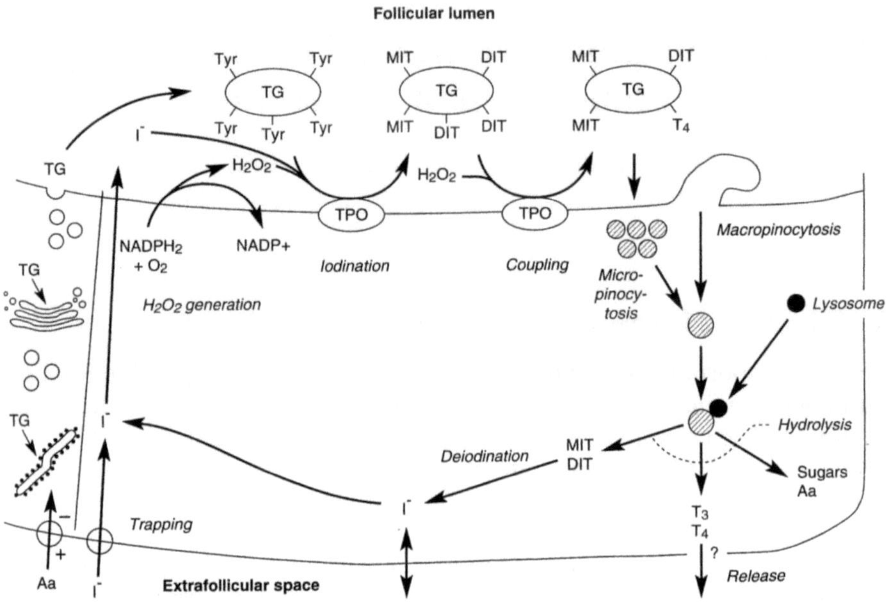

Fig. 1. Major steps in thyroid hormone synthesis. (Courtesy of Prof. J. Dumont, Brussels, with modifications)

transport process. Its uptake is increased in hyperthyroidism and in some types of congenital dyshormogenesis but is decreased in hypothyroidism. The site of iodide transport in thyroid epithelial cells is most likely the basal membrane (CHAMBARD et al. 1983). The interior of the thyroid follicular cell maintains a negative potential with respect to the extracellular space and the follicular lumen (WOODBURY and WOODBURY 1963). Both compartments are 40–50 mV positive with respect to the intracellular compartment. The iodide that is concentrated against the electrical gradient at the basal membrane flows downhill with the electrical gradient across the apical membrane into the follicular lumen.

Cloning and characterization of the thyroid iodide transporter, using the expression system of *Xenopus laevis* oocytes, was recently reported (DAL et al. 1996). The cDNA is 2893 bp in length and codes for a protein of 618 amino acids with a molecular weight of 65 kDa. The characteristics of this protein suggest an intrinsic membrane protein with 12 putative transmembrane domains. Iodide is ultimately translocated via the apical cell membrane into the follicular lumen and an apical I^- transporter has also been proposed to exist. The iodide trapping mechanism is stimulated by thyroid-stimulating hormone (TSH) and other stimulators of the cAMP cascade, and inhibited by the mitogens epidermal growth factor (EGF) and 12-*O*-tetradecanoylphorbol 13-acetate (TPA), a phosphatidylinositol pathway agonist. Both latter substances dedifferentiate thyroid follicular cells (RASPÉ and DUMONT 1995). A biphasic effect of TSH on iodide transport has been observed in in vivo studies in the rat. During the first 4h after TSH stimulation the thyroid/serum ratio (T/S) of iodide decreased, but then gradually increased to above normal levels after 8–10h. This phenomenon was explained on the basis that TSH stimulation rapidly decreased efflux of iodide from the thyroid cell and that stimulation of influx required synthesis of the iodide transporter (HALMI et al. 1960). This biphasic effect was later also found in thyroid preparations in vitro from different species including mouse, canine, cow and FRTL-5 cells. When hypophysectomized rats are fed a low-iodine diet, thyroidal radioactive iodide uptake increases. Thus, in areas with iodine deficiency not only the elevated serum TSH, but also the iodine deficiency per se, stimulates transport of iodide into the thyroid gland.

II. Biosynthesis of T_4 and T_3

After uptake of iodide in the follicular cell, it is oxidized and bound to tyrosyl residues of the thyroglobulin (TG) molecule, forming monoiodotyrosine (MIT) and diiodotyrosine (DIT) residues (Fig. 2). The essential steps in this process require, apart from the presence of iodide and TG, a peroxidase and supply of H_2O_2.

III. Thyroid Peroxidase

Thyroid peroxidase (thyroperoxidase, TPO, EC 1.11.18) has been cloned and two different cDNAs have been found (KIMURA et al. 1989): one of 3048bp

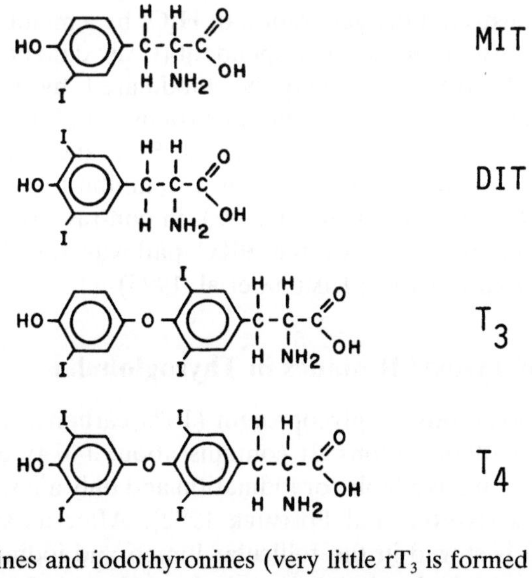

Fig. 2. Iodotyrosines and iodothyronines (very little rT_3 is formed in the thyroid, see text)

coding for a protein of 933 amino acids and a molecular weight of 103026 daltons (TPO-1) and the other of 2877 bp coding for a protein lacking 57 amino acids (exon 10 spliced out) with a molecular weight of 96744 daltons (TPO-2). Both TPOs are found in normal and abnormal thyroid tissue. The TPO gene is located on chromosome 2 p25 → p24, spans over 115 kb and has 17 exons (DE VIJLDER et al. 1988; BARNETT et al. 1993). TSH, forskolin and $(Bu)_2cAMP$ induce TPO gene expression, which is, however, inhibited by retinoic acid (NAMBA et al. 1993). Two thyroid-specific proteins, TTF-1 and TTF-2, have been cloned which bind to the promoter of the TPO gene (FRANCIS-LANG et al. 1990). The cAMP cascade induces TTF-2 expression which is inhibited by the protein kinase-C (PKC) pathway. TPO mRNA contains the code for a signal peptide and is synthesized in the rough endoplasmic reticulum (RER) and transported to the Golgi apparatus, where it is glycosylated. There are five characteristic N-glycosylation sites in the TPO molecule, four being occupied by mannose-rich oligosaccharides (RAWITCH et al. 1990). After glycosylation, peroxidase along with TG is packaged in exocytotic vesicles and fuses with the apical membrane of the follicular cell (ERICSON et al. 1990).

IV. H_2O_2 Generation

Peroxidase requires H_2O_2 for oxidation. The microsomal enzyme NADPH-cytochrome C reductase is probably not responsible for H_2O_2 generation in thyroid particles such as mitochondria, endoplasmic reticulum, lysosomes and other organelles (CARVALHO et al. 1996). Transfer of reducing equivalents from NADH to NADH-cytochrome B_5 reductase and cytochrome B_5 are possibly another source of H_2O_2 generation in the thyroid (OHTAKI et al. 1973). Others have demonstrated the generation of H_2O_2 by a membrane-associated NADPH-oxidase system that is Ca^{2+} dependent (CARVALHO et al. 1996; DUPUY et al. 1991). H_2O_2 availability may be modulated by the presence of glutathione-reductase and glutathione peroxidase and by catalase. TSH stimulates H_2O_2 generation in the dog thyroid. EGF and phorbol esters that stimulate the PKC pathway have been shown to inhibit the effects of chronic TSH stimulation (RASPÉ and DUMONT 1995), in contrast to results of others who find a stimulatory effect of the PKC pathway on H_2O_2 generation (BJÖRKMAN and ECKHOLM 1992; KIMURA et al. 1995).

V. Iodination of Tyrosyl Residues in Thyroglobulin

Human TG is a homodimeric glycoprotein (10% carbohydrate) with a molecular weight of 670000 daltons. It contains about 140 tyrosyl residues of which about only 40 are available for iodination and only a few are involved in hormone synthesis (NUNEZ and POMMIER 1982). After its synthesis in the follicular cell, TG is stored in the follicular lumen and iodination of tyrosyl residues takes place at the border of the apical membrane of the follicular cell.

The mechanism of tyrosyl iodination has been studied by several laboratories. Iodide is oxidized by peroxidase to a reactive intermediate which then reacts with tyrosine in a peptide linkage: I_2 is probably not the reactive iodine intermediate (TAUROG 1970). The possibility that the intermediate is the free radical of iodine (NUNEZ and POMMIER 1982) is also unlikely because, although peroxidase-catalysed reactions may involve a free radical mechanism, there is evidence that peroxidase-catalysed oxidation of I^- is a two-electron reaction and not a radical reaction, favouring the view that I^+ is the intermediate in both TPO- and lactoperoxidase-catalysed iodination (NAKAMURA et al. 1983). Another possibility is that hypoiodite is the intermediate (MAGNUSSON et al. 1984). (For review, see BJÖRKMAN and EKHOLM 1990.) The thioureylene antithyroid drugs propylthiouracil (PTU) and methimazole probably inhibit iodination by multiple mechanisms (see Chap. 9, this volume). Iodination of tyrosyl residues in TG results in the formation of MIT and DIT residues.

VI. Coupling of Iodotyrosines

Iodothyronines are formed by joining the iodinated hydroxyphenyl group of one iodotyrosine residue to the phenolic hydroxyl group of another (Fig. 2). The coupling is catalysed by thyroperoxidase that is also involved in tyrosyl iodination. When human TG is iodinated in vitro then, depending on the amount of iodine added, 5–15 iodotyrosyls are produced; by contrast, the formation of iodothyronines is absent at low iodine concentrations, but occurs at five sites at high iodine concentrations. The sequences around the iodotyrosyls fall into three consensus groups: (1) Glu/Asp-Tyr, associated with synthesis of T_4 (residues 24, 2572 and 1309), or iodotyrosine (residues 2586 and 991), (2) Ser/Thr-Tyr-Ser, associated with synthesis of iodothyronines (residue 2765) and iodotyrosines (residues 1466 and 883), and (3) Glu-X-Tyr (LAMAS et al. 1989). The amino acid sequence Ser-Tyr-Ser (residue 5) is possibly involved in T_3 formation (PALUMBO et al. 1990). When MIT couples with DIT, T_3 is formed and when DIT couples with DIT, T_4 is formed (Fig. 2). After injection of ^{131}I in vivo, the formation of MIT and DIT occurs within minutes. The coupling to T_3 and T_4 proceeds slowly and hours or days are required to reach a steady state of the reaction. The distribution of iodoamino acids is dependent on the degree of iodination of TG. MIT is represented most abundantly followed by DIT except at high iodination concentrations, when DIT is the predominant iodoamino acid. T_4 and lastly T_3 are synthesized at a much lower rate. The iodothyronine content in porcine TG increases linearly between 0.7% and 1.6% iodine. At 1.6% it contains six residues of T_4 and two of T_3 (MARRIQ et al. 1980). In poorly iodinated TG, T_3 is preferentially synthesized over T_4 and MIT/DIT ratios are increased (NUNEZ and POMMIER 1982). Only minimal quantities of free iodinated amino acids are present in the thyroid. In resting glands, bound ^{131}I first appears at the periphery of the colloid but then diffuses rapidly through the colloid in the follicular lumen. Excessive amounts of iodide decrease iodination and thyroid hormone synthesis. This effect is known as the Wolff-Chaikoff effect (see Chap. 8, this volume).

VII. Endocytosis of Iodinated Thyroglobulin

In principle, two mechanisms exist for the endocytosis of TG from the follicular lumen into the follicular cell, i.e. macropinocytosis or pseudopod-dependent endocytosis leading to colloid droplet formation, and micropinocytosis or coated vesicle-dependent endocytosis. Macropinocytosis enables the cell to engulf large amounts of TG and has clearly been demonstrated to be predominantly present in the rat thyroid. In this process pseudopods (Fig. 3) are formed at the apical membrane upon TSH stimulation, enabling uptake of colloid droplets from the follicular lumen. Micropinocytosis is predominantly present in the human thyroid, although excessive TSH stimulation may trigger the process of macropinocytosis (ROUSSET and MORNEX 1991). The process of micropinocytosis is a receptor-mediated process. Elegant studies by KOSTROUCH et al. (1993) have shown that, in contrast to earlier notions, the endocytotic process does not exhibit selectivity towards different iodination grades of engulfed TG, but that the thyrocyte possesses a sorting machinery for endocytosed TG. Internalized TG molecules that have a low degree of iodination are recycled back into the follicular lumen for completion of iodina-

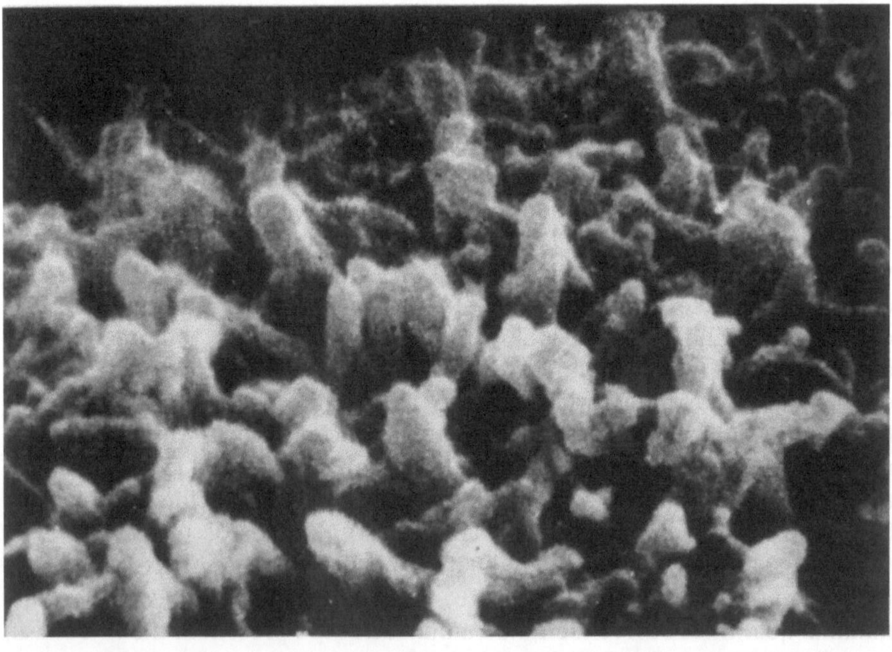

Fig. 3. Pseudopods at the apical membrane of the follicular cell. (Courtesy of Prof. J. Dumont, Brussels)

tion and hormone synthesis. Highly iodinated TG is conveyed to lysosomal compartments for further processing, i.e. hydrolysis.

VIII. Release of T_3 and T_4

In order to liberate T_4 and T_3 from peptide linkage to TG after endocytosis, TG molecules are first transported to early endosomes and then to late endosomes, also called prelysosomes. Fusion of late endosomes with lysosomes yields phagolysosomes that contain proteolytic enzymes (Kostrouch et al. 1991). The full complement of proteases and peptidases has been shown to be present in lysosomes for release of thyroid hormone residues and degradation of TG. Selectivity of cleavage for liberation of T_4 and T_3 has been suggested on the basis of the presence of proteolytic enzymes involved in cleavage at terminal regions of TG. Indeed, T_4 and T_3 are preferentially located at both ends of the amino acid sequence of the TG molecule (see above). It has been suggested that degradation of TG involves two main steps, i.e. early selective proteolytic cleavage resulting in release of T_4 and T_3 and delayed, nonselective proteolysis leading to extensive degradation of the TG backbone (Rousset et al. 1989). T_3 secreted by the thyroid is not only derived from hydrolysed TG, but also from 5′-deiodination of hydrolysed T_4 by type I deiodinase (Ishii et al. 1981). Although the exact contribution of this T_3 pathway versus the novo T_3 synthesis to total T_3 secreted by the human thyroid gland in vivo is not known, it has been demonstrated that enzyme activity is much enhanced in Graves' thyroid tissue (Ishii et al. 1981). Type I deiodinase activity due to increased protein synthesis is also affected by TSH and by Graves' IgG in human thyrocytes and in FRTL-5 rat thyroid cells (Ishii et al. 1983; Toyoda et al. 1990). Type I 5′-deiodinase activity is also present in thyroid cells of the dog (Lauerberg and Boye 1982), mouse, guinea pig and rat, but not in cattle, pig, sheep, goat, rabbit, deer and llama (Beech et al. 1993). Type I deiodinase activity, however, is present in the livers of all these species (Beech et al. 1993) (see Sect. D).

After hydrolysis of TG, MIT and DIT are deiodinated within the thyroid cell by a dehalogenase which is NADPH dependent and is found in the thyroid, but also in peripheral tissues (Stanbury and Morris 1958). The liberated iodide is re-utilized for hormone synthesis ("intrathyroidal iodide cycle"), but is partly lost from the thyroid gland ("iodide leak"). Although the process of release of T_3 and T_4 into the blood is commonly described to be by passive diffusion, it is at present not at all certain that this is correct. Abundant evidence has been presented that transport of thyroid hormones across plasma membranes of target cells into the cellular compartment is an active, stereospecific, often energy and sodium-dependent process (Docter and Krenning 1990) (see below). Efflux of intracellularly located thyroid hormones from rat hepatocytes appears to be carrier mediated but independent of energy (Hennemann et al., unpublished). No studies have been reported in recent years concerning the crossing of thyroid hormones over the plasma membrane of follicular thyroid cells, but the presence of a carrier-mediated process is certainly a possibility.

B. Thyroid Hormone Plasma Membrane Transport

After release from the thyroid gland, thyroid hormones are bound in plasma by thyroid hormone binding-proteins (see Chap. 5) and transported to the tissues. Before metabolism of thyroid hormones can take place, they have to be transported through the plasma membrane of target cells. In the following sections, plasma membrane transport will be discussed as studied in isolated cells and in the intact liver as well as the (patho)physiological significance of this process in humans.

I. Studies of Plasma Membrane Thyroid Hormone Transport in Isolated Cells

Although it has been assumed for a long time that thyroid hormones transverse the lipid-rich plasma membrane by diffusion because of their lipophilic properties, it has now clearly been established that transport into target cells is a carrier-mediated, mostly energy- and Na^+-dependent process. Even only on theoretical grounds it is improbable that the transport process is that of passive diffusion. Thus, it has been calculated that the pore radius of the plasma membrane varies between 3.5 and 5.5 Å (STITZER and JACQUEZ 1975). The mean radius, however, of for instance T_3 has been reported to vary between 7.2 and 7.5 Å (STITZER and JACQUEZ 1975). Furthermore, as thyroid hormones are in a charged state, it is even more difficult to passively cross the plasma membrane. This has been shown using the electron spin resonance stop-flow technique, demonstrating that T_3 does not "flip-flop" at any appreciable rate in prepared phospholipid bilayers, as after partitioning into the membrane it remains in the outer half of the bilayer (LAI et al. 1985). Stereospecific carrier-mediated transport has been found in a variety of cells in different species such as mouse neuroblastoma cells, human glioma cells, rat astrocytes, rat and human red blood cels, choriocarcinoma cells, rat myoblasts, human white blood cells, mouse and rat thymocytes, mouse and human fibroblasts, human hepatoma cells, rat and human hepatocytes, rat anterior pituitary tumour cells and rat anterior pituitary cells (for review see KRAGIE 1994).

The most studied cell is the rat hepatocyte. Two saturable binding sites are found for T_3 (Fig. 4) and T_4 in rat and human hepatocytes, i.e. a low-affinity site (LAS) and a high-affinity site (HAS). The LAS does not show temperature or energy dependency and probably represents binding to the outer surface of the cell membrane. The HAS, however, is highly dependent on temperature and the presence of energy and is also dependent on the Na^+ gradient. Uptake of thyroid hormone is inhibited by ouabain, a specific inhibi-

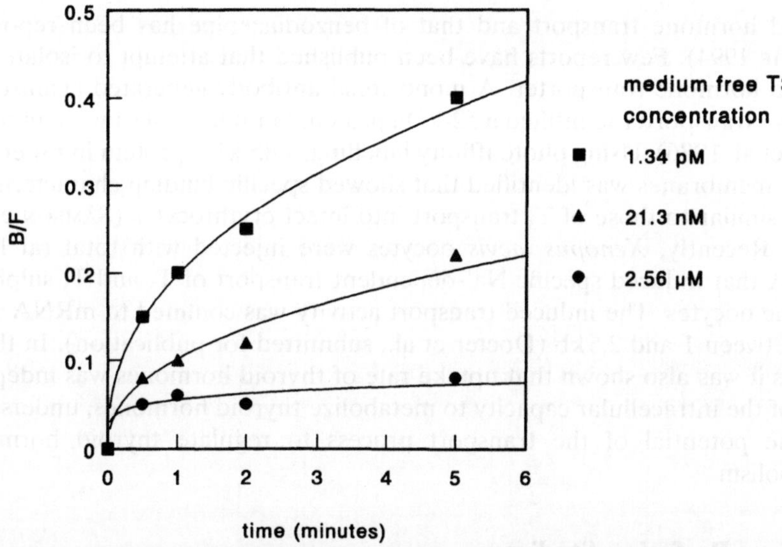

Fig. 4. Saturability of initial T_3 uptake by rat hepatocytes in primary culture. *B*, amount of T_3 bound by hepatocytes; *F*, free T_3 in incubation medium)

tor of Na^+, K^+-ATPase, showing indeed that the Na^+ gradient is important for thyroid hormone transport. Transport is also inhibited by metabolic inhibitors such as KCN, DNP and oligomycin. The K_m value of the HAS in rat hepatocytes at 21°C is around 20 n*M* for T_3 and 1.2 n*M* for T_4, and for the LAS 1800 n*M* and 1000 n*M*, respectively (see for review BEECH et al. 1993). The rat hepatocyte has separate putative transporters, one for T_4 and rT_3 and one for T_3, although T_4 and T_3 do inhibit each other's transport mechanisms (Krenning et al. 1981, 1982; DOCTER and KRENNING 1990; DE JONG et al. 1994a). Transport of thyroid hormones into target cells has shown to be rate limiting on subsequent metabolism and nuclear binding (HENNEMANN et al. 1986; HALPERN and HINKLE 1982; PONTECORVI et al. 1987). Uptake characteristics with regard to K_m values, Na^+ and temperature dependency, and sensitivity to ouabain and metabolic blockers are similar in rat hepatocytes, human hepatocytes and human fibroblasts (DOCTER et al. 1987; DE JONG et al. 1993). Many authors only find high-affinity binding sites in the different cell types studied that are stereospecific, temperature dependent, mostly energy dependent and often Na^+ dependent. The absence of LAS may be attributed not only to differences in cell types and species but also in techniques used.

Rat anterior pituitary cells, in contrast to rat hepatocytes, seem to have only one transporter for both T_3 and T_4, which is dependent on temperature, energy and the Na^+ gradient (EVERTS et al. 1993, 1994a). Thyroid hormones and aromatic amino acids (tryptophan, phenylalanine, tyrosine) competitively inhibit each other's transport, but so far no convincing evidence has been presented that they share common transporters. Also, competition between thyroid hormone transport and that of benzodiazepine has been reported (KRAGIE 1994). Few reports have been published that attempt to isolate the thyroid hormone transporter. A monoclonal antibody generated against the putative transporter identified a 52-kDa protein in rat liver plasma membrane (MOL et al. 1986). Using photoaffinity labelling, a 45-kDa protein in rat erythrocyte membranes was identified that showed specific binding characteristics for T_3 similar to those of T_3 transport into intact erythrocytes (SAMSON et al. 1993). Recently, *Xenopus laevis* oocytes were injected with total rat liver mRNA that induced specific Na^+-dependent transport of T_3 and T_3 sulphate into the oocytes. The induced transport activity was confined to mRNA species between 1 and 2.5 kb (Docter et al., submitted for publication). In these studies it was also shown that uptake rate of thyroid hormones was independent of the intracellular capacity to metabolize thyroid hormones, underscoring the potential of the transport process to regulate thyroid hormone metabolism.

II. Liver Perfusion Studies

Probably the first evidence that, also in the intact organ, uptake of thyroid hormone is rate limiting for subsequent metabolism came from a study in which uptake of T_4 was measured in livers of fed rats and of 3-day fasted rats (JENNINGS et al. 1979; JENNINGS 1984). Thyroxine uptake in livers from fasted rats was only 42% of that in fed rats and resulted in a proportionate decrease in T_3 production. Subsequent studies, using the system of the isolated perfused rat liver, were performed to obtain more insight into the mechanism of the decrease in thyroid hormone uptake after fasting in the rat. Forty-eight hours of fasting resulted in a decrease of about 40% of plasma membrane T_3 transport, while intrahepatic T_3 metabolism remained unaltered. Addition to the circulating medium of insulin and cortisol and/or glucose, 30 min prior to the transport studies, normalized T_3 transport in fasted rat livers but had no influence on transport in fed livers (DE JONG et al. 1992). As uptake was normalized within 30 min, it was concluded that this was probably caused by restoration of intracellular ATP rather than normalization of intracellular thyroid hormone-binding protein levels that hypothetically might have decreased during fasting. In another series of rat liver perfusion experiments, fructose added to the medium resulted in a substantial decrease in intracellular ATP that was paralleled by a similar reduction in T_4 transport (DE JONG et al. 1994b) (Fig. 5). In addition, studies in humans showed that i.v. fructose induced inhibition of T_4 transport into the liver (see below).

As a general conclusion it can be said that thyroid hormone transport into the liver is not only dependent on intracellular ATP when studied in vitro, but also when studied in the intact liver. Transport of thyroid hormone into the intracellular compartment of the liver is dependent on the free hormone concentration, but not on the thyroid hormone binding-protein concentration

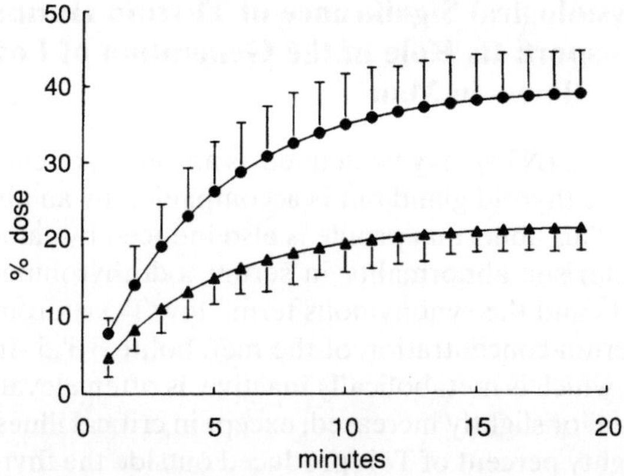

Fig. 5. Uptake of ^{125}I-thyroxine by the perfused rat liver without (○) and with (▲) fructose in the circulating medium

of the medium (DOCTER et al. 1990). This study confirms the so-called free hormone hypothesis stating that it is the free but not the total thyroid hormone concentration that determines the rate of entry into the hepatocyte. However, in addition to the free hormone concentration, cellular factors such as ATP concentration influence uptake rate. These and other factors (see below) play a role in the overall determination of thyroid hormone entry into target tissues. Results of transport studies of T_3 in livers of hypo- and hyperthyroid rats showed that adaptive mechanisms were generated, favouring tissue euthyroidism (DE JONG et al. 1994c). Thus, in hypothyroid rat livers, transport was not changed, but metabolism of thyroid hormone was decreased, so that intracellular thyroid hormone bioavailability was increased. In hyperthyroid rat livers, however, transport of thyroid hormone into the liver was decreased, but intracellular metabolism was increased, both effects thus decreasing bioavailability. Similar to the results of in vitro studies, analysis of transport of T_4 and T_3 in livers of rats treated with amiodarone showed that T_4 and T_3 were transported by different carriers. Although transport of T_4 into the liver and subsequent metabolism were inhibited by pretreatment with amiodarone, uptake and metabolism of T_3 were unaffected (DE JONG et al. 1994a). Energy-dependent transport of a compound is usually against a concentration gradient. Thus, a higher concentration of the free compound would be expected to be present in the intracellular compartment versus the extracellular compartment. To study this aspect, experiments were conducted using the isolated rat liver perfusion model. Both influx and efflux from the liver and metabolic parameters of T_4 and T_3 were determined. The free T_4 and T_3 intracellular concentrations were determined in diluted liver cytosol. It appeared that the calculated intracellular versus extracellular ratio for free T_4 was 18.2 and for free T_3 18.8 (DOCTER et al. 1993).

III. (Patho)physiological Significance of Thyroid Hormone Plasma Membrane Transport: Its Role in the Generation of Low Serum T_3 in Non-thyroidal Illness in Man

Non-thyroidal illness (NTI) may be defined as any acute or chronic illness that is not related to the thyroid gland but is accompanied by an abnormal thyroid hormone profile. This abnormal profile is also induced by caloric deprivation. The most characteristic abnormality in serum iodothyronine levels is a decrease in serum T_3 and the synonymous term "low T_3 syndrome" is therefore also used. The serum concentration of the metabolite 3,3′,5′-triiodothyronine (reverse T_3, rT_3), which is metabolically inactive, is often elevated while serum T_4 is mostly normal or slightly increased, except in critical illness, where it may be decreased. Eighty percent of T_3 is produced outside the thyroid gland by 5′-deiodination of T_4, in which process the liver plays a dominant role. The decrease in serum T_3 in NTI and starvation in humans is caused by a diminution in plasma T_3 production, while metabolic clearance rate (MCR) of T_3 remains about the same (HENNEMANN 1986). The elevation of plasma rT_3, which is virtually all produced outside the thyroid gland (predominantly in the brain; see Sect. C) is caused by a decreased MCR by the liver, while rT_3 production rate remains unaltered (HENNEMANN 1986). The decrease in serum T_4 in critical illness is caused by decreased serum binding and also by a lowered production rate (HENNEMANN 1986). It should be noted that the low T_3 syndrome in rats is predominantly caused by an initial fall in TSH secretion followed by roughly parallel decreases in plasma T_4 and T_3, while rT_3 is hardly detectable (KAPLAN and UTIGER 1978; ROSENBAUM et al. 1980; KINLAW et al. 1985). In addition, peripheral 5′ deiodination of iodothyronines is also decreased (HENNEMANN 1986). By contrast, the low T_3 syndrome in caloric deprivation and in NTI in the human is predominantly caused by alterations in peripheral thyroid hormone metabolism, while thyroid gland activity is mostly normal except that it may be modestly decreased in critical illness. In man, the described abnormalities in production rates and MCR of iodothyronines can be either explained by inhibition of transport of thyroid hormones into tissues and/or by inhibition of deiodination. It is obviously not possible to obtain direct information about these two aspects in humans during caloric deprivation and illness. Indirect evidence may be obtained by performing plasma iodothyronine tracer kinetics that are analysed on the basis of compartmental analysis. In this way unidirectional influx and efflux rates into and from tissues respectively can be separately measured. On the basis of these and other parameters, the process of transport into tissues and of intracellular metabolism can be assessed. Using this technique, studies during caloric deprivation in obese but otherwise healthy volunteers revealed that T_4 transport into tissues was inhibited by about 50% and that of T_3 by about 25% (VAN DER HEYDEN et al. 1986). The difference in transport inhibition was at least partly explained by different sensitivity of the T_4 and T_3 transport process to decreases in intracellular ATP induced by starvation (see below). In contrast to previous studies

(HENNEMANN 1986), a decrease in T_4 production rate was noted of 20%, while T_3 production rate dropped by 40%. Inhibition of peripheral T_4 to T_3 conversion could only partly explain the marked decrease in plasma T_3 production, and it was concluded that T_4 transport inhibition into T_3-producing tissues (predominantly the liver) plays an important role in the generation of the low T_3 syndrome in caloric deprivation. KAPTEIN et al. (1982, 1987) studied T_4 transfer into tissues during critical non-thyroidal illness and also found marked inhibition of T_4 transport into tissues. However, no inhibition of T_3 transport was noted in these studies. That T_4 transport inhibition into the liver is not only rate limiting for subsequent deiodination to T_3 in vitro, but also in vivo, was also substantiated by a study in a human subject who appeared to have a subnormal plasma T_3 production rate due to selective inhibition of T_4 transport into the liver (HENNEMANN et al. 1993) (Fig. 6).

As to the cause of transport inhibition, *cellular* and *extracellular* factors have to be considered. One of the intracellular factors is most probably ATP. It has been shown in isolated hepatocytes, as well as in liver perfusion studies (see above), that the transport rate of thyroid hormones is dependent on the intracellular ATP concentration. In vitro studies indicate that T_4 transport is more sensitive to a lowered intracellular ATP than T_3 transport (KRENNING et al. 1982). There is also evidence that in starvation and in NTI intracellular energy stores may be reduced (KRENNING et al. 1983). In agreement with the different effects of intracellular ATP decreases on T_4 and T_3 transport are the findings in humans that, in caloric restriction and in NTI, T_4 transport into tissues is more profoundly affected than that of T_3 (see above). More direct evidence that a decrease in hepatic ATP in humans affects T_4 transport negatively has been reported in studies in volunteers injected with an intravenous bolus of fructose. Although liver ATP measurement could obviously not be performed, a decrease was indirectly evidenced by an increase in serum lactate and uric acid (SAMSON et al. 1993). Other cellular factors that may interfere with thyroid hormone uptake into tissues in starvation and in NTI are possible changes in membrane fluidity by dietary manipulation or in disease or by changes in the sodium gradient over the plasma membrane (SCHACHTER 1984).

Regarding extracellular factors, it was found that serum of patients with NTI inhibited T_4 and T_3 uptake in rat hepatocytes in culture. The effect on T_4 uptake was more pronounced than on that of T_3 and inhibition was progressive with increasing severity of NTI (VOS et al. 1995) (Fig. 7). It was also reported that serum of critically ill patients inhibited T_4 entry into the isolated intact rat liver by more than 50% (VOS et al. 1991). Analysis of serum of patients with NTI revealed that in uraemia two substances that inhibit T_4 uptake in rat hepatocytes are present in increased concentrations. These substances are a furanic acid, 3-carboxy-4-methyl-5-propyl-2-furanpropanoic acid, and indoxyl sulphate (LIM et al. 1993a). In patients with non-uraemic critical illness both bilirubin and non-esterified fatty acids, circulating in increased concentrations, also inhibited T_4 uptake into rat hepatocytes (LIM et al. 1993b). It was also found that in caloric restriction as in NTI, non-esterified fatty acids were

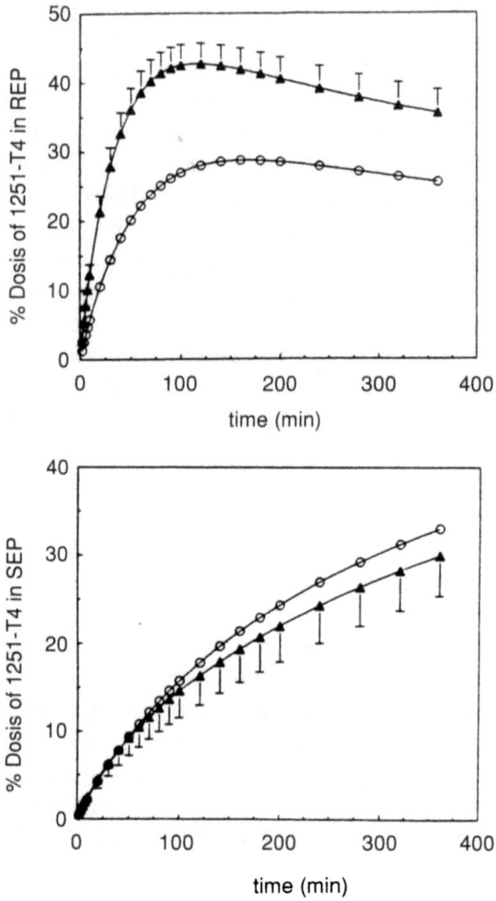

Fig. 6. Uptake of thyroxine into rapidly equilibrating compartment (*REP*), i.e. predominantly the liver, and into slowly equilibrating compartment (*SEP*), i.e. rest of the body, in a subject with selective inhibition of T_4 transport into the liver (○) and in controls (▲)

elevated to the extent that serum of such patients exerted inhibitory effects on T_4 transport into rat hepatocytes (LIM et al. 1994).

Thus, both intracellular and extracellular factors may contribute to transport inhibition of T_3 and particularly of T_4 into tissues, notably the liver. As plasma rT_3 is cleared by the liver and rT_3 and T_4 share the same transport mechanism in the liver [which is different from that of T_3 (KRENNING et al. 1982)], a decrease in MCR of rT_3 in starvation and in NTI (see above) readily explains an increased plasma rT_3 in these conditions. It seems possible that variations in composition of diet and of amount of calories consumed, and more generally in energy turnover, may be of influence on cellular and extracellular factors that regulate thyroid hormone transport into tissues

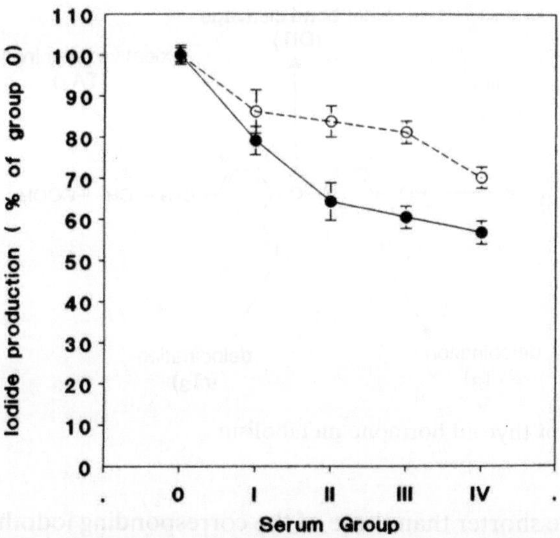

Fig. 7. Transport, as reflected by iodide production in the medium, of T_4 (●) and T_3 (○) into rat hepatocytes in primary culture, in the presence of serum of healthy controls (group 0) and of patients with increasing severity of disease (group I → IV)

and thus play a role in the physiological regulation of thyroid hormone bioavailability.

Lowered T_3 production in starvation and in NTI is considered to be a defence mechanism in situations of stress as it results in conservation of energy and of protein, i.e. organ function (GARDNER et al. 1979; HENNEMANN 1986).

C. Thyroid Hormone Metabolism

Thyroxine undergoes multiple metabolic reactions (Fig. 8) (ENGLER and BURGER 1984; VISSER 1988; KÖHRLE et al. 1991; LARSEN and BERRY 1995): the most important of these is deiodination, not only in quantitative terms but especially because of its role in the regulation of thyroid hormone bioactivity. Thus, T_4 is converted by 5′-deiodination (outer ring deiodination, ORD) to the bioactive hormone T_3 or by 5-deiodination (inner ring deiodination, IRD) to the inactive metabolite rT_3. T_3 is inactivated by IRD to 3,3′-diiodothyronine (3,3′-T_2), a metabolite that is also generated by ORD of rT_3.

In addition to deiodination, iodothyronines are metabolized by conjugation of the phenolic hydroxyl group with sulphate or glucuronic acid (VISSER 1994a), and, to a minor extent, by ether bond cleavage (GREEN 1994) and oxidative deamination of the alanine side chain (SIEGRIST-KAISER and BURGER 1994) (Fig. 8). The latter converts T_4 to Tetrac (TA_4) and T_3 to Triac (TA_3). TA_4 and TA_3 bind with higher affinity to plasma proteins than T_4 and T_3, respectively. However, both in rats and humans the half-lives of circulating

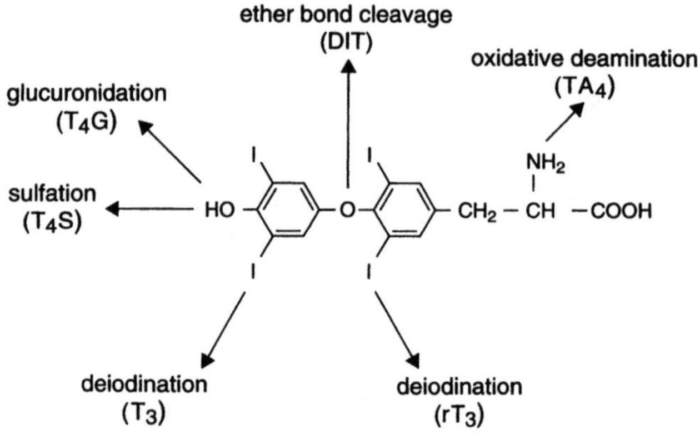

Fig. 8. Pathways of thyroid hormone metabolism

TA_4 and TA_3 are shorter than those of the corresponding iodothyronines. This explains the low in vivo bioactivity of TA_3, although it has a higher affinity than T_3 for, in particular, the β-type T_3 receptor (SIEGRIST-KAISER and BURGER 1994).

Sulphation and glucuronidation are so-called phase II detoxication reactions, the general purpose of which is to increase the water solubility of the substrates and thus to facilitate their urinary and biliary clearance. However, only small amounts of iodothyronine sulphates normally appear in bile, urine or serum, because they are rapidly deiodinated by the type I iodothyronine deiodinase. In particular, the IRD of T_4 sulphate (T_4S) and T_3 sulphate (T_3S) is strongly enhanced, suggesting that sulphate conjugation is a primary step leading to the irreversible inactivation of thyroid hormone (VISSER 1994a, 1994b). When ID-I activity is low, e.g. during fetal development, NTI and fasting, these sulphates accumulate in serum and active T_3 may be recovered by hydrolysis of T_3S by tissue sulphatases and bacterial sulphatases in the intestine (VISSER 1994b; CHOPRA 1994; POLK 1995). In contrast to the sulphates, iodothyronine glucuronides are rapidly excreted in the bile. However, this is not an irreversible pathway of hormone disposal, since after hydrolysis of the glucuronides by bacterial β-glucuronidases in the intestine at least part of the liberated iodothyronines are reabsorbed, constituting an enterohepatic cycle (VISSER 1994a). In the following sections the biochemical aspects of the deiodination, sulphation and glucuronidation pathways in particular will be reviewed.

D. Deiodination

ORD is regarded as an activating pathway by which the prohormone T_4 is converted to active T_3, whereas IRD is regarded as an inactivating pathway by which both T_4 and T_3 are converted to inactive metabolites. Also, physicochemically, ORD and IRD are distinct processes, since the C-I bonds are much stronger in the inner (tyrosyl) than in the outer (phenolic) ring. Three types of iodothyronine deiodinases have been identified (Table 1) (Visser 1988; Köhrle et al. 1991; Larsen and Berry 1995), the structures of which have recently been characterized (Table 2). They are homologous, integral membrane proteins which all require thiols as cofactor. However, they have distinct tissue distributions, catalytic specificities, physiological functions and regulatory aspects (Visser 1988; Köhrle et al. 1991; Larsen and Berry 1995).

The type I iodothyronine deiodinase (ID-I) is located predominantly in liver, kidney and thyroid (Visser 1988; Köhrle et al. 1991; Larsen and Berry 1995). Evidence has been presented that the enzyme is associated in rat liver with the endoplasmic reticulum and in rat kidney with the plasma membranes. It catalyses the ORD and/or IRD of a variety of iodothyronine derivatives, in particular sulphates (see below). In the presence of dithiothreitol (DTT) as cofactor, ID-I displays high K_m and V_{max} values (Table 3). Among the non-sulphated iodothyronines, rT_3 is by far the preferred substrate, the ORD of which is orders of magnitude faster than the deiodination of any other iodothyronine (Table 3). Therefore, it is not surprising that ID-I is probably the primary site for the clearance of plasma rT_3. Although it catalyses the conversion of T_4 to T_3 much less effectively, ID-I is supposed to be the major source of circulating T_3 (Visser 1988; Köhrle et al. 1991; Larsen and Berry 1995). ID-I activity in liver and kidney is stimulated in hyperthyroidism and decreased in hypothyroidism, representing the regulation of ID-I activity by T_3 at the transcriptional level (O'Mara et al. 1993). ID-I activity in cultured thyroid cells is stimulated by both T_3 and TSH (Toyoda et al. 1992). (For an extensive review of ID-I, see Berry and Larsen 1994.)

The type II iodothyronine deiodinase (ID-II) is expressed primarily in the brain, the anterior pituitary gland and brown adipose tissue (Visser 1988; Köhrle et al. 1991; Leonard and Safran 1994). However, expression of ID-II mRNA has recently also been shown in human heart and skeletal muscle (Croteau et al. 1996; Salvatore et al. 1996). It has been reported that in rat brain ID-II is expressed in neurons, in particular in nerve terminals, although the enzyme can also be induced in cultured glial cells by a variety of factors (Leonard and Safran 1994). ID-II has only ORD activity, exhibiting low K_m

Table 1. Characteristics of the three types iodothyronine deiodinases

Type	I	II	III
	↙T_4↘ T_3 rT_3 ↘T_2↙	↙T_4 T_3 rT_3 T_2↙	T_4↘ T_3 rT_3 ↘T_2
Tissues	liver, kidney, thyroid	brain, BAT, pituitary	brain, skin, placenta
PTU	inhibition	no effect	no effect
Hypothyroidism	decrease	increase	decrease
Hyperthyroidism	increase	decrease	increase

Table 2. Alignment of the amino acid sequences of rat ID-I, ID-II and ID-III. Data derived from [96, 102, 105] (Courtesy Dr. D.L. St. Germain)

I	M--GL--SQL	WL------WL	KRLVIFLQ--	VALEVATGKV	LMTLF-----	PERVKQNILA	43
II	M--GLLSVDL	LI------TL	QILPVFFSNC	LFLALYDSVI	LLKHV-----	ALLLSRSKST	47
III	MLRSLLLHSL	RLCAQTASCL	VLFPRFLGTA	FMLWLLDFLC	IRKHFLRRRH	PDHPEPEVEL	60
I	MGQKTGMTRN	PRFAPDNWVP	TFFSIQYFWF	VLKVRWQRLE	DRAEYGGLAP	NCTVVRLSGQ	103
II	RGEWRRMLTS	EGLRCVWNSF	LLDAYKQVKL	GEDAPNSSVV	HVSNPEAGNN	CASEKTADGA	107
III	NSEGEEMPPD	DPPICVSDDN	RLCTLASLKA	VMHGQKLDFF	KQAHEGGPAP	NSEVVRPDGF	120
I	KCN-VWDFIQ	GSRPLVLNFG	SCT$PSFLLK	FDQFKRLVDD	FASTADFLII	YIEEAHATDG	162
II	ECH-LLDFAS	AERPLVVNFG	SAT$PPFTRQ	LPAFRQLVEE	FSSVADFLLV	YIDEAHPSDG	166
III	QSQRILDYAQ	GTRPLVLNFG	SCT$PPFMAR	MSAFQRLVTK	YQRDVDFLII	YIEEAHPSDG	180
I	WAFKNNVDIR	Q----HRSLQ	DRLRAAHLLL	AR---SPQCP	VVVDTMQNQS	SQLYAALPER	215
II	WAVPGDSSMS	FEVKKHRNQE	DRCAAAHQLL	ERFSLPPQCQ	VVADRMDNNA	NVAYGVAFER	226
III	WVTTDSPVVI	PQ---HRSLE	DRVSAARVLQ	QG---APGCA	LVLDTMANSS	SSAYGAYFER	234
I	LYVIQEGRIC	YKGKPGPWNY	NPEEVRAVLE	KLCIP-PGHM	P-QF		257
II	VCIVQRRKIA	YLGGKGPFSY	NLQEVRSWLE	KNFSK-R$IL	D		266
III	LYVIQSGTIM	YQGGRGPDGY	QVSELRTWLE	RYDEQLHGTR	PRRL		278

$ – Selenocysteine (Sec).

Table 3. Kinetic parameters of iodothyronine deiodinases

Substrate	Reaction	Product	K_m	V_{max}	V_{max}/K_m
ID-I (rat liver)[a]			*μM*	*pmol*	
T_4	ORD	T_3	2.3	30	13
T_4	IRD	rT_3	1.9	18	9
rT_3	ORD	3,3′-T_2	0.06	559	8730
T_3	IRD	3,3′-T_2	6.2	36	6
ID-II (hypothyroid rat brain)[b]			*nM*	*fmol*	
T_4	ORD	T_3	1.1	11	10
rT_3	ORD	3,3′-T_2	2.8	6	2
ID-III (rat brain)[c]			*nM*	*fmol*	
T_4	IRD	rT_3	37	144	4
T_3	IRD	3,3′-T_2	5.5	134	24

V_{max}, per min and per mg protein.
[a] VISSER TJ, FEKKES D, DOCTER R, HENNEMANN G (1979) Kinetics of enzymic reductive deiodination of iodothyronines. Biochem J 179:489–495.
[b] VISSER TJ, LEONARD JL, KAPLAN MM, LARSEN PR (1982) Kinetic evidence suggesting two mechanisms for iodothyronine 5′-deiodination in rat cerebral cortex. Proc Natl Acad Sci USA 79:5080–5084.
[c] KAPLAN MM, VISSER TJ, YASKOSKI KA, LEONARD JL (1983) Characteristics of iodothyronine tyrosyl ring deiodination by rat cerebral cortical microsomes. Endocrinology 112:35–42.

and V_{max} values, and a slight preference for T_4 over rT_3 as substrate (Table 3). In contrast to ID-I, it does not catalyse the deiodination of sulphated iodothyronines (Visser et al., unpublished). The amount of T_3 in tissues expressing ID-II is derived to a large extent from local conversion of T_4 by this enzyme and to a minor extent from plasma T_3 (LARSEN et al. 1981). In general, ID-II activity is increased in hypothyroidism and decreased in hyperthyroidism. Part of this negative control is explained by substrate-induced inactivation of the enzyme by T_4 and rT_3 (LEONARD and SAFRAN 1994). However, a presumably receptor-mediated inhibition of ID-II activity by T_3 has been demonstrated in pituitary tumour cells (HALPERIN et al. 1994).

The type III iodothyronine deiodinase (ID-III) is located predominantly in brain, especially fetal brain, neonatal skin, placenta and fetal intestine (VISSER 1988; KÖHRLE et al. 1991; ST. GERMAIN 1994). High ID-III activities are also found in embryonic chicken liver (DARRAS et al. 1992). The subcellular localization of the enzyme has not been assessed, but highest activities are associated with the microsomal fractions of the tissues. ID-III has only IRD activity, catalysing the inactivation of T_4 and T_3 with intermediate K_m and V_{max} values (Table 3). ID-III in tissues such as the brain is thought to play a role in the regulation of intracellular T_3 levels, while its presence in placenta and fetal tissues may protect developing tissues against exposure to high levels of active thyroid hormone (ST. GERMAIN 1994). In adult subjects, ID-III may be an important site for clearance of plasma T_3 and production of plasma rT_3. In brain and skin, but not in placenta, ID-III activity is increased in hyperthyroidism and decreased in hypothyroidism (VISSER 1988; KÖHRLE et al. 1991; ST. GERMAIN 1994). Little is known at present about the mechanism of this regulation.

E. Characterization of Iodothyronine Deiodinases

The first report on the structural characterization of an iodothyronine deiodinase was published by the group of BERRY and LARSEN in 1991, who cloned rat ID-I cDNA using *Xenopus laevis* oocytes as an expression system (BERRY et al. 1991a). In the subsequent 5 years not only ID-I but also ID-II and ID-III have been cloned from several species, with major contributions also of ST. GERMAIN and coworkers (MANDEL et al. 1992; TOYODA et al. 1995b; MAIA et al. 1995; ST. GERMAIN et al. 1994; BECKER et al. 1995; CROTEAU et al. 1995; SALVATORE et al. 1995; DAVEY et al. 1995; CROTEAU et al. 1996). The deduced amino acid sequences of rat ID-I, ID-II and ID-III are given in Table 2. These developments have greatly advanced our understanding of the molecular mechanisms of thyroid hormone deiodination. Thus, it has been shown that the three types of iodothyronine deiodinases are homologous proteins, consisting of ≈250 amino acids. Although they are all basic and hydrophobic proteins, a particulary lipophilic sequence is present at the N terminus of all three deiodinases, which probably represents a membrane-spanning region (TOYODA et al. 1995a). Studies of the topography of rat ID-I have suggested that the major part of the protein is exposed on the cytoplasmic surface of the membrane, with only a short N-terminal tail sticking out of the other side of the membrane (TOYODA et al. 1995a). Analysis of detergent extracts of rat liver or kidney membranes have indicated an apparent molecular weight of 50–60 kDa for native ID-I (LEONARD and VISSER 1986), which is about twice the molecular weight of the protein encoded by the cDNA, suggesting that ID-I is a dimer of two identical subunits. Analysis of detergent extracts of brain cell membranes have indicated an apparent molecular weight of ≈200 kDa, suggesting a multimeric complex of different subunits (SAFRAN and LEONARD 1991). Supposedly, one of these is the ≈30-kDa protein shown in Table 2, while another ≈30-kDa subunit appears to be involved with the substrate-induced internalization and inactivation of ID-II in brain cells (LEONARD and SAFRAN 1994; SAFRAN and LEONARD 1991). The subunit composition of ID-III has not been investigated.

The most remarkable feature of all three types of iodothyronine deiodinase is that they are selenoproteins, i.e. they contain selenocysteine (Sec) residues. Sec is encoded by the TGA (UGA) codon, which is called an opal stop codon because it usually signals termination of translation. However, if the 3′ untranslated region of the mRNA contains a particular stem loop structure, termed Sec-insertion (SECIS) element, the UGA codon specifies the insertion of Sec (for reviews of the synthesis of selenoproteins, see BERRY and LARSEN 1992; LARSEN and BERRY 1995.) Table 2 shows the amino acid sequences of the three iodothyronine deiodinases in the rat. All three cDNAs feature roughly halfway through the coding sequence, in a particularly conserved domain, a TGA codon which encodes a Sec residue. However, in contrast to the amphibian enzyme (DAVEY et al. 1995), both rat and human ID-II have at the C terminus a second TGA codon, just upstream of a TAA stop codon (CROTEAU et al. 1996). It remains to be determined if this second TGA codon specifies the incorporation of a second Sec residue or if it acts as a translation termination codon.

Before ID-I was identified as a selenoprotein, this was suspected based on findings of strongly reduced ID-I activities in homogenates of liver and kidney, but not of thyroid, from rats reared on a selenium (Se)-deficient diet (BECKETT et al. 1987). This is associated with a minor decrease in serum T_3 and a marked increase in serum T_4. Such studies have produced equivocal data regarding the Se dependence of the type II and type III deiodinases. ID-II activities have been shown to be decreased in brown adipose tissue and brain of Se-deficient rats (BECKETT et al. 1989; ARTHUR et al. 1991; MEINHOLD et al. 1993). However, this Se deficiency-induced decrease in brain ID-II activity is not observed in hypothyroid animals (CHANOINE et al. 1992). Together with other observations, this suggested that the decrease in brain D-II activity in Se-deficient euthyroid animals is due, at least in part, to an increased substrate-induced enzyme inactivation resulting from the increased serum T_4 levels (CHANOINE et al. 1992). In addition, it has been found that ID-II activity in rat glial cell cultures is not affected by Se depletion, in contrast to an almost complete disappearance of glutathione peroxidase (GPx), another selenoenzyme (SAFRAN et al. 1991). As for ID-III, the activity of the brain enzyme was found to decrease only slightly while enzyme activities in placenta and skin are not affected at all in Se-deficient rats (MEINHOLD et al. 1993; CHANOINE et al. 1993). These unexpected minor effects of Se deficiency on ID-II and ID-III activities, despite the fact that their cDNA sequences appear to code for Sec-containing proteins, may be explained by the findings that the selenium state of different tissues varies greatly in Se-deficient animals (BERRY and LARSEN 1992; LARSEN and BERRY 1995). In addition, the efficiency of the SECIS element to assist in the read-through of the UGA codon may vary between the different selenoproteins, which could result in the preferred incorporation of Sec into some selenoproteins (e.g. deiodinases) over others (e.g. GPx) (BERRY and LARSEN 1992; LARSEN and BERRY 1995).

ID-I catalyses the deiodination of iodothyronines by DTT by a "ping pong" mechanism, suggesting that the enzyme alternates between two distinct forms (LEONARD and VISSER 1986). The native form is thought to be converted by reaction with the iodothyronine substrate into an intermediate form, which is converted back to native enzyme by reaction with the cofactor (DTT). Another remarkable feature of ID-I is its extreme sensitivity to inactivation by the SH group-blocking reagent iodoacetate (IAc) (LEONARD and VISSER 1986). This inactivation requires only micromolar concentrations of IAc, and is prevented competitively by substrate, which was initially explained by assuming the carboxymethylation of a highly reactive SH group in the enzyme-active centre. This explanation seemed to fit with the findings that 6-*n*-propyl-2-thiouracil (PTU) is a potent inhibitor of ID-I, where the inhibition is uncompetitive with substrate and competitive with cofactor, suggesting that PTU and cofactor react with the same intermediate enzyme form. Since thiouracil derivatives have been found to be highly reactive towards protein sulphenyl iodide (SI) groups, it was only natural to assume the generation of such an enzyme intermediate in the catalytic cycle of ID-I (LEONARD and VISSER 1986). However, as soon as ID-I was identified as a selenoprotein it was realized that it is perhaps the Sec residue which in the reduced (SeH) form is modified by IAc and in the selenenyl iodide (SeI) form is the target for inhibition by PTU, resulting in the putative reaction mechanism shown in Fig. 9. The active participation of Sec in the catalytic process is supported by the findings that mutation of Sec into Cys results in a hundredfold decrease in deiodinase activity, while replacement of Sec by Leu yields an enzymatically inactive protein (BERRY et al. 1991a, 1992). Furthermore, ID-I activity is inhibited by very low concentrations ($\approx 10^{-8}\,M$) of gold thioglucose (GTG), which is know to form a highly stable complex with reduced Sec (BERRY et al. 1991b, 1992) (Fig. 9). Therefore, Sec is probably the catalytic centre of ID-I.

Figure 10 compares the effects of PTU, IAc and GTG on the activities of the three types of iodothyronine deiodinases from rat, determined at substrate levels roughly equal to their K_m values. ID-I is clearly most sensitive to these inhibitors, with IC_{50} values of $\approx 5\,\mu M$ for PTU, $\approx 2\,\mu M$ for IAc and $\approx 0.05\,\mu M$ for GTG. Both ID-II and ID-III are much less sensitive to inhibition by these compounds: IC_{50} values of PTU are $>1000\,\mu M$ and of IAc $\approx 1000\,\mu M$ for both enzymes. The IC_{50} value of GTG amounts to $\approx 1\,\mu M$ for ID-II and to $\approx 5\,\mu M$ for ID-III. Not only the presence of Sec in all three deiodinases, but also that of other conserved domains, in particular around this catalytically important Sec

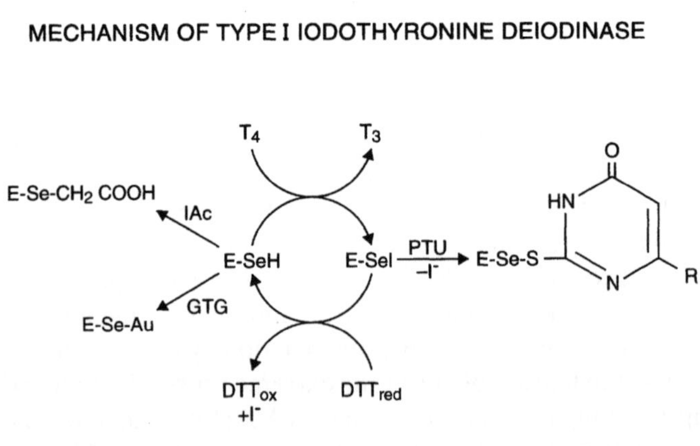

Fig. 9. Putative catalytic mechanism of ID-I and inhibition by PTU, IAc and GTG

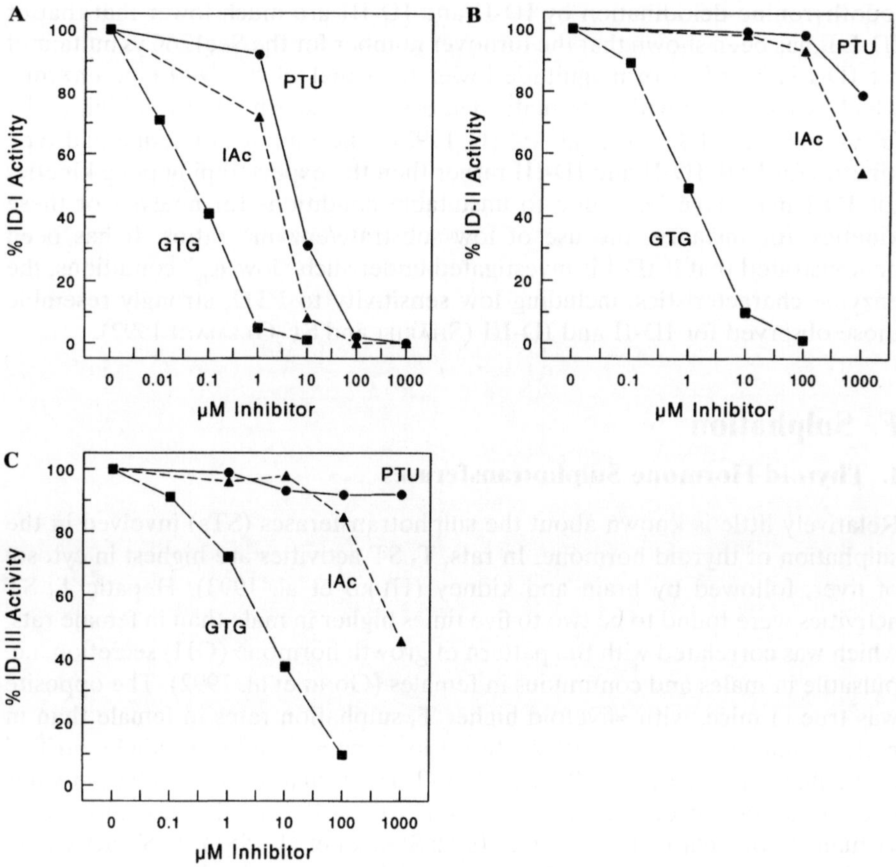

Fig. 10A–C. Dose-dependent inhibition of iodothyronine deiodinases by PTU, IAc and GTG. **A** ID-I activity of rat liver microsomes tested with 0.1 μM rT_3 and 10 m*M* DTT. **B** ID-II activity of hypothyroid brain microsomes tested with 0.25 n*M* T_4 and 25 m*M* DTT. **C** ID-III activity of rat placenta microsomes tested with 10 n*M* T_3 and 10 m*M* DTT

residue, strongly suggests the same mechanism of deiodination for the different enzymes. This seems to be contradicted by the widely different susceptibilities of ID-I vs. ID-II and ID-III to the different mechanism-based inhibitors PTU, IAc and GTG (see also Mol et al. 1993; Berry et al. 1991c; Santini et al. 1992a). This conclusion also seems to be in conflict with previous findings that, in contrast to the ping pong kinetics of ID-I, the other two enzymes appear to follow sequential-type kinetics, suggesting the formation of a ternary enzyme-substrate-cofactor complex during catalysis (Leonard and Visser 1986). A possible explanation for this apparent discrepancy is to assume that the low susceptibility of ID-II and ID-III to especially IAc and GTG indicates that the reactivity of the selenol group in these enzymes is much less than that in ID-I. This would imply that the turnover numbers for iodothyronine deiodination by ID-II and ID-III are much lower that that of ID-I. It has been shown that the turnover number for the Sec126Cys mutant of rat ID-I is 2 orders of magnitude lower than that of the wild-type enzyme, which is associated with a dramatic decrease in its sensitivity for inhibition by GTG and PTU (BERRY et al. 1991b, 1992). The findings of sequential-type kinetics for both ID-II and ID-III rather than the expected ping pong kinetics for ID-I may have been due to unsuitable conditions for analysis of these kinetics, for instance, the use of low substrate/enzyme ratios. It has been demonstrated that if ID-I is investigated under such "low-K_m" conditions, the enzyme characteristics, including low sensitivity to PTU, strongly resemble those observed for ID-II and ID-III (SHARIFI and ST. GERMAIN 1992).

F. Sulphation

I. Thyroid Hormone Sulphotransferases

Relatively little is known about the sulphotransferases (STs) involved in the sulphation of thyroid hormone. In rats, T_3 ST activities are highest in cytosol of liver, followed by brain and kidney (HURD et al. 1993). Hepatic T_3 ST activities were found to be two to five times higher in male than in female rats, which was correlated with the pattern of growth hormone (GH) secretion, i.e. pulsatile in males and continuous in females (GONG et al. 1992). The opposite was true in mice, with ≈fivefold higher T_3 sulphation rates in female than in male animals (GONG et al. 1992). In rat liver cytosol and in partially purified aryl sulphotransferase (AST) I and AST IV preparations, sulphation rates decreased in the order $3,3'\text{-}T_2 \gg TA_3 > T_3 > rT_3 > T_4$, with T_4 sulphation being virtually undetectable (GONG et al. 1992; SEKURA et al. 1981). T_3 ST activity in rat liver is relatively heat stable, shows a high K_m value for T_3 ($\approx 100\,\mu M$) and is inhibited by low concentrations of DCNP (IC_{50} 5.5 μM) and pentachlorophenol (IC_{50} 0.065 μM) (HURD et al. 1993; GONG et al. 1992). Inconsistent effects of thyroid state on T_3 ST activity in rat liver have been reported (HURD et al. 1993; GONG et al. 1992). Hepatic T_3 ST activity in fetal rats shows a strong increase between 17 and 20 days of gestation. Enzyme activities in liver and kidney of 20-day fetal rats are about half of those in the mother, while brain T_3 ST activity is still very low at this stage (HURD et al. 1993).

T_3 is a substrate for at least three phenol sulphotransferases (PSTs) in human tissues, i.e. for two forms of thermostable, phenol-preferring PST (P-PST) as well as for a thermolabile, monoamine-preferring PST (M-PST) (YOUNG et al. 1988). P-PST is especially abundant in liver and is also most important for T_3 sulphation in this tissue, while M-PST is more prevalent in the intestine. T_3 sulphation in human liver is inhibited by low concentrations of 2,6-dichloro-4-nitrophenol (DCNP; $IC_{50} \approx 5\,\mu M$), a selective inhibitor of the P-PST isoenzyme. K_m values amount to ≈100–200 μM for T_3 and to ≈0.1–0.4 μM for PAPS with the different enzyme preparations. No sex dependence was found for human liver T_3 ST activity (GONG et al. 1992).

II. Deiodination of Iodothyronine Sulphates

Although ID-I is capable of converting T_4 with similar efficiency by ORD to T_3 and by IRD to rT_3, this is changed dramatically after sulphate conjugation (VISSER 1994a, 1994b). The IRD of T_4S by rat ID-I is accelerated ≈200-fold while ORD of T_4S becomes undetectable (Fig. 11), excluding conversion of T_4 to T_3 via their sulphates. IRD of T_3 by rat and human ID-I is also markedly stimulated (≈ 40-fold) by sulphation (Fig. 11) (VISSER 1994a, 1994b). The acetic acid analogue TA_3 is also deiodinated in the inner ring by ID-I, and is in fact a better substrate than T_3. IRD of TA_3 is further strongly facilitated (≈ 50-fold) by sulphate conjugation. Thus, the combined effects of the acetic acid side chain and the phenolic sulphate group ensure that TA_3S is deiodinated $\approx 10^3$ more efficiently than T_3 (VISSER 1994a, 1994b). As mentioned before, rT_3 is the preferred ID-I substrate; its ORD to 3,3′-T_2 is catalysed >100-fold more effectively than the deiodination of any other non-sulphated iodothyronine (Table 3). Deiodination of rT_3 is not influenced by sulphation, suggesting that the catalytic efficiency of ID-I is already optimal with non-sulphated rT_3 (Fig. 11). While sulphation inhibits ORD of T_4 and is without effect on ORD of rT_3, it markedly stimulates ORD of 3,3′-T_2 (Fig. 11) (VISSER 1994a, 1994b).

Thus, sulphation facilitates the IRD of T_4, T_3 and TA_3, while it either inhibits (T_4), does not affect (rT_3) or markedly stimulates (3,3′-T_2) the ORD of other substrates. The mechanism by which sulphation especially stimulates the IRD of the various substrates remains unclear. In some cases sulphation primarily effects an increase in V_{max}, while in others there is a predominant

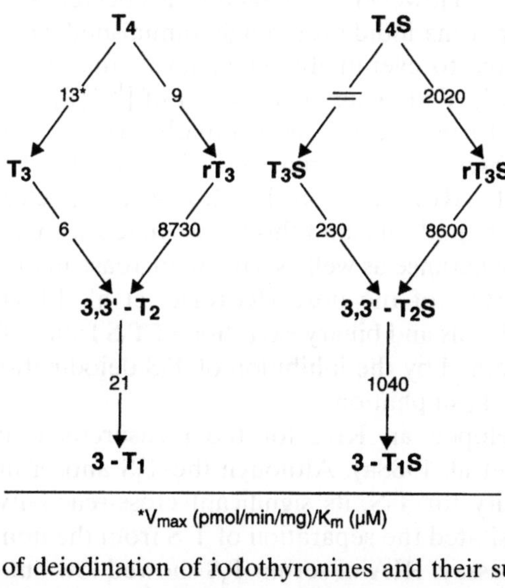

Fig. 11. Efficiency of deiodination of iodothyronines and their sulphates by rat liver ID-I

decrease in apparent K_m value (VISSER 1994a, 1994b). The facilitated deiodination of sulphated iodothyronines by rat liver ID-I is due to interaction of the negatively charged sulphate group with protonated residues in the active centre of this basic protein. The effect depends both on the site and the nature of the conjugating group. Type I deiodination of different iodothyronines is only moderately stimulated by sulphonation of the α-NH_2 group, in contrast with the pronounced effects of sulphonation of the 4′-OH group (RUTGERS et al. 1991). We have also found that ID-I does not catalyse the deiodination of T_3G (EELKMAN ROODA et al. 1989c). The effects of sulphation appear specific for ID-I, since deiodination of sulphated substrates is not observed with either ID-II (VISSER et al., unpublished) or ID-III (SANTINI et al. 1992c).

III. Occurrence of Iodothyronine Sulphates

After IV injection of $[^{125}I]T_3$ to control bile duct-cannulated rats, $[^{125}I]T_3G$ was found to be the predominant radioactive product excreted in the bile (DE HERDER et al. 1987). Pretreatment of rats with PTU had little effect on the biliary excretion of T_3G, but excretion of T_3S and 3,3′-T_2S was strongly increased. While treatment of rats with DCNP alone did not affect biliary excretion of T_3 metabolites as compared with untreated rats, DCNP greatly diminished the PTU-induced excretion of T_3S and 3,3′-T_2S. This is in agreement with the above-mentioned in vitro findings, suggesting an important contribution of DCNP-sensitive PSTs to hepatic T_3 sulphation.

T_3S may also be detected in blood. After i.v. administration of $[^{125}I]T_3$ to untreated rats, iodide is the predominant radioactive metabolite in plasma (RUTGERS et al. 1987). However, if labelled T_3 is injected in PTU-treated rats, the appearance of plasma iodide is strongly diminished, and T_3S and 3,3′-T_2S accumulate in plasma to eventually higher levels than that of remaining T_3 (RUTGERS et al. 1987). Following i.v. injection of $[^{125}I]T_3S$ to control rats, the conjugate is cleared from plasma more rapidly than T_3. Iodide is again the main metabolite observed in plasma, and ≈20% of the dose is excreted as intact T_3S in the bile (RUTGERS et al. 1987). Plasma T_3S clearance is strongly decreased in PTU-treated rats, and this is associated with a marked decrease in plasma iodide appearance as well as with an increase in the biliary excretion of intact T_3S to ≈80% of the dose (RUTGERS et al. 1987). Therefore, the increase in plasma levels and biliary excretion of T_3S from injected T_3 in PTU-treated rats is explained by the inhibition of T_3S deiodination by ID-I rather than an increase in T_3 sulphation.

We have developed an RIA for the measurement of T_3S in serum (EELKMAN ROODA et al. 1988a). Although the T_3S antiserum showed a relatively high specificity for T_3S, its significant cross-reactivity with T_3 and in particular T_4 necessitated the separation of T_3S from the non-conjugated hormones prior to the assay. RIA of serum T_3S showed low but detectable levels in normal rats and markedly increased levels after treatment with PTU, but not with methimazole, which does not inhibit ID-I (EELKMAN ROODA et al. 1989a). Similar results were obtained in animals treated with the X-ray contrast agent iopanoic acid (IOP), which also inhibits ID-I (EELKMAN ROODA et al. 1988b).

Analysis of human serum with this RIA demonstrated that T_3S levels in normal subjects were mostly undetectable (<0.1 nmol/l) (EELKMAN ROODA et al. 1989b). Serum T_3S just reached the lower limit of detection of the RIA in healthy volunteers treated with T_3 (1 μg/kg body weight per day). Serum T_3S in these T_3-treated subjects showed a minimal increase after administration of PTU but they were markedly elevated after administration of IOP (EELKMAN ROODA et al. 1989b). The effects of these drugs on serum T_3S were strongly correlated with those on serum rT_3, which is also largely cleared by type I deiodination. LOPRESTI et al. (1991) have reported on the extremely rapid clearance of circulating T_3S in normal humans, which is inhibited moderately by PTU administration but markedly by IOP administration. Therefore, the increase in serum T_3S observed after administration of PTU and especially IOP to T_3-treated subjects appears to be due primarily to a decrease in T_3S deiodination and not to an increase in T_3S production.

The groups of WU and CHOPRA have been able to develop improved RIAs for serum T_3S, which can be applied directly to ethanol extracts without further prepurification. In agreement with our findings, CHOPRA et al. (1992) showed that serum T_3S levels are low in normal subjects (<0.1 nmol/l), and that they increase significantly after treatment of patients with IOP. They further noted that the serum T_3S/T_3 ratio is decreased in hyperthyroid patients and strongly increased in hypothyroid patients and in patients with non-thyroidal illness (NTI). In addition, they found high T_3S levels in fetal cord serum of healthy newborns. These findings may be explained by a low ID-I activity in hypothyroidism and NTI and during fetal development and an increased enzyme activity in the hyperthyroid state. The increased serum T_3S in NTI may also be due to decreased hepatic reuptake of the conjugate. Therefore, these recent data demonstrate that also in humans serum T_3S levels accumulate to high levels if its deiodination by ID-I is impaired.

After i.v. injection of $[^{125}I]T_4$ to normal rats, T_4G was found to be the predominant radioactive compound in bile together with smaller amounts of T_3G, rT_3G and T_4S (RUTGERS et al. 1989b). Treatment of rats with PTU resulted in a decrease in T_3G excretion, reflecting the decreased T_4 to T_3 conversion, and large increases in rT_3G and T_4S excretion, due to inhibited degradation of rT_3 and T_4S by ID-I. These findings suggested that sulphation is a significant pathway of hepatic T_4 metabolism in rats, and that T_4S is predominantly cleared by type I deiodination. However, serum radioactive T_4S was undetectable even in PTU-treated rats (RUTGERS et al. 1989b).

Using very sensitive and specific RIAs for T_4S, WU et al. (1992a) and CHOPRA et al. (1993) have recently reported on the measurement of low concentrations of T_4S in human serum, i.e. 100 and 19 pmol/l, respectively.

Compared with serum of normal adults, T_4S levels were increased in human amniotic fluid and in fetal cord serum obtained at the time of delivery (WU et al. 1992a; CHOPRA et al. 1993). Both groups observed an increase in serum T_4S after administration of IOP to hyperthyroid patients. Together, these findings indicate that sulphation is a significant pathway for metabolism of T_4 in humans and rats, and that serum T_4S accumulates in conditions associated with low ID-I activity.

WU et al. (1993a) have recently also reported on the measurement of rT_3S in human serum using a newly developed RIA for this sulphoconjugate. Although rT_3S concentrations were low in normal human subjects (mean 40 pmol/l), and no significant changes were noted in hypothyroid, hyperthyroid or pregnant subjects, marked elevations were observed after administration of IOP to hyperthyroid patients (WU et al. 1993a). Striking increases in rT_3S levels were also observed in fetal cord serum relative to serum rT_3S in adults (WU et al. 1993a). Therefore, rT_3 appears to be sulphated to some extent in humans, although this may be significant only if ID-I, the principal site of rT_3 and rT_3S metabolism, is inhibited.

Finally, the development of a specific RIA for 3,3′-T_2S was recently reported by WU et al. (1994). Serum T_2S was undetectable in normal subjects, but significant T_2S immunoreactivity was observed in cord serum and in the serum of pregnant women. However, high-performance liquid chromatography (HPLC) analysis demonstrated that only part of T_2S immunoreactivity in cord serum represented authentic T_2S. The remainder of the immunoreactivity in cord serum and all immunoreactivity in maternal serum was accounted for by a cross-reacting substance, termed compound W, which as yet has not been identified (WU et al. 1994).

Very high levels of T_4S, T_3S, rT_3S and 3,3′-T_2S have been measured in plasma, bile and meconium of fetal sheep as well as in the amniotic and allantoic fluids (WU et al. 1992b, 1993b, 1995). This is explained by the low hepatic ID-I activity, which develops mostly after birth. However, kinetic studies suggest that not only the clearance of these sulphates is decreased in fetal sheep but also that their production is increased compared with neonatal sheep (POLK et al. 1994).

IV. Possible Role of Iodothyronine Sulphation

T_3 is inactivated by sulphation; T_3S does not bind to the T_3 receptor and is devoid of thyromimetic activity in several systems (SPAULDING 1994; EVERTS et al. 1994b). Furthermore, T_3S is rapidly degraded by ID-I. It has been postulated that T_3 sulphation has an important function when ID-I activity is low, such as in hypothyroidism and during fetal development (SANTINI et al. 1992b). Under these conditions, T_3S is not degraded in tissues which normally have high ID-I activity, while the hormone is also protected by sulphation against degradation by ID-III. Active T_3 could then be recovered from T_3S by sulphatases in tissues where hormone action is required (SANTINI et al. 1992b).

Desulphation of T_3S in vivo has recently been observed after injection of the conjugate to hypothyroid rats (SANTINI et al. 1993). However, the exact biological function of the different iodothyronine sulphates, in particular during fetal development, remains to be fully explored.

G. Glucuronidation

Glucuronidation is a major metabolic pathway for thyroid hormone in rats (VISSER 1994a), but much less is known about the importance of thyroid hormone glucuronidation in humans. In rats equilibrated with radioiodinated T_4 or T_3, roughly similar amounts of radioactivity are excreted as iodide in the urine and in the form of iodothyronines in the faeces (MORREALE DE ESCOBAR and ESCOBAR DEL REY 1967). The latter are mainly derived from the biliary excretion of glucuronides, which are subsequently hydrolysed in the intestine, although there is also evidence for direct secretion of thyroid hormone from the mesenteric veins into the intestinal lumen (DISTEFANO et al. 1993). Irrespective of its origin, part of the non-conjugated hormone is reabsorbed from the intestine, and the remainder is excreted with the faeces (VISSER 1990). Intestinal hydrolysis of iodothyronine glucuronides is mediated largely by bacterial β-glucuronidases, since rats in which the intestinal microflora was eliminated with antibiotics excrete iodothyronines in the faeces largely as conjugates (RUTGERS et al. 1989a; DE HERDER et al. 1989).

A large number of drugs and xenobiotics have been found to stimulate peripheral thyroid hormone metabolism due to the induction of iodothyronine UDP-glucuronyltransferase (UGT) activities (CURRAN and DEGROOT 1991). The resultant compensatory increase in thyroid function may lead to thyroid hyperplasia and after chronic treatment in rats even to thyroid neoplasia (MCCLAIN 1989). Inducers of hepatic thyroid hormone glucuronidation are classified as (1) polyaromatic and polyhalogenated aromatic compounds, such as 3-methylcholanthrene (MC), benzpyrene, polychlorobiphenyls (PCBs), dioxin, α-naphtoflavone and hexachlorobenzene (HCB) (BEETSTRA et al. 1991; DE SANDRO et al. 1991, 1992; SAITO et al. 1991; BARTER and KLAASSEN 1992a, 1992b; VAN RAAY et al. 1993; VISSER et al. 1993c); (2) the anticonvulsant drug phenobarbital (DE SANDRO 1991; MCCLAIN et al. 1989); (3) the hypolipidemic phenoxyisobutyrate (fibrate) derivatives clofibrate, ciprofibrate and nafenopine (KAISER et al. 1988; VISSER et al. 1991, 1993c), and other peroxisome proliferators, such as dehydroepiandrosterone (MCINTOSH and BERDANIER 1992), polychlorinated paraffins (WYATT et al. 1993), perfluorodecanoic acid (LANGLEY and PILCHER 1985) and phthalates (HINTON et al. 1986); and (4) various other compounds, including pregnenolone-16α-carbonitrile (BARTER and KLAASSEN 1992a, 1992b), spironolactone (SEMLER et al. 1989), the leukotriene antagonist L-649,923 (SANDERS et al. 1988) and the cardiac inotropic drug OPC 8212 (LUEPRASITSAKUL et al. 1991). For reviews of the thyroid hormone glucuronidation pathway and its response to microsomal enzyme inducers, the reader is referred to VISSER (1990) and CURRAN and DEGROOT (1991).

I. Thyroid Hormone UDP-Glucuronyltransferases

Previous work in our laboratory has suggested that at least three UGT isoenzymes are involved with the glucuronidation of iodothyronines in rat liver (Table 4). This was based on the following findings: (1) parallel with an increase in phenol UGT activity, using *p*-nitrophenol (PNP) as substrate, hepatic T_4 and rT_3 UGT activities, but not T_3 UGT activity, are strongly induced by treatment of rats with MC-type inducers (BEETSTRA et al. 1991; VAN RAAY et al. 1993; VISSER et al. 1993c); (2) parallel with an increase in bilirubin UGT activity, hepatic T_4 and rT_3 UGT activities, but not T_3 UGT activity, are strongly induced by treatment of rats with clofibrate or ciprofibrate (VISSER et al. 1991, 1993c); (3) hepatic T_4 and rT_3 UGT activities, but not T_3 UGT activity, are strongly decreased in Gunn rats which have a defect in the *UGT1* gene coding for multiple bilirubin and phenol UGTs (see below) (VISSER et al. 1993b; EMI et al. 1995); and (4) relative to normal Wistar HA (high-activity) rats, T_3 UGT activity, but not T_4 and rT_3 UGT activities, is strongly decreased in Wistar LA (low-activity), Fischer and WAG rats which have a defect in the gene coding for androsterone UGT (BEETSTRA et al. 1991; VAN RAAY et al. 1993; VISSER et al. 1991, 1993b; HOMMA et al. 1992). These results, thus, suggest that T_4 is predominantly glucuronidated in rat liver by both bilirubin UGT and phenol UGT, while T_3 is primarily conjugated by androsterone UGT. This is supported by studies with V79 cell lines transfected with cDNA of different human UGT isoenzymes, showing significant glucuronidation of T_4 and rT_3, but not T_3, by the bilirubin UGT HP3 as well as the phenol UGT HP4 (VISSER et al. 1993a). However, in contrast to the latter "bulky" phenol-preferring isoenzyme, little or no glucuronidation of iodothyronines was observed with the planar phenol-preferring isoenzyme HP1, which glucuronidates substrates such as PNP. Therefore, the parallel increase in iodothyronine and PNP UGT activities in response to MC-type inducers does not reflect the induction of a common enzyme but rather the simultaneous induction of different isoen-

Table 4. Characteristics of three types of iodothyronine UDP-glucuronyltransferases

Type	I	II	III
hUGT	HP3	HP4	?
Substrates	Bili	Phenols	Andro
	rT_3, T_4	rT_3, T_4	T_3
Fibrates	↑	≈	≈
MC inducers	≈	↑↑	≈
LA, Fischer, WAG rats	≈	≈	↓↓
Gunn rats	↓↓	↓↓	≈

zymes, i.e. one for PNP (HP1-like) and one for iodothyronines (HP4-like) (VISSER et al. 1993c).

Hepatic bilirubin UGT activity is increased and PNP UGT activity is decreased in thyroidectomized rats, and the opposite changes are observed in hyperthyroid animals (ROY CHOWDHURY et al. 1983; VAN STEENBERGEN et al. 1989; MASMOUDI et al. 1996). At least two bilirubin UGTs and at least two phenol UGTs are encoded by the *UGT1* gene, a gene complex comprising multiple unique exons (exons I) and a set of four common exons (exons II-V) (EMI et al. 1995). Transcription may start at any of the different unique exons, each under control of its own promoter, yielding primary transcripts of varying length depending on the location of the relevant exon I in the *UGT1* gene. By differential splicing of these primary transcripts, multiple mRNA species are produced that each combine a unique exon I, coding for the substrate-binding domain, with the common exons II-V, coding for the cofactor-binding domain of the enzyme (OWENS and RITTER 1992; BURCHELL et al. 1994; EMI et al. 1995). An attractive explanation of the effects of thyroid status on bilirubin and PNP UGT activities is that the promoter of one or more bilirubin UGT-specific exons I is under negative control by the T_3 receptor, whereas the promoter of one or more phenol UGT-specific exons I is under positive control by the T_3 receptor (MASMOUDI et al. 1996). Thyroid status has little effect on liver androsterone UGT activity in rats (VISSER et al. 1996). Considering the opposite effects of thyroid hormone on bilirubin and phenol UGT activities and the lack of effect on androsterone UGT activities, it is not surprising that hepatic UGT activities for T_4 and T_3 show little change in hypo- or hyperthyroid rats (VISSER et al. 1996). It should be mentioned that treatment of rats with methimazole results in a marked induction of a hepatic PNP UGT isoenzyme not involved with thyroid hormone glucuronidation, which is independent of the thyrostatic activity of methimazole (VISSER et al. 1996).

II. Role of Thyroid Hormone Glucuronidation in Humans

On the basis of the smaller proportion of hormone undergoing faecal excretion, it is generally assumed that glucuronidation is less important in humans (VISSER 1994a). This seems to be supported by the findings that UGT activities for T_4 and especially T_3 are much lower in human liver than in rat liver microsomes (VISSER et al. 1993a). However, type I deiodinase activity is also much lower in human than in rat liver (VISSER et al. 1988), although the enzyme is undoubtedly a prominent site for peripheral T_4 to T_3 conversion in humans. Furthermore, glucuronidation is not an irreversible pathway of thyroid hormone metabolism, since biliary-excreted glucuronides are hydrolysed in the intestine and the liberated iodothyronines are partially reabsorbed (RUTGERS et al. 1989a; DE HERDER et al. 1989), and the efficiency of such an enterohepatic cycle may be greater in humans than in rats. Increased faecal loss may arise also in humans if this cycle is interrupted due to administration of drugs or gastrointestinal disease, which interfere with the deconjugation and resorption processes (HAYS 1988). In addition, T_4 glucuronidation may also be markedly increased in humans by the same drugs and xenobiotics which have been shown to induce T_4 UGT activity in rats.

Significant decreases in serum T_4 and FT_4 levels have been documented in patients treated with anticonvulsant drugs, in particular phenytoin and carbamazepine (ISOJÄRVI et al. 1992), or the antituberculosis drug rifampicin (OHNHAUS and STUDER 1983), while serum T_3 and TSH levels are usually unchanged. Where this was studied, an increase in T_4 clearance was observed, in particular via the faecal route. These changes are compatible with the selective induction of hepatic T_4 UGT activity, similar to observations in rats. Treatment of human subjects with such drugs even results in a significant increase in thyroid volume (HEGEDÜS et al. 1985). Lowering of serum T_4 would be most pronounced in subjects in whom the increased T_4 disposal cannot be compensated by an increased T_4 secretion, e.g. in cases of (subclinical) thyroid failure, insufficient iodine intake or, in particular, T_4 replacement therapy. However, the exact role of thyroid hormone glucuronidation in humans under different pathophysiological conditions remains to be established.

III. Glucuronidation of Iodothyroacetic Acid Analogues

Since there is evidence suggesting that the acetic acid metabolites TA_3 and TA_4 are rapidly cleared in rats and humans by glucuronidation, we have tested liver microsomes from both species for TA_3 and TA_4 UGT activities (MORENO et al. 1994). The results were quite remarkable with respect to both the rate and type of glucuronidation of these compounds. In rat liver, TA_3 and TA_4 were glucuronidated at the phenolic hydroxyl group like the parent iodothyronines (Fig. 12), but at rates which were >40 times higher than

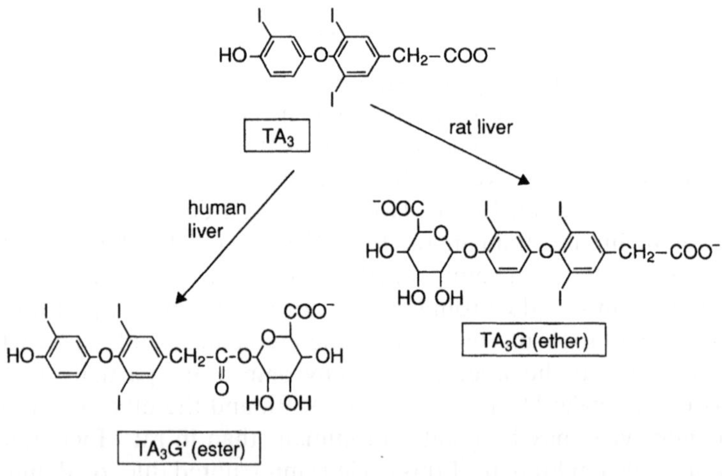

Fig. 12. Glucuronidation of Triac (TA_3) in human and rat liver

glucuronidation of T_3 and T_4 (MORENO et al. 1994). Even greater differences were found in human liver, where glucuronidation of TA_3 and TA_4 was ≈600 and 60 times faster than glucuronidation of T_3 and T_4, respectively (MORENO et al. 1994). Furthermore, unlike the stable ether glucuronides produced in rat liver microsomes, TA_3 and TA_4 were conjugated in human liver primarily at the carboxyl group to labile ester glucuronides (Fig. 12). In general, the latter conjugates (1) are rapidly hydrolysed, in particular under alkaline conditions, (2) undergo rearrangement by acyl migration to the 2, 3 and 4 position of the glucuronic acid moiety, and (3) form covalent adducts with proteins (SPAHN-LANGGUTH and BENET 1992). It could be speculated that the latter may contribute to the formation of covalent, radioactive complexes with plasma proteins (so-called non-extractable iodine) after injection of labelled T_4 or T_3 in humans (HAYS et al. 1980).

Acknowledgement. The authors would like to thank Prof. J.J.M. De VIJLDER, Amsterdam, for critically reading the section on thyroid hormone synthesis, and Prof. D.L. St. GERMAIN for providing us with sequence information before publication.

References

Arthur JR, Nicol F, Beckett GJ, Trayhurn P (1991) Impairment of iodothyronine 5′-deiodinase activity in brown adipose tissue and its acute stimulation by cold in selenium deficiency. Can J Physiol Biochem 69:782–785

Barnett PS, Jones TH, McGregor AM, Banga JP, Sheer D (1993) Regional sublocalization of the human peroxidase gene (TPO) by tritium and fluorescence in situ hybridization to chromosome 2p25-p24. Cytogenet Cell Genet 62:188–189

Barter RA, Klaassen CD (1992a) UDP-glucuronosyltransferase inducers reduce thyroid hormone levels in rats by an extrathyroidal mechanism. Toxicol Appl Pharmacol 113:36–42

Barter RA, Klaassen CD (1992b) Rat liver microsomal UDP-glucuronosyltransferase activity toward thyroxine: characterization, induction and form specificity. Toxicol Appl Pharmacol 115:261–267

Becker KB, Schneider MJ, Davey JC, Galton VA (1995) The type III 5-deiodinase in Rana catesbeiana tadpoles is encoded by a thyroid hormone-responsive gene. Endocrinology 136:4424–4431

Beckett GJ, Beddows SE, Morrice PC, Nicol F, Arthur JR (1987) Inhibition of hepatic deiodination of thyroxine is caused by selenium deficiency in rats. Biochem J 248:443–447

Beckett GJ, MacDougall DA, Nicol F, Arthur JR (1989) Inhibition of type I and type II iodothyronine deiodinase activity in rat liver, kidney and brain produced by selenium deficiency. Biochem J 259:887–892

Beech SG, Walker SW, Dorrance AM, Arthur JR, Nicole F, Lee D, Beckett GJ (1993) The role of thyroidal type-I iodothyronine deiodinase in tri-iodothyronine production by human and sheep thyrocytes in primary culture. J Endocrinol 136:361–370

Beetstra JB, Van Engelen JGM, Karels P, Van der Hoek HJ, De Jong M, Docter R, Krenning EP, Hennemann G, Brouwer A, Visser TJ (1991) Thyroxine and 3,3′,5-triiodothyronine are glucuronidated in rat liver by different uridine diphosphate-glucuronyltransferases. Endocrinology 128:741–746

Berry MJ, Larsen PR (1992) The role of selenium in thyroid hormone action. Endocr Rev 13:207–219

Berry MJ, Larsen PR (1994) Molecular structure and biochemistry of type I iodothyronine deiodinase. In: Wu SY, Visser TJ (eds) Thyroid hormone metabo-

lism: molecular biology and alternate pathways. CRC Press, Baco Raton, pp 1–21
Berry MJ, Banu L, Larsen PR (1991a) Type I iodothyronine deiodinase is a selenocysteine-containing enzyme. Nature 349:438–440
Berry MJ, Kieffer JD, Harney JW, Larsen PR (1991b) Selenocysteine confers the biochemical properties characteristic of the type I iodothyronine deiodinase. J Biol Chem 266:14155–14158
Berry MJ, Kieffer JD, Larsen PR (1991c) Evidence that cysteine, not selenocysteine, is the catalytic site of type II iodothyronine deiodinase. Endocrinology 129:550–552
Berry MJ, Maia AL, Kieffer JD, Harney JW, Larsen PR (1992) Substitution of cysteine for selenocysteine in type I iodothyronine deiodinase reduces the catalytic efficiency of the protein but enhances its translation. Endocrinology 131:1848–1852
Björkman U, Ekholm R (1990) Biochemistry of thyroid hormone formation and secretion. In: Greer MA (ed) The thyroid gland, Raven Press, New York, pp 83–125
Björkman U, Eckholm R (1992) Hydrogen peroxide generation and its regulation in FRTL-5 and porcine thyroid cells. Endocrinology 130:393–399
Burchell B, Coughtrie MWH, Jansen PLM (1994) Function and regulation of UDP-glucuronosyltransferase genes in health and disease. Hepatology 20:1622–1630
Carvalho DP, Dupuy C, Goren Y, Legue O, Pommier J, Haye B, Virion A (1996) The Ca^{2+}- and reduced nicotinamide adenine dinucleotide phosphate-dependent hydrogen peroxide generating system is induced by thyrotropin in porcine thyroid cells. Endocrinology 137:1007–1012
Chambard M, Verrier B, Gabrion J, Mochant J (1983) Polarization of thyroid cells in culture: evidence for the basolateral localization of iodide "pumps" and of the thyroid-stimulating hormone receptor-adenylcyclase complex. J Cell Biol 96:1172–1177
Chanoine JP, Safran M, Farwell AP, Tranter P, Ekenbarger DM, Dubord S, Alex S, Arthur JR, Beckett GJ, Braverman LE, Leonard JL (1992) Selenium deficiency and type II 5′-deiodinase regulation in the euthyroid and hyperthyroid rat: evidence of a direct effect of thyroxine. Endocrinology 130:479–484
Chanoine JP, Alex S, Stone S, Fang SL, Veronikis I, Leonard JL, Braverman LE (1993) Placental 5-deiodinase activity and fetal thyroid hormone economy are unaffected by selenium deficiency in the rat. Pediat Res 34:288–292
Chopra IJ (1994) The role of sulfation and desulfation in thyroid hormone metabolism. In: Wu SY, Visser TJ (eds) Thyroid hormone metabolism: molecular biology and alternate pathways. CRC Press, Baco Raton, pp 119–138
Chopra IJ, Wu SY, Chua Teco GN, Santini F (1992) A radioimmunoassay of 3,5,3′-triiodothyronine sulfate: studies in thyroidal and nonthyroidal diseases, pregnancy, and neonatal life. J Clin Endocrinol Metab 75:189–194
Chopra IJ, Santini F, Hurd RE, Chua Teco GN (1993) A radioimmunoassay for measurement of thyroxine sulfate. J Clin Endocrinol Metab 76:145–150
Croteau W, Whittemore SL, Schneider MJ, St.Germain DL (1995) Cloning and expression of a cDNA for a mammalian type III iodothyronine deiodinase. J Biol Chem 270:16569–16575
Croteau W, Davey JC, Galton VA, St.Germain DL (1996) Cloning of the mammalian type II iodothyronine deiodinase: a selenoprotein differentially expressed and regulated in human and rat brain and other tissues. J Clin Invest 98:405–417
Curran PG, DeGroot LJ (1991) The effect of hepatic enzyme-inducing drugs on thyroid hormones and the thyroid gland. Endocr Rev 12:135–150
Dal G, Levy O, Carrasco N (1996) Cloning and characterization of the thyroid iodide transporter. Nature 379:458–460
Darras VM, Visser TJ, Berghman LR, Kühn ER (1992) Ontogeny of type I and type III deiodinase activities in embryonic and posthatch chicks: relationship with changes in plasma triiodothyronine and growth hormone levels. Comp Biochem Physiol 103A:131–136
Davey JC, Becker KB, Schneider MJ, St.Germain DL, Galton VA (1995) Cloning of a cDNA for the type II iodothyronine deiodinase. J Biol Chem 270:26786–26789

DeGroot LJ, Larsen PR, Hennemann G (1996) The thyroid and its diseases, 6th edn. Churchill Livingstone, New York, p 33

De Herder WW, Bonthuis F, Rutgers M, Otten MH, Hazenberg MP, Visser TJ (1987) Effects of inhibition of type I iodothyronine deiodinase and phenol sulfotransferase on the biliary clearance of triiodothyronine in rats. Endocrinology 122:153–157

De Herder WW, Hazenberg MP, Pennock-Schröder AM, Oosterlaken AC, Rutgers M, Visser TJ (1989) On the enterohepatic cycle of triiodothyronine in rats: importance of the intestinal microflora. Life Sci 45:849–856

De Jong M, Docter R, Van der Hoek HJ, Vos RA, Krenning EP, Hennemann G (1992) Transport of T_3 into the perfused rat liver and subsequent metabolism are inhibited by fasting. Endocrinology 131:463–470

De Jong M, Visser TJ, Bernard BF, Docter R, Vos RA, Hennemann G, Krenning EP (1993) Transport and metabolism of iodothyronines in cultured human hepatocytes. J Clin Endocrinol Metab 77:139–143

De Jong M, Docter R, Van der Hoek H, Krenning EP, Van der Heide H, Quero, Plaisier P, Vos RA, Hennemann G (1994a) Different effects of amiodarone on transport of T_4 and T_3 into the perfused rat liver. Am J Physiol 266:E44–E49

De Jong M, Docter R, Bernard BF, Van der Heyden JTM, Van Toor H, Krenning EP, Hennemann G (1994b) T_4 uptake into the perfused rat liver and liver T_4 uptake in humans are inhibited by fructose. Am J Physiol 266:E768–E775

De Jong M, Docter R, Van der Hoek HJ, Krenning EP, Hennemann G (1994c) Adaptive changes in transmembrane transport and metabolism of triiodothyronine in perfused livers of fed and fasted hypothyroid and hyperthyroid rats. Metabolism 43:1355–1361

De Sandro V, Chevrier M, Boddaert A, Melcion C, Cordier A, Richert L (1991) Comparison of the effects of propylthiouracil, amiodarone, diphenylhydantoin, phenobarbital, and 3-methylcholanthrene on hepatic and renal T_4 metabolism and thyroid gland function in rats. Toxicol Appl Pharmacol 111:263–278

De Sandro V, Catinot R, Kriszt W, Cordier A, Richert L (1992) Male rat hepatic UDP-glucuronosyltransferase activity toward thyroxine. Activation and induction properties – relation with thyroxine plasma disappearance rate. Biochem Pharmacol 43:1563–1569

De Vijlder JJM, Dinsart C, Libert F, Geurts van Kessel A, Bikker H, Bolhuis PA, Vassart G (1988) Regional localization of the gene for thyroid peroxidase to human chromosome 2pter → p 12. Cytogenet Cell Genet 47:170–172

DiStefano JJ, Nguyen TT, Yen YM (1993) Transfer kinetics of 3,5,3′-triiodothyronine and thyroxine from rat blood to large and small intestines, liver, and kidneys in vivo. Endocrinology 132:1735–1744

Docter R, Krenning EP (1990) Role of cellular transport systems in the regulation of thyroid hormone bioactivity. In: Greer MA (ed) The thyroid gland. Raven Press, New York, pp 233–254

Docter R, Krenning EP, Bernard HF, Hennemann G (1987) Active transport of iodothyronines into human cultured fibroblasts. J Clin Endocrinol Metab 65:624–628

Docter R, De Jong M, Van der Hoek HJ, Krenning EP, Hennemann G (1990) Development and use of a mathematical two-pool model of distribution and metabolism of 3,3′,5-triiodothyronine in a recirculating rat liver perfusion system: albumin does not play a role in cellular transport. Endocrinology 126:451–459

Docter R, Bernard HF, Van Toor H, Krenning EP, De Jong M (1993) The presence of a gradient of free T_4 and T_3 over the rat liver cell membrane. J Endocrinol Invest 16 (Suppl 2–6):10

Docter R, Friesema ECH, Van Stralen PGJ, Krenning EP, Everts ME, Visser TJ, Hennemann G (1997) Expression of triiodothyronine and triiodothyronine sulfate transport in *Xenopus laevis* oocytes Endocrinology (in press)

Dupuy C, Virion A, Ohayon R, Kaniewski J (1991) Mechanism of H_2O_2 formation

catalyzed by NADPH oxidase in thyroid plasma membrane. J Biol Chem 266:3739–3743
Eelkman Rooda SJ, Kaptein E, Van Loon MAC, Visser TJ (1988a) Development of a radioimmunoassay for triiodothyronine sulfate. J Immunoassay 9:125–134
Eelkman Rooda SJ, Van Loon MAC, Bonthuis F, Heusdens FA, Kaptein E, Visser TJ (1988b) Effects of iopanoic acid on the metabolism of T_3 in rats. Ann Endocrinol 49:182
Eelkman Rooda SJ, Kaptein E, Rutgers M, Visser TJ (1989a) Increased plasma 3,5,3′-triiodothyronine sulfate in rats with inhibited type I iodothyronine deiodinase activity, as measured by radioimmunoassay. Endocrinology 124:740–745
Eelkman Rooda SJ, Kaptein E, Visser TJ (1989b) Serum triiodothyronine sulfate in man measured by radioimmunoassay. J Clin Endocrinol Metab 69:552–556
Eelkman Rooda SJ, Otten MH, Van Loon MAC, Kaptein E, Visser TJ (1989c) Metabolism of T_3 by rat hepatocytes. Endocrinology 125:2187–2197
Emi Y, Ikushiro SI, Iyanagi T (1995) Drug-responsive and tissue-specific alternative expression of multiple first exons in rat UDP-glucuronosyltransferase family 1 (UGT1) gene complex. J Biochem 117:392–399
Engler D, Burger AG (1984) The deiodination of iodothyronines and their derivatives in man. Endocr Rev 5:151–184
Ericson LE, Johanson V, Molne J et al (1990) Intracellular transport and cell surface expression of thyroperoxidase. In: Carayon P, Ruf J (eds) Thyroperoxidase and thyroid autoimmunity. John Libbey Eurotext, London, pp 107–116
Everts ME, Docter R, Van Buuren JCJ, Van Koetsveld PM, Hofland LJ, De Jong M, Krenning EP, Hennemann G (1993) Evidence for carrier-mediated uptake of triiodothyronine in cultured anterior pituitary cells of euthyroid rats. Endocrinology 131:1278–1285
Everts ME, Docter R, Moerings EPCM, Van Koetsveld PM, Visser TJ, De Jong M, Krenning EP, Hennemann G (1994a) Uptake of thyroxine in cultured anterior pituitary cells of euthyroid rats. Endocrinology 134:2490–2497
Everts ME, Visser TJ, Van Buuren JCJ, Docter R, Krenning EP, Hennemann G (1994b) Uptake of triiodothyronine sulfate and suppression of thyrotropin secretion in cultured anterior pituitary cells. Metabolism 43:1282–1286
Francis-Lang H, Brice M, Martin U, DiLauro R (1990) The thyroid specific nuclear factor, TTF-1, binds to the rat thyroperoxidase promotor. In: Carayon P, Ruf J (eds) Thyroperoxidase and thyroid autoimmunity. John Libbey Eurotext, London, pp 25–32
Gardner DF, Kaplan MM, Stanley CA, Utiger RD (1979) Effect of triiodothyronine replacement on the metabolic and pituitary responses to starvation. N Engl J Med 300:579–584
Gong DW, Murayama N, Yamazoe Y, Kato R (1992) Hepatic triiodothyronine sulfation and its regulation by growth hormone and triiodothyronine in rats. J Biochem. 112:112–116
Green WL (1994) Ether-link cleavage of iodothyronines. In: Wu SY, Visser TJ (eds) Thyroid hormone metabolism: molecular biology and alternate pathways. CRC Press, Baco Raton, pp 199–221
Halmi NS, Granner DK, Doughman DJ, Peters BH, Müller G (1960) Biphasic effect of TSH on thyroidal iodide collection in rats. Endocrinology 67:70–81
Halperin Y, Shapiro LE, Surks MI (1994) Down-regulation of type II L-thyroxine 5′-monodeiodinase in cultured GC cells: different pathways of regulation by L-triiodothyronine and 3,3′,5′-triiodo-L-thyronine. Endocrinology 135:1464–1469
Halpern J, Hinkle PM (1982) Evidence for an active step in thyroid hormone transport to nuclei: drug inhibition of L-^{125}I-triiodothyronine binding to nuclear receptors in rat pituitary tumor cells. Endocrinology 110:1070–1075
Hays MT (1988) Thyroid hormone and the gut. Endocr Res 14:203–224
Hays MT, McGuire RA, Hoogeveen JT, Diezeraad KN (1980) Measurement method for radioactive thyroxine, triiodothyronine, iodide, and iodoprotein in samples with low activity. J Nucl Med 21:225–232

Hegedüs L, Hansen JM, Lühdorf K, Perrild H, Feldt-Rasmussen U, Kampmann JP (1985) Increased frequency of goitre in epileptic patients on long-term phenytoin or carbamazepine treatment. Clin Endocrinol 23:423–429
Hennemann G, Krenning EP, Polhuis M, Mol JA, Bernard HF, Visser TJ, Docter R (1986) Carrier-mediated transport of thyroid hormones into rat hepatocytes is rate limiting in total cellular uptake. Endocrinology 119:1870–1872
Hennemann G (ed) (1986) Thyroid hormone metabolism. Marcel Dekker, New York
Hennemann G, Vos RA, De Jong M, Krenning EP, Docter R (1993) Decreased peripheral 3,5,3′-triiodothyronine (T_3) production from thyroxine (T_4): a syndrome of impaired thyroid hormone activation due to transport inhibition of T_4 into T_3-producing tissues. J Clin Endocrinol Metab 77:1431–1435
Hinton RH, Mitchell FE, Mann A, Chescoe D, Price SC, Nunn A, Grasso P, Bridges JW (1986) Effects of phthalic esters on the liver and thyroid. Environ Health Perspect 70:195–210
Homma H, Kawai H, Kubota M, Matsui M (1992) Large deletion of androsterone UDP-glucuronosyltransferase gene in the inherited deficient strain of Wistar rats. Biochim Biophys Acta 1138:34–40
Hurd RE, Santini F, Lee B, Naim P, Chopra IJ (1993) A study of the 3,5,3′-triiodothyronine sulfation activity in the adult and the fetal rat. Endocrinology 133:1951–1955
Ishii H, Inada M, Tanaka K, Mashio Y, Naito K, Nishikawa M, Imura H (1981) Triiodothyronine generation from thyroxine in human thyroid: enhanced conversion in Graves' thyroid tissue. J Clin Endocrinol Metab 52:1211–1217
Ishii H, Inada M, Tanaka K, Mashio Y, Naito K, Nishikawa M, Matsuzuka F, Kuma K, Imura H (1983) Induction of outer and inner ring monodeiodinases in human thyroid gland by thyrotropin. J Clin Endocrinol Metab 57:500–505
Isojärvi JIT, Pakarinen AJ, Myllylä VV (1992) Thyroid function with antiepileptic drugs. Epilepsia 33:142–148
Jennings AS (1984) Regulation of hepatic triiodothyronine production in the streptozotocin-induced diabetic rat. Am J Physiol 247:E526–E533
Jennings AS, Ferguson DC, Utiger RD (1979) Regulation of the conversion of thyroxine to triiodothyronine in the perfused rat liver. J Clin Invest 64:1614–1623
Kaiser CA, Seydoux J, Giacobino JP, Girardier L, Burger AG (1988) Increased plasma clearance rate of thyroxine despite decreased 5′-monodeiodination: study with a peroxisome proliferator in the rat. Endocrinology 122:1087–1093
Kaplan MM, Utiger RD (1978) Iodothyronine metabolism in rat liver homogenates. J Clin Invest 61:459–471
Kaplan MM, Visser TJ, Yaskoski KA, Leonard JL (1983) Characteristics of iodothyronine tyrosyl ring deiodination by rat cerebral cortical microsomes. Endocrinology 112:35–42
Kaptein EM, Robinson WJ, Grieb D, Nicoloff JT (1982) Peripheral serum thyroxine, triiodothyronine and reverse triiodothyronine kinetics in the low-thyroxine state of acute non-thyroidal illnesses. J Clin Invest 69:526–535
Kaptein EM, Kaptein JS, Chang EI, Egodage PM, Nicoloff JT, Massry SG (1987) Thyroxine transfer and distribution in critical non-thyroidal illnesses, chronic renal failure, and chronic ethanol abuse. J Clin Endocrinol Metab 65:606–623
Kimura S, Hong YS, Kotani I, Ohtaki S, Kikkawa F (1989) Structure of the human thyroid peroxidase gene: comparison and relationship to the human myeloperoxidase gene. Biochemistry 28:4481–4489
Kimura T, Okajima F, Sho K, Kobayashi I, Kondo Y (1995) Thyrotropin-induced hydrogen peroxide production in FRTL-5 thyroid cells is mediated not by adenosine 3′,5′-monophosphate, but by Ca^{2+} signalling followed by phospholipase-A2 activation and potentiated by an adenosine derivative. Endocrinology 136:116–123
Kinlaw WB, Schwartz HL, Oppenheimer JH (1985) Decreased serum triiodothyronine in starving rats is due primarily to diminished thyroidal secretion of thyroxine. J Clin Invest 75:1238–1241
Köhrle J, Hesch RD, Leonard JL (1991) Intracellular pathways of iodothyronine

metabolism. In: Braverman LE, Utiger RD (eds) The thyroid. Lippincott, Philadelphia, pp 144–189

Kostrouch Z, Munari-Silem Y, Rajas F, Bernier-Valentin F, Rousset B (1991) Thyroglobulin internalized by thyrocytes passes through early and late endosomes. Endocrinology 129:2202–2211

Kostrouch Z, Bernier-Valentin F, Munari-Silem Y, Rajas F, Rabilloud R, Rousset B (1993) Thyroglobulin molecules internalized by thyrocytes are sorted in early endosomes and partially recycled back to the follicular lumen. Endocrinology 132:2645–2653

Kragie L (1994) Membrane iodothyronine transporters, part I: Review of physiology. Endocrinol Res 20:319–341

Krenning EP, Docter R, Bernard HF, Visser TJ, Hennemann G (1981) Characteristics of active transport of thyroid hormone into rat hepatocytes. Biochim Biophys Acta 676:314–32

Krenning EP, Docter R, Bernard HF, Visser TJ, Hennemann G (1982) Decreased transport of thyroxine (T_4), 3,3′,5-triiodothyronine (T_3) and 3,3′,5′-triiodothyronine (rT_3) into rat hepatocytes in primary culture due to decrease of cellular ATP content and various drugs. FEBS Lett 140:229–233

Krenning EP, Docter R, Visser TJ, Hennemann G (1983) Plasma membrane transport of thyroid hormone: its possible pathophysiological significance. J Endocrinol Invest 6:59–66

Lai C-S, Korytowski W, Niu C-H, Cheng S-Y (1985) Transverse motion of spin-labeled 3,3′,5-triiodo-L-thyronine in phospholipid bilayers. Biochem Biophys Res Commun 131:408–412

Lamas L, Anderson PC, Fox JW, Dunn JT (1989) Consensus sequences for early iodination and hormogenesis in human thyroglobulin. J Biol Chem 264:13541–13545

Langley AE, Pilcher GD (1985) Thyroid, bradycardic and hypothermic effects of perfluoro-n-decanoic acid. J Toxicol Environ Health 15:485–491

Larsen PR, Berry MJ (1995) Nutritional and hormonal regulation of thyroid hormone deiodinases. Annu Rev Nutr 15:323–352

Larsen PR, JE Silva, Kaplan MM (1981) Relationship between circulating and intracellular thyroid hormones: physiological and clinical implications. Endocr Rev 2:87–102

Laurberg PM, Boye N (1982) Outer and inner ring monodeiodination of thyroxine by dog thyroid and liver: a comparative study using a particulate cell fraction. Endocrinology 110:2124–2130

Leonard JL, Visser TJ (1986) Biochemistry of deiodination. In: Hennemann G (ed) Thyroid hormone metabolism. Marcel Dekker, New York, pp 189–229

Leonard JL, Safran M (1994) Hormonal regulation of type II iodothyronine deiodinase in the brain. In: Wu SY, Visser TJ (eds) Thyroid hormone metabolism: molecular biology and alternate pathways. CRC Press, Baco Raton, pp 23–44

Lim C-F, Bernard BF, De Jong M, Docter R, Krenning EP, Hennemann G (1993a) A furan fatty acid and indoxyl sulphate are the putative inhibitors of thyroxine hepatocytes transport in uremia. J Clin Endocrinol Metab 76:318–324

Lim C-F, Docter R, Visser TJ, Krenning EP, Bernard BF, Van Toor H, De Jong M, Hennemann G (1993b) Inhibition of thyroxine transport into cultured rat hepatocytes by serum of non-uremic critically-ill patients: effects of bilirubin and nonesterified fatty acids. J Clin Endocrinol Metab 76:1165–1172

Lim C-F, Docter R, Krenning EP, Van Toor H, Bernard BF, De Jong M, Hennemann G (1994) Transport of thyroxine into cultured hepatocytes: effects of mild nonthyroidal illness and calorie restriction in obese subjects. Clin Endocrinol 40:79–85

LoPresti JS, Mizuno L, Nimalysuria A, Anderson KP, Spencer CA, Nicoloff JT (1991) Characteristics of 3,5,3′-triiodothyronine sulfate metabolism in euthyroid man. J Clin Endocrinol Metab 73:703–709

Lueprasitsakul W, Fang SL, Alex S, Braverman LE (1991) Effect of the cardiac inotropic drug, OPC 8212, on pituitary-thyroid function in the rat. Endocrinology 128:2709–2714

Magnusson RP, Taurog A, Dorris ML (1984) Mechanism of iodide-dependent catalytic activity of thyroid peroxidase and lactoperoxidase. J Biol Chem 259:197–205

Maia AL, Berry MJ, Sabbag R, Harney JW, Larsen PR (1995) Structural and functional differences in the dio1 gene in mice with inherited type 1 deiodinase deficiency. Mol Endocrinol 9:969–980

Mandel SJ, Berry MJ, Kieffer JD, Harney JW, Warne RL, Larsen PR (1992) Cloning and in vitro expression of the human selenoprotein, type I iodothyronine deiodinase. J Clin Endocrinol Metab 75:1133–1139

Marriq C, Arnand C, Rolland M, Lissitsky S (1980) An approach to the structure of thyroglobulin. Hormone-forming sequences in porcine thyroglobulin. Eur J Biochem 111:33–47

Masmoudi T, Planells R, Mounie J, Artur Y, Magdalou J, Goudonnet H (1996) Opposite regulation of bilirubin and 4-nitrophenol UDP-glucuronosyltransferase mRNA levels by 3,3′,5-triiodo-L-thyronine in rat liver. FEBS Lett 379:181–185

McClain RM (1989) The significance of hepatic microsomal enzyme induction and altered thyroid function in rats: implications for thyroid gland neoplasia. Toxicol Pathol 17:294–306

McClain RM, Levin AA, Posch R, Downing JC (1989) The effect of phenobarbital on the metabolism and excretion of thyroxine in rats. Toxicol Appl Pharmacol 99:216–228

McIntosh K, Berdanier CD (1992) Influence of dehydroepiandrosterone (DHEA) on the rat thyroid hormone status of BHE/cdb rats. J Nutr Biochem 3:194–199

Meinhold H, Campos-Barros A, Walzog B, Köhler R, Müller F, Behne D (1993) Effects of selenium and iodine deficiency on type I, type II and type III iodothyronine deiodinases and circulating thyroid hormones in the rat. Exp Clin Endocrinol 101:87–93

Mol JA, Krenning EP, Docter R, Rozing J, Hennemann G (1986) Inhibition of iodothyronine transport into rat liver cells by a monoclonal antibody. J Biol Chem 261:7640–7643

Mol K, Kaptein E, Darras VM, De Greef WJ, Kühn E, Visser TJ (1993) Different thyroid hormone-deiodinating enzymes in tilapia (*Oreochromis niloticus*) liver and kidney. FEBS Lett 321:140–143

Moreno M, Kaptein E, Goglia F, Visser TJ (1994) Rapid glucuronidation of tri- and tetraiodothyroacetic acid to ester glucuronides in human liver and to ether glucuronides in rat liver. Endocrinology 135:1004–1009

Morreale de Escobar G, Escobar del Rey F (1967) Extrathyroid effects of some antithyroid drugs and their metabolic consequences. Rec Progr Horm Res 23:87–137

Nakamura M, Yamazaki I, Nakagawa H, Ohtaki S (1983) Steady state kinetics and regulation of thyroid peroxidase-catalyzed iodination. J Biol Chem 258:3837–38421

Namba H, Yamashita S, Morita S, Villadolid MC, Kimura H, Yokoyama N, Izumi M, Ishikawa N, Ito K, Nagataki S (1993) Retinoic acid inhibits human thyroid peroxidase and thyroglobulin gene expression in cultured human thyrocytes. J Endocrinol Invest 16:87–93

Nunez J, Pommier J (1982) Formation of thyroid hormones. Vitam Horm 39:175–229

Ohnhaus EE, Studer H (1983) A link between liver microsomal enzyme activity and thyroid hormone metabolism in man. Br J Clin Pharmacol 15:71–76

Ohtaki S, Mashimo K, Yamazaki I (1973) Hydrogen peroxide generating system in hog thyroid microsomes. Biochim Biophys Acta 292:825–833

O'Mara BA, Dittrich W, Lauterio TJ, St. Germain DL (1993) Pretranslational regulation of type I 5′-deiodinase by thyroid hormones and in fasted and diabetic rats. Endocrinology 133:1715–1723

Owens IS, Ritter JK (1992) The novel bilirubin/phenol UDP-glucuronosyltransferase

UGT1 gene locus: implications for multiple nonhemolytic familial hyperbilirubinemia phenotypes. Pharmacogenetics 2:93–108
Palumbo G, Gentil F, Condorelli GL, Salvatore G (1990) The earliest site of iodination in thyroglobulin is residue number 5. J Biol Chem 265:8887–8892
Polk DH (1995) Thyroid hormone metabolism during development. Reprod Fertil Dev 7:469–477
Polk D, Wu SY, Fisher DA (1994) Alternate pathways of thyroid hormone metabolism in developing mammals. In: Wu SY, Visser TJ (eds) Thyroid hormone metabolism: molecular biology and alternate pathways. CRC Press, Baco Raton, pp 223–243
Pontecorvi A, Lakshmanan M, Robbins J (1987) Intracellular transport of 3,5,3′-triiodo-L-thyronine in rat skeletal myoblasts. Endocrinology 121:2145–2152
Raspé E, Dumont JE (1995) Tonic modulation of dog thyrocyte H_2O_2 generation and I-uptake by thyrotropin through the cyclic adenosine 3′5′-monophosphate cascade. Endocrinology 136:965–973
Rawitch AB, Pollock G, Yang SX, Taurog A (1990) The location and nature of the N-linked oligosaccharide units in porcine thyroid peroxidase: studies on the tryptic glycopeptides. In: Carayon P, Ruf J (eds) Thyroperoxidase and thyroid autoimmunity. John Libbey Eurotext, London, pp 69–76
Rosenbaum RL, Maturlo SJ, Surks MI (1980) Changes in thyroidal economy in rat bearing transplantable Walker 256 carcinomas. Endocrinology 106:1386–1391
Rousset B, Mornex R (1991) The thyroid hormone secretory pathway – current dogmas and alternative hypotheses. Mol Cell Endocrinol 78:C89–C93
Rousset B, Selmi S, Bornet H, Bourgeat P, Rabilloud R, Munari-Silem Y (1989) Thyroid hormone residues are released from thyroglobulin with only limited alteration of the thyroglobulin structure. J Biol Chem 254:12620–12626
Roy Chowdhury J, Roy Chowdhury N, Moscioni AD, Tukey R, Tephley TR, Arias IM (1983) Differential regulation by triiodothyronine of substrate-specific uridine diphosphoglucuronate glucuronosyl transferases in rat liver. Biochim Biophys Acta 761:58–65
Rutgers M, Bonthuis F, De Herder WW, Visser TJ (1987) Accumulation of plasma triiodothyronine sulfate in rats treated with propylthiouracil. J Clin Invest 80:758–762
Rutgers M, Heusdens FA, Bonthuis F, De Herder WW, Hazenberg MP, Visser TJ (1989a) Enterohepatic circulation of triiodothyronine (T_3) in rats: importance of the microflora for the liberation and reabsorption of T_3 from biliary T_3 conjugates. Endocrinology 125:2822–2830
Rutgers M, Pigmans IGAJ, Bonthuis F, Docter R, Visser TJ (1989b) Effects of propylthiouracil on the biliary clearance of thyroxine (T_4) in rats: decreased excretion of 3,5,3′-triiodothyronine glucuronide and increased excretion of 3,3′,5′-triiodothyronine glucuronide and T_4 sulfate. Endocrinology 125:2175–2186
Rutgers M, Heusdens FA, Visser TJ (1991) Deiodination of iodothyronine sulfamates by rat liver microsomes. Endocrinology 129:1375–1381
Safran M, Leonard JL (1991) Comparison of the physicochemical properties of type I and type II iodothyronine 5′-deiodinase. J Biol Chem 266:3233–3238
Safran M, Farwell AP, Leonard JL (1991) Evidence that type II 5′ deiodinase is not a selenoprotein. J Biol Chem 266:13477–13480
Saito K, Kaneko H, Sato K, Yoshitake A, Yamada H (1991) Hepatic UDP-glucuronyltransferase(s) activity toward thyroid hormones in rats: induction and effects on serum thyroid hormone levels following treatment with various enzyme inducers. Toxicol Appl Pharmacol 111:99–106
Salvatore D, Low SC, Berry MJ, Maia AL, Harney JW, Croteau W, St.Germain DL, Larsen PR (1995) Type 3 iodothyronine deiodinase: cloning, in vitro expression, and functional analysis of the placental selenoenzyme. J Clin Invest 96:2421–2430

Salvatore D, Bartha T, Harney JW, Larsen PR (1996) Molecular biological and biochemical characterization of the human type 2 selenodeiodinase. Endocrinology 137:3308–3315

Samson M, Osty J, Blondeau JP (1993) Identification by photoaffinitylabeling of a membrane thyroid hormone-binding protein associated with the triiodothyronine transport system in rat erythrocytes. Endocrinology 132:2470–2476

Sanders JE, Eigenberg DA, Bracht LJ, Wang WR, Van Zwieten MJ (1988) Thyroid and liver trophic changes in rats secondary to liver microsomal enzyme induction caused by an experimental leukotriene antagonist (L-649,923). Toxicol Appl Pharmacol 95:378–387

Santini F, Chopra IJ, Hurd RE, Solomon DH, Chua Teco GN (1992a) A study of the characteristics of the rat placental iodothyronine 5-monodeiodinase: evidence that it is distinct from the rat hepatic iodothyronine 5′-monodeiodinase. Endocrinology 130:2325–2332

Santini F, Chopra IJ, Wu SY, Solomon DH, Chua Teco GN (1992b) Metabolism of 3,5,3′-triiodothyronine sulfate by tissues of the fetal rat: a consideration of the role of desulfation of 3,5,3′-triiodothyronine sulfate as a source of T_3. Pediatr Res 31:541–544

Santini F, Hurd RE, Chopra IJ (1992c) A study of metabolism of deaminated and sulfoconjugated iodothyronines by rat placental iodothyronine 5-monodeiodinase. Endocrinology 131:1689–1694

Santini F, Hurd RE, Lee B, Chopra IJ (1993) Thyromimetic effects of 3,5,3′-triiodothyronine sulfate in hypothyroid rats. Endocrinology 133:105–110

Schachter D (1984) Fluidity and function of hepatocyte plasma membranes. Hepatology 4:140–151

Sekura RD, Sato K, Cahnmann HJ, Robbins J, Jakoby WB (1981) Sulfate transfer to thyroid hormones and their analogs by hepatic aryl sulfotransferase. Endocrinology 108:454–456

Semler DE, Chengelis CP, Radzialowsky FM (1989) The effects of chronic ingestion of spironolactone on serum thyrotropin and thyroid hormone in the male rat. Toxicol Appl Pharmacol 98:263–268

Sharifi J, St.Germain DL (1992) The cDNA for the type I iodothyronine 5′-deiodinase encodes an enzyme manifesting both high K_m and low K_m activity. J Biol Chem 267:12539–12544

Siegrist-Kaiser CA, Burger AG (1994) Modification of the side chain of thyroid hormone. In: Wu SY, Visser TJ (eds) Thyroid hormone metabolism: molecular biology and alternate pathways. CRC Press, Baco Raton, pp 175–198

Spahn-Langguth H, Benet LZ (1992) Acyl glucuronides revisited: is the glucuronidation process a toxification as well as a detoxification mechanism? Drug Metab Rev 24:5–48

Spaulding SW (1994) Bioactivities of conjugated iodothyronines. In: Wu SY, Visser TJ (eds) Thyroid hormone metabolism: molecular biology and alternate pathways. CRC Press, Baco Raton, pp 139–153

Stanbury BJ, Morris ML (1958) Deiodination of diiodotyrosine by cell-free systems. J Biol Chem 233:106–108

St.Germain DL (1994) Biochemical study of type III iodothyronine deiodinase. In: Wu SY, Visser TJ (eds) Thyroid hormone metabolism: molecular biology and alternate pathways. CRC Press, Baco Raton, pp 45–66

St.Germain DL, Schwartzman RA, Croteau W, Kanamori A, Wang Z, Brown DD, Galton VA (1994) A thyroid hormone-regulated gene in Xenopus laevis encodes a type III iodothyronine 5-deiodinase. Proc Natl Acad Sci USA 91:7767–7771,11282

Stitzer LK, Jacquez JA (1975) Neutral amino acid transport pathways in uptake of L-thyroxine by Ehrlich ascites cells. Am J Physiol 229:172–177

Taurog A (1970) Thyroid peroxidase-catalyzed iodination of thyroglobulin: inhibition of excess iodide. Arch Biochem Biophys 139:212–220

Toyoda N, Nishikawa M, Horimoto M, Yoshikawa N, Mori Y, Yoshimora M, Masaka M, Tanaka K, Inada M (1990) Graves' immunoglobulin G stimulates iodothyronine 5′ deiodinating activity in FRTL-5 rat thyroid cells. J Clin Endocrinol Metab 70:1506–1511

Toyoda N, Nishikawa M, Mori Y, Gondou A, Ogawa Y, Yonemoto T, Yoshimara M, Masaki H, Inada M (1992) Thyrotropin and triiodothyronine regulate iodothyronine 5′-deiodinase messenger ribonucleic acid levels in FRTL-5 rat thyroid cells. Endocrinology 131:389–394

Toyoda N, Berry MJ, Harney JW, Larsen PR (1995a) Topological analysis of the integral membrane protein, type I iodothyronine deiodinase. J Biol Chem 270:12310–12318

Toyoda N, Harney JW, Berry MJ, Larsen PR (1995b) Identification of critical amino acids for 3,3′,5′-triiodothyronine deiodination by human type I deiodinase based on comparative functional-structural analyses of the human, dog and rat enzymes. J Biol Chem 269:20329–20334

Van der Heyden JTM, Docter R, Van Toor H, Wilson JHP, Hennemann G, Krenning EP (1986) Effects of caloric deprivation on thyroid hormone tissue uptake and generation of low T_3 syndrome. Am J Physiol 251:E156–E163

Van Raaij JAGM, Kaptein E, Visser TJ, Van den Berg KJ (1993) Increased glucuronidation of thyroid hormone in hexachlorobenzene-treated rats. Biochem Pharmacol 45:627–631

Van Steenbergen W, Fevery J, De Vos R, Leyten R, Heirwegh KPM, De Groote J (1989) Thyroid hormones and the hepatic handling of bilirubin. I. Effects of hypothyroidism and hyperthyroidism on the hepatic transport of bilirubin mono- and diconjugates in the Wistar rat. Hepatology 9:314–321

Visser TJ (1988) Metabolism of thyroid hormone. In: Cooke BA, King RJB, Van der Molen HJ (eds) Hormones and their actions, part I. Elsevier, Amsterdam, pp 81–103

Visser TJ (1990) Importance of deiodination and conjugation in the hepatic metabolism of thyroid hormone. In: Greer MA (ed) The thyroid gland. Raven Press, New York, pp 255–283

Visser TJ (1994a) Sulfation and glucuronidation pathways of thyroid hormone metabolism. In: Wu SY, Visser TJ (eds) Thyroid hormone metabolism: molecular biology and alternate pathways. CRC Press, Baco Raton, pp 85–117

Visser TJ (1994b) Role of sulfation in thyroid hormone metabolism. Chem Biol Interact 92:293–303

Visser TJ, Fekkes D, Docter R, Hennemann G (1979) Kinetics of enzymic reductive deiodination of iodothyronines. Biochem J 179:489–495

Visser TJ, Leonard JL, Kaplan MM, Larsen PR (1982) Kinetic evidence suggesting two mechanisms for iodothyronine 5′-deiodination in rat cerebral cortex. Proc Natl Acad Sci USA 79:5080–5084

Visser TJ, Kaptein E, Terpstra OT, Krenning EP (1988) Deiodination of thyroid hormone by human liver. J Clin Endocrinol Metab 67:17–24

Visser TJ, Kaptein E, Harpur ES (1991) Differential expression and ciprofibrate induction of hepatic UDP-glucuronyltransferases for thyroxine and triiodothyronine in Fischer rats. Biochem Pharmacol 42:444–446

Visser TJ, Kaptein E, Gijzel AL, De Herder WW, Ebner T, Burchell B (1993a) Glucuronidation of thyroid hormone by human bilirubin and phenol UDP-glucuronyltransferase isoenzymes. FEBS Lett 324:358–360

Visser TJ, Kaptein E, Van Raaij JAGM, Tjong Tjin Joe C, Ebner T, Burchell B (1993b) Multiple UDP-glucuronyltransferases for the glucuronidation of thyroid hormone with preference for 3,3′,5′-triiodothyronine (reverse T_3). FEBS Lett 315:65–68

Visser TJ, Kaptein E, Van Toor H, Van Raaij JAGM, Van den Berg KJ, Tjong Tjin Joe C, Van Engelen JGM, Brouwer A (1993c) Glucuronidation of thyroid hormone in rat liver: effects of in vivo treatment with microsomal enzyme inducers and in vitro assay conditions. Endocrinology 133:2177–2186

Visser TJ, Kaptein E, Gijzel A, De Herder WW, Cannon ML, Bonthuis F, De Greef WJ (1996) Effects of thyroid status and thyrostatic drugs on hepatic glucuronidation of iodothyronines and other substrates in rats. Induction of phenol UDP-glucuronyltransferase by methimazole. Endocrine 4:79–85

Vos RA, De Jong M, Docter R, Van Toor H, Bernard BF, Krenning EP, Hennemann G (1991) Morbidity-dependent thyroid hormone transport inhibition by serum of patients with non-thyroidal illness (NTI) in rat hepatocytes and in the perfused rat liver. In: Gordon A, Gross J, Hennemann G (eds) Progress in thyroid research. Balkema AA, Rotterdam, The Netherlands, pp 693–696

Vos RA, De Jong M, Bernard BF, Docter R, Krenning EP, Hennemann G (1995) Impaired thyroxine and 3,5,3′-triiodothyronine handling by rat hepatocytes in the presence of serum of patients with non-thyroidal illness. J Clin Endocrinol Metab 80:2364–2370

Wolff J (1960) Thyroidal iodide transport. I. Cardiac glycosides and the role of potassium. Biochim Biophys Acta 38:316–324

Woodbury DM, Woodbury JW (1963) Correlation of micro-electrode potential recordings with histology of rat and guinea pig thyroid glands. J Physiol (London) 169:553–567

Wu SY, Huang WS, Polk D, Florsheim WH, Green WL, Fisher DA (1992a) Identification of thyroxine sulfate (T_4S) in human serum and amniotic fluid by a novel T_4S radioimmunoassay. Thyroid 2:101–105

Wu SY, Polk D, Wong S, Reviczky A, Vu R, Fisher DA (1992b) Thyroxine sulfate is a major thyroid hormone metabolite and a potential intermediate in the monodeiodination pathways in fetal sheep. Endocrinology 131:1751–1756

Wu SY, Huang WS, Polk D, Chen WL, Reviczky A, Williams J, Chopra IJ, Fisher DA (1993a) The development of a radioimmunoassay for reverse triiodothyronine sulfate in human serum and amniotic fluid. J Clin Endocrinol Metab 76:1625–1630

Wu SY, Polk DH, Huang WS, Reviczky A, Wang K, Fisher DA (1993b) Sulfate conjugates of iodothyronines in developing sheep; effect of fetal hypothyroidism. Am J Physiol 265:E115–E120

Wu SY, Polk DH, Chen WL, Fisher DA, Huang WS, Yee B (1994) A 3,3′-diiodothyronine sulfate cross-reactive compound in serum from pregnant women. J Clin Endocrinol Metab 1505–1509

Wu SY, Polk D, Fisher DA, Huang WS, Reviczky AL, Chen WL (1995) Identification of 3,3′-T_2S as a fetal thyroid hormone derivative in maternal urine in sheep. Am J Physiol 268:E33–E39

Wyatt I, Coutts CT, Elcombe CR (1993) The effect of chlorinated paraffins on hepatic enzymes and thyroid hormones. Toxicology 77:81–90

Young WF, Gorman CA, Weinshilboum RM (1988) Triiodothyronine: a substrate for the thermostable and thermolabile forms of human phenol sulfotransferase. Endocrinology 122:1816–1824

CHAPTER 5

Thyroid Hormone Transport

J.R. STOCKIGT, C-F. LIM, J.W. BARLOW, and D.J. TOPLISS

A. Introduction

It is now over half a century since it was shown that circulating thyroid hormones bind non-covalently to plasma proteins (TREVORROW 1938). The identity of these binding proteins in various species, the relationship of the free and bound hormone fractions to biological activity, the diagnostic importance of total or free hormone measurements, and the effects of other ligands which compete for specific hormone-binding sites have been extensively studied. Numerous hereditary variations in the three major human thyroid hormone-binding proteins have been described (see REFETOFF 1989, 1994; BARTALENA 1990, 1994, for detailed reviews). In addition, the validity of the free hormone hypothesis, which holds that hormone delivery to tissues is a function of the free hormone concentration at equilibrium, has been extensively discussed (PARDRIDGE 1981; MENDEL 1989a; EKINS 1990).

There is generally close correlation between the free hormone concentration and the biological activity of thyroid hormones, with the bound component (more than 99% in the case of T_4 and T_3) having a fundamental reservoir function that serves to replenish the free concentration. The relationships between total and free T_4 and T_3 concentrations are shown in Table 1. The various bound moieties are in rapid equilibrium with the free hormone, and any tendency for the minute free concentration to fall as a result of tissue uptake or clearance is "buffered" by dissociation. In an autoradiographic study, MENDEL et al. (1987a) demonstrated much more even distribution of labelled T_4 within perfused hepatic tissues in the presence of binding proteins than in buffer alone. In addition to their interaction with T_4 and T_3, the thyroid hormone-binding proteins have a high affinity for many natural and synthetic analogues of iodothyronines. Detailed studies of these interactions will not be reviewed here (see SNYDER et al. 1976; ROBBINS et al. 1978; ANDREA et al. 1980).

As emphasised by EKINS (1990), a valid in vitro measurement of the free T_4 or free T_3 concentration at equilibrium at 37°C does not imply that this concentration applies to all tissues, at all positions across the axes of capillaries, or at various points during tissue transit. In some instances, after extensive irreversible exit of free hormone from the circulation, the bound hormone may ultimately contribute substantially to the quantity of hormone that is

Table 1. Relationship between total and free concentrations of thyroxine (T_4) and triiodothyronine (T_3) in normal human serum

	T_4	*T_3
Total concentration nM	60–140	1.1–2.7
Free concentration pM	10–25	3–8
Unbound fraction	1:3000–1:4000	1:300–1:400

* Higher values in childhood; probable minor decline in old age.

taken up by the tissues. Because of differences in dissociation rate (MENDEL 1989a), various protein-bound fractions can contribute disproportionately to the free hormone concentration under non-steady-state conditions during tissue transit. The studies of HILLIER (1971) demonstrate that the albumin-bound fraction, because of its more rapid dissociation, is likely to make a contribution greater than its proportional hormone carriage at equilibrium during tissue transit. Nevertheless, studies which inferred that the albumin-bound moiety was virtually as readily available as the free component (PARDRIDGE et al. 1981) appear to have overestimated this effect (see MENDEL 1989a).

In the numerous types of hereditary binding abnormalities, it is notable that the free hormone concentration (when measured in vitro by fully validated methods such as equilibrium dialysis) shows a high degree of inverse correlation with the plasma concentration of thyroid-stimulating hormone (TSH), which currently gives the best available objective index of thyroid hormone action. This relationship strongly supports the free hormone hypothesis, regardless of theoretical arguments as to its limitations. However, a rigid distinction between bound and free hormone moieties is perhaps of little relevance, in view of the estimate by HILLIER (1975) that hormone molecules from these two components are in rapid interchange up to several million times per day.

B. Serum Binding in Humans

The three major T_4- and T_3-binding proteins in human serum are thyroxine-binding globulin (TBG), transthyretin (TTR, prealbumin), and albumin (Table 2). Normally, about 70% of the circulating T_4 is bound to TBG, 10%–20% to TTR and 10%–20% to albumin (PRINCE and RAMSDEN 1977; ROBBINS and JOHNSON 1979). In defining the kinetics of protein carriage of thyroid hormones, it is important to distinguish between the dissociation constant (K_d expressed as M/l) or its reciprocal K_a (l/M), which define the free hormone concentration at which a particular binding site is half occupied, and the dissociation rate (expressed as $t_{1/2}$, s) or the rate constant (sec^{-1}), which defines

Table 2. Approximate concentrations, occupancy and kinetics of thyroid hormone binding proteins in normal human serum at 37°C

Protein	Concentration M	Occupancy by T_4	Proportion of T_4 carried	Dissociation constant K_d M.L^{-1}		Off rate $t^1/_2$ sec	
				T_4	T_3	T_4	T_3
Thyroxine binding globulin	3×10^{-7}	30%	70%	10^{-10}	2×10^{-9}	20–40	5–10
Transthyretin	2×10^{-6}	0.5%	10–20%	10^{-3}	6×10^{-8}	8	<2
Albumin	6×10^{-4}	<0.01%	10–20%	10^{-6}*	10^{-5}*	<2	<1

* Highest affinity site.

Table 3. Known human variants of thyroid hormone binding proteins

Protein	Circulating concentration	T_4 binding affinity	Number of variants
TBG	Undetectable	–	3
	Low	Low	6
	Normal	Normal	5
	Normal	Undetectable	1
	High	Normal	1
TTR	? Normal	Undetectable	1
	? Normal	Low	5
	? Normal	Normal	3
	Normal ? high	Increased	3
Albumin	Normal	Increased	1
	Undetectable	–	1

Compiled from REFETOFF (1994) and BARTALENA (1994).

the rate of unidirectional dissociation, or delivery, of hormone from that binding site. The former parameter describes an equilibrium between association and dissociation which, together with the number of binding sites, determines the proportion of hormone carried on each of several classes of binding protein at equilibrium. The dissociation rate, a unidirectional maximum rate of hormone delivery, is relevant under non-steady-state conditions, as for example when free hormone is rapidly removed from the circulating compartment during tissue transit. The relationship between dissociation rate and tissue transit times determines whether the free hormone concentration will remain uniform at various tissue sites. Both K_d and dissociation rate are highly temperature dependent. Free T_4 fraction is higher at 37°C than at room temperature by a factor of up to 2 (KORCEK and TABACHNIK 1976), and dissociation is much faster (HILLIER 1975).

Minor T_4 binding has also been described to lipoproteins which may carry as much as 3% of the circulating T_4 (BENVENGA et al. 1988; BENVENGA et al.

1993), but the significance of this fraction remains unclear. Gamma-globulin binding of T_4 has been reported in some patients with autoimmune thyroid disease and may reflect thyroglobulin autoantibodies that cross-react with T_3 or T_4 (BENVENGA et al. 1987). Such antibodies cause potent diagnostic artefacts in free hormone assays (BECK-PECCOZ et al. 1984; VYAS and WILKIN 1994) and may occasionally be important as binders of thyroid hormone in vivo (SAKATA et al. 1985).

The numerous hereditary variants due to molecular changes in each of the three major binding proteins are summarised in Table 3. These variants have been extensively reviewed (REFETOFF 1994, SARAIVA 1995) and will be considered only briefly here.

I. Thyroxine-Binding Globulin

1. Normal Structure

Thyroxine-binding globulin (TBG) is a single polypeptide chain a-globulin, with molecular weight of about 54 kDa (REFETOFF 1989). Cloning and sequencing of a cDNA for human TBG (FLINK et al. 1986) has shown that it is synthesised as a 415 amino acid protein. The first 20 amino acid residues of the TBG peptide are hydrophobic in nature and probably represent the signal peptide which is removed in the endoplasmic reticulum, leaving a mature protein of 395 amino acids as a single chain. This mature protein has a molecular weight of 44 180, in close agreement with the 45 kDa previously reported for non-glycosylated TBG (BARTALENA et al. 1984). There are five potential glycosylation sites, although only four are used, at amino acid residues 16, 79, 145, and 391 (FLINK et al. 1986), giving an average of ten terminal sialic acid moieties. BARTALENA (1990), in evaluating the importance of the carbohydrate moieties of TBG, estimated that their principal influence was on protein half-life in blood, stability in vitro, and microheterogeneity on electrophoresis, with only minor effects on immunoreactivity and T_4 binding.

The amino acid sequence of human TBG shares a high degree of sequence homology with rat TBG (70%), human corticosteroid-binding globulin (CBG, 55%) and the members of the serine protease inhibitor family (SERPINS), which includes α-antitrypsin (53% homology) and α_1-antichymotrypsin (58% homology) (FLINK et al. 1986; HAMMOND et al. 1987). The possible significance of the structural similarity between human TBG, CBG and the SERPINS remains unclear, since the hormone-binding proteins appear to be devoid of antiprotease activity.

The normal concentration of human serum TBG measured by radioimmunoassay is between 10 and 30 mg/l (0.2–0.6 μM). TBG is normally 20%–40% occupied by T_4 and <1% occupied by T_3. Occupancy may increase markedly in hyperthyroidism, due to both an increase in total T_4 and a decrease in TBG concentration, leading to a disproportionate rise in free T_4 relative to the increase in total T_4 (see below).

Before the advent of radioimmunoassay, the concentration of TBG was estimated from the maximum binding capacity of this protein for T_4, based on the assumption of one T_4-binding site on every TBG molecule. These estimates are in general agreement with subsequent direct assays.

2. Inherited Variants

Multiple inherited TBG variants, often designated geographically, can result in an increased TBG concentration or a partial or complete TBG deficiency in serum (Table 3). Of about 16 known X-linked TBG mutants, three cause complete TBG deficiency, while at least 6 other types result in a reduced affinity for T_4, and are associated with subnormal serum TBG concentrations (REFETOFF 1994). In numerous instances, variants of TBG show increased or decreased heat lability in vitro. TBG deficiency (complete or partial) has been attributed to a single amino acid deletion or double amino acid substitution which may lead to frame shift and premature termination of the protein (REFETOFF 1994). In the face of total TBG deficiency, the concentration of total T_4 is about $25\,nM$, with normal free T_4 and TSH, suggesting that normal thyroid hormone regulation can occur in the complete absence of the major circulating binding protein.

Alterations in serum TBG concentrations may result from either altered synthesis or degradation related to the primary amino acid sequence, or to the glycosylation of the secreted protein. As emphasised by REFETOFF (1994), intracellular retention and breakdown of defective TBG molecules, rather than extracellular degradation, is usually the cause of low serum concentrations. Diminished TBG binding of T_4 is especially prevalent in some ethnic groups, for example among Australian aborigines, up to 30% of whom have low serum total T_4 concentrations associated with subnormal serum concentrations of an abnormally heat-labile TBG (MURATA et al. 1985) that shows subnormal affinity for T_4 (MOHR et al. 1987). Of particular interest is a recently described variant TBG with normal physical and electrophoretic properties and normal serum concentration, but negligible binding affinity for T_4 (JANSSEN et al. 1994).

The binding of T_4 to TBG from patients with inherited X-linked TBG excess is indistinguishable from the common type of TBG. In some cases at least, the excess is due to gene duplication (MORI et al. 1995). In general, each of the various methods for serum free T_4 estimation, as well as binding corrections based on T_3-uptake measurements, give a useful semiquantitative correction for TBG abnormalities, whether hereditary or acquired.

3. Acquired Variants

Acquired variations in TBG concentrations have been attributed to pathophysiological, environmental and nutritional factors and to drug effects (Table 4). The molecular mechanisms responsible for the effect of numerous drugs

Table 4. Drug effects on serum TBG concentrations

Increase	Oestrogens Tamoxifen Heroin Methadone 5-fluouracil Perphenazine Clofibrate Mitotane
Decrease	Thyroid hormone excess Androgens, anabolic steroids Glucocorticoids L-asparaginase Interleukin-6

(e.g. androgen, clofibrate, perphenazine) and pathological conditions (such as oat cell carcinoma) remain unresolved (BARTALENA 1993).

The commonest acquired change in TBG is an increase in concentration due to exogenous or endogenous oestrogen excess. Increases in total T_4 and T_3 are associated with increased concentrations of TBG that show a greater proportion of bands with anodal mobility on isoelectric focusing, due to increase in sialic acid content of the side chains (AIN et al. 1987). Reduced TBG degradation rate due to oligosaccharide modification appears to be the major mechanism of oestrogen-induced TBG excess (AIN et al. 1988).

Concentrations of TBG correlate inversely with thyroid hormone levels in human hyper- and hypothyroidism (KONNO 1985), and in experimental primate studies (GLINOER et al. 1979). Using human hepatocytes in culture, CROWE et al. (1995) showed a T_3-induced decrease in TBG secretion into the cell medium, with concordant changes in mRNA. In humans, serum TBG concentrations are decreased by glucocorticoid excess (OPPENHEIMER and WERNER 1966). Adrenalectomy in rats increases serum binding-capacity and increases hepatic TBG mRNA levels (EMERSON et al. 1993).

Unlike human TBG, rat TBG is strongly repressed during adult life but actively expressed during postnatal development (SAVU et al. 1987), in senescence (SAVU et al. 1991), and in the face of malnutrition (ROUAZE-ROMET et al. 1992) and hypothyroidism (VRANCKX et al. 1990).

II. Transthyretin

1. Normal Structure

Transthyretin (TTR, thyroxine-binding prealbumin; previously known as prealbumin), a protein of approximately 55 kDa which circulates in the serum of a wide range of vertebrates (RICHARDSON et al. 1994), is a tetramer consisting of four identical polypeptide chains held together by non-covalent bonds. The tetrameric structure of TTR is symmetrical about a central cavity which completely penetrates the molecule. There are two T_4-binding sites on TTR, one at each end of the central cavity (FERGUSON et al. 1975; ROBBINS et al. 1978), which display the phenomenon of negative cooperativity in which the binding of T_4 at one site inhibits T_4 binding at the other (FERGUSON et al. 1975). However, this phenomenon is probably of little physiological significance because it has been demonstrated only at unphysiologically high free T_4 concentrations.

The normal serum concentration of TTR is in the range of 100–400 mg/l (2–8 μM). TTR is a negative acute-phase reactant and its serum concentration decreases rapidly during acute illness or malnutrition as a result of reduced hepatic synthesis (SCHREIBER 1987). At normal concentrations, TTR is <1% occupied by T_4, with an affinity for T_4 and a rate of dissociation intermediate between TBG and albumin (Table 1). The desamino analogues of T_3 and T_4, triiodothyroacetic acid and tetraiodothyroacetic acid, generally have higher affinity for TTR than their parent compounds (ANDREA et al. 1980).

In absolute terms, the liver is the principal site of synthesis of TTR (JORNVALL et al. 1981; DICKSON et al. 1982), but the choroid plexus (SCHREIBER et al. 1990) and the pancreatic islets (JACOBSSON et al. 1990) are additional sites of TTR synthesis. In evolutionary terms, TTR synthesis at the choroid plexus precedes the ontogeny of TTR synthesis in the liver (RICHARDSON et al. 1994). It is of interest that the T_4-binding domain of TTR appears to have been conserved over the past 350 million years (RICHARDSON et al. 1994).

An unusual feature of TTR is that it also binds retinol-binding protein, the carrier of vitamin A. Each TTR molecule is able to bind four molecules of retinol-binding protein, but only one molecule of retinol-binding protein is normally complexed with one molecule of TTR (HELLER and HOROWITZ 1974). The binding sites for T_4 and retinol-binding protein on TTR are separate, and while there is no evidence that T_4 affects retinol binding, a recent study suggests that retinol can impair T_4 binding to TTR (SMITH et al. 1994).

2. Inherited Variants

Numerous TTR variants characterised by single amino acid substitutions have been described in man, many of which have been found in patients with familial amyloidosis (see SARAIVA 1995 for review). Complete deficiency of TTR has never been described in man, suggesting that a deficiency of this protein might be lethal. However, a line of transthyretin-null mice produced by gene knock-out show no obvious abnormality of thyroid hormone metabolism or action (PALHA et al. 1994).

It is notable that increased binding of T_4 to the [Thr^{109}]TTR variant (MOSES et al. 1990) can give rise to mild hyperthyroxinaemia, with a raised total concentration of T_4 of 160–200 nM (MOSES et al. 1982; LALLOZ et al. 1984). Kinetic studies with this variant protein show a T_4-binding affinity about sevenfold higher than the normal TTR (LALLOZ et al. 1984). In the face of normal TBG and albumin concentrations, this variant TTR probably binds about 50% of circulating T_4 in euthyroid subjects. The [Met^{119}] variant of TTR has been shown to have about double normal affinity for T_4, but total T_4 is usually not outside the reference range (CURTIS et al. 1994).

Of at least 30 mutations described for TTR, many have now been examined for T_4 affinity. In a study comparing the interaction of T_4 with ten different naturally occurring human TTR variants, a wide spectrum of T_4 affinities was observed (ROSEN et al. 1993). Relative to the wild-type TTR, three show increased affinity for T_4, one [Thr^{109}] of sufficient affinity to cause euthyroid hyperthyroxinaemia, while three have approximately normal affinity, and five TTR variants show reduced affinity for T_4 (BARTALENA 1994).

III. Albumin

1. Normal Structure

As well as being the principal carrier of numerous hydrophobic compounds in serum, albumin also binds T_4 in its region 2, which is shared with ligands such as D- and L-tryptophan, octanoate, chlorazepate, *p*-iodobenzoate, and chloride ion (KRAGH-HANSEN 1981). A non-glycoprotein, with a carbohydrate content of less than 0.05% in normal plasma (PETERS 1985), albumin normally carries 10%–20% of circulating T_4 (Table 2), and has one moderate affinity binding site in region 2 and numerous sites of lower affinity that are probably of little physiological relevance.

Human serum albumin, a highly conserved 66-kDa protein (PETERS 1985), has a molar concentration of approximately 600 μM, corresponding to about 40 g/l. The proportion of albumin occupied by T_4 is less than 0.002%. Such low occupancy dictates that other ligands that bind to this region will have a negligible direct influence on T_4 binding. The importance of albumin as a determinant of T_4 binding, in vivo and in vitro, relates not to direct hormone carriage, but to its role in determining the free concentration of other ligands that compete for T_4 binding to TBG (see below).

2. Inherited Variants

Hyperthyroxinaemia can result from a variant albumin with increased affinity for T_4, the total albumin concentration being unchanged. In this disorder, now termed familial dysalbuminaemic hyperthyroxinaemia (FDH), the total T_4 concentration in affected individuals is about 200 nM (HENNEMANN et al. 1979; STOCKIGT et al. 1981a). Scatchard analysis of albumin binding showed two T_4-binding sites on the variant molecule, a normal site with K_d 4.3 μM and an abnormal site with 50- to 100-fold higher affinity, K_d 52 nM (DOCTER et al. 1981; BARLOW et al. 1982). The capacity of the higher affinity T_4-binding site was approximately 200 μM, suggesting that relative to the molar concentration of albumin, at least one-third of the albumin molecule appears to contain the extra binding site. Based on its affinity and capacity, the additional site binds about 50% (i.e. 100 nM) of the total circulating T_4 (200 nM), thus accounting for the observed hyperthyroxinaemia (BARLOW et al. 1982). Some studies suggest that this component is also present in trace quantities in normal serum (DOCTER et al. 1984). This variant is due to an Arg-His substitution at position 218 of the human albumin molecule (PETERSEN et al. 1994). A recent study reported that the recombinant mutant protein has a T_4 affinity 65-fold greater than normal (PETERSEN et al. 1995), similar to the affinity reported for the natural protein more than a decade before (BARLOW et al. 1982).

In FDH, because of a markedly increased affinity of the variant protein for numerous T_4-analogue tracers as well as T_4 itself, serum total T_4 and free T_4 index values and free T_4 measured by analogue-based methods give results suggestive of hyperthyroidism. In contrast, serum total T_3, free T_3 and TSH values, and free T_4 measured by valid methods are normal (STOCKIGT et al. 1983). As in other binding variations that show enhanced affinity or capacity, the increased concentration of total circulating T_4 appears to be an appropriate response in the face of increased T_4 binding so as to maintain a normal free T_4 concentration.

Only a few cases of total hereditary analbuminaemia have been described in man, but in a report of one kindred (KALLEE 1996) there was evidence of mild TSH excess, consistent with impaired thyroid hormone delivery. In contrast, the Nagase strain of analbuminaemic rat showed no evidence of any abnormality of thyroid hormone action or distribution (MENDEL et al. 1989b).

IV. Thyroxine Binding in Other Vertebrates

Plasma binding of thyroid hormones shows widespread variation between species. Comparative studies have been hampered by the conventional classification of binding proteins mainly on the basis of their electrophoretic mobility, rather than functional binding properties. As noted by LARSSON et al. 1985), a protein with the binding characteristics of TTR may not migrate in a pre-albumin position. In many non-human species, concentrations of binding proteins, particularly TBG, have been shown to vary widely during development or reproductive cycle, in response to food intake and seasonal cycles (VRANKX et al. 1994; SAVU et al. 1987).

In contrast to humans and other eutherians such as horse, goat, and sheep, in which TBG is the dominant binding protein, many vertebrate species show highly variable binding. On the basis of extensive studies of the functional rather than electrophoretic properties of T_4-binding proteins in 15 vertebrate species, LARSSON et al. (1985) suggested that TTR might be present in the serum of all vertebrates, but that inference is now in doubt. In other studies, binding of T_4 by both TTR and albumin was observed in avian species (chicken duck, goose, and ostrich), and the diprotodont marsupials (kangaroo, wallaby, possum, wombat, and koala), but TTR could not be identified in the blood of fish, toads, reptiles, monotremes, or Australian polyprotodont marsupials (RICHARDSON et al. 1994). The free concentration of thyroid hormone showed much less variation between species than the total concentration (REFETOFF et al. 1970), in general agreement with the free hormone hypothesis of thyroid hormone delivery.

V. Role of Binding Proteins

The probable physiological importance of binding proteins has been inferred autoradiographically by MENDEL et al. (1987a). When rat hepatic lobules were perfused with $[^{125}I]T_4$ in the absence of protein, virtually all of the T_4 was taken up by the periportal cells. With either 4% human serum albumin alone, or human serum, the labelled hormone was taken up uniformly by all cells within the lobule. When oleic acid was added to albumin at concentrations that displaced T_4, the redistributive effect of albumin was eliminated, although oleic acid did not have this effect with whole serum, where T_4 would be carried predominantly on TBG and TTR. This finding suggests that circulating binding proteins facilitate uniform distribution of T_4 within tissues.

It is notable that the normal free concentration of T_4 is close to its K_d for TBG; at half occupancy of the protein this relationship favours effective "buffering" of the free T_4 concentration as total T_4 changes. However, since the free concentration of T_3 is several orders of magnitude lower than its K_d for TBG, this stabilising effect will be less effective for T_3. With marked increases in total T_4, the corresponding increase in free T_4 becomes amplified as the occupancy of TBG approaches or exceeds its capacity (ROBBINS and JOHNSON 1982).

Additional possible functions of thyroid hormone-binding proteins include protection from iodine depletion due to urinary loss of hormone and provision of a large extrathyroidal pool of preformed hormone. It has not been established that thyroid hormone-binding proteins have a role in targeted hormone delivery via receptors specific for these proteins, as has been suggested for CBG (ROSNER 1990) and TTR (DIVINO and SCHUSSLER 1990). Notably, MENDEL and WEISIGER (1990) found no evidence that T_4-binding proteins, either human or rat, facilitated the uptake of T_4 perfused by rat liver.

Paradoxically, the highest levels of TBG in rats are associated with the lowest total serum of levels of thyroid hormone through the life cycle (SAVU et al. 1991), for example in response to nutritional deprivation, or in hypothyroidism (VRANCKX et al. 1994), thus further tending to lower the free hormone concentration at these times.

C. Binding Kinetics

I. Binding Kinetics, Capacity and Affinity

Thyroid hormone-binding sites merit detailed investigation, either as isolated proteins or in mixed biological fluids, for a number of reasons. First, alternations in serum binding may cause diagnostically confusing changes in total circulating or apparent free hormone levels. Second, hormone delivery to tissues may be altered by changes in binding proteins. Third, it may be possible, using serum-binding sites as a model, to develop competitors that interact with specific tissue-binding sites as hormone agonists or antagonists.

The analysis that follows will show how knowledge of the relationships between binding affinity, binding capacity, sample dilution, and hormone addition in vitro can be used to: (1) characterise a specific high-affinity binding protein in a heterogeneous system or mixed biological fluid, (2) establish a highly sensitive assay for the minute amounts of TBG secreted by cultured hepatocytes, and (3) develop simple diagnostic tests for hereditary high-capacity binding abnormalities.

First, it is relevant to question and refute the widely held assumption that sample dilution has little influence on the distribution, or *proportional* carriage, of a ligand among multiple sites that differ widely in affinity and capacity.

The interaction of a ligand with a single binding site is an equilibrium reaction that obeys the law of mass action. Concentrations of bound and free hormone are directly related:

$$B = K_a \cdot F(R_0 - B) \tag{1}$$

Where B is the concentration of bound hormone, K_a is a temperature-dependent constant, F is the concentration of free hormone, $R_0 - B$ is the concentration of unoccupied binding sites, and R_0 is the total number of sites. By definition, a binding protein is 50% occupied when F is the inverse of K_a. If the total number of binding sites is fixed, the degree of occupancy at any given F is dependent on the affinity, K_a. It is notable that no part of the above equation contains the total hormone concentration (although in practice many binding reactions are expressed as a function of the total hormone concentration, particularly for radioimmunoassays and studies of serum binding).

In any equilibrium binding reaction, there will be a sigmoidal relationship between the fraction of bound hormone (B/T) and the concentration of binding sites at any given fixed concentration of free ligand (Fig. 1). For optimal characterisation of any binding site, its concentration should be chosen to allow the greatest fluctuation in B/T with changes in free hormone. For a value of about 50% B/T, the concentration of binding sites that allows optimal quantitation can be estimated by rearranging the mass action equation:

$$K_a(R_0 - B) = B/F \tag{2}$$

$$R_0 = B/F \cdot K_d + B \tag{3}$$

$$\text{At } 50\%\ B/T,\ B = F = K_d \text{ and } R_0 = 2K_d \tag{4}$$

That is, changes in B/T are analytically optimal when the concentration of a binding site is approximately double the K_d. In this way a solution containing multiple binding sites of sufficiently different affinities can be adjusted by

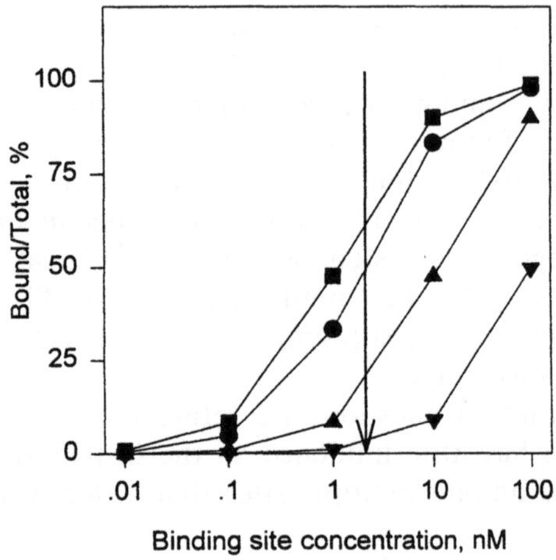

Fig. 1. Calculated changes in hormone binding (*B/T*) wth variable concentrations of a binding site of K_d 1 *nM* at constant free hormone concentrations of 0.1 *nM* (■), 1 *nM* (●), 10 *nM* (▲), and 100 *nM* (▼). Measured changes in binding are greatest when the concentration of binding sites is approximately twice the free hormone concentration *as designated by the arrow*. At higher or lower binding site concentrations, responses in *B/T* become progressively obscured

dilution to give the desired 50% *B/T* for each site. At the relevant dilution for one site, others may be virtually unoccupied or almost saturated, depending on their relative affinities, and will have little influence on *B/T* with changes in *F*. Thus, high-affinity binding can be "dissected" from low-affinity sites at high dilution; conversely, low-affinity binding is best examined with little dilution, if necessary by increasing the free hormone concentration with labelled or unlabelled preparations.

From the affinity and capacity of each major T_4-binding protein, as summarised in Table 2, occupancy and proportional ligand carriage can be adjusted by dilution and/or hormone addition so that other binding proteins with higher or lower affinities make little contribution to total binding. For example, at a serum dilution of 1:4000, chosen so that approximately half the total T_4 (~10 p*M* with total concentration ~20 p*M*) is bound to TBG, only a small proportion is bound to each of the lower affinity proteins.

Conversely, if the endogenous hormone is raised markedly and binding is studied at 1:100 dilution, both TBG and TTR are virtually saturated and contribute less than 1% to measured *B/T*. Under these conditions, fluctuations in *B/T* reflect predominantly changes in T_4 binding to albumin (Fig. 2).

The above calculations assume that the separation of bound and free hormone at equilibrium is instantaneous and perfect, but this is unlikely for any physical separation, especially for low-affinity binding where rapidly dissociating ligand is adsorbed by a non-specific matrix (Munro et al. 1989).

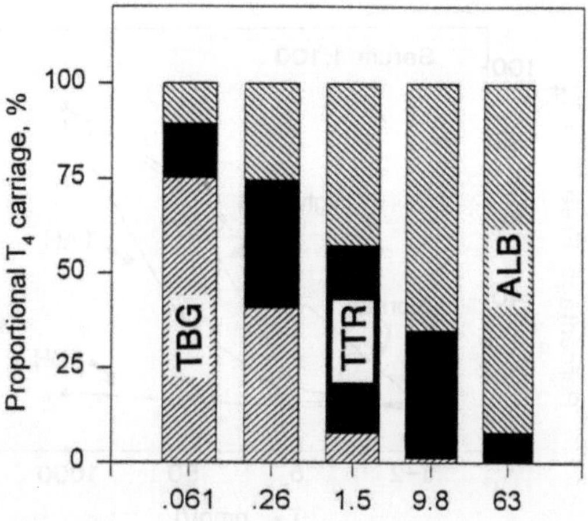

Fig. 2. Calculated effect of hormone addition on proportional occupancy of serum binding proteins in vivo. In normal human serum with total T_4 97 n*M* and free T_4 20 p*M*, the hormone is bound in the proportions TBG (69%), TTR (18%), and albumin (13%). Addition of hormone to raise the free level by tenfold increments progressively accentuates proportional hormone carriage on lower affinity sites

Hence, such abbreviated separation systems give a qualitative rather than quantitative estimate of low-affinity binding. In studies of high-affinity binding sites, the contribution of low-affinity binding sites can be further diminished or eliminated by inclusion of a competitor which saturates a particular binding site. For example, when TBG binding is measured in diluted serum, the contribution of TTR can be reduced to a negligible fraction by the use of barbitone, which inhibits T_4 binding to TTR (INGBAR 1963).

II. Characterisation of High-Capacity, Low-Affinity Binding

The abnormal high-capacity T_4-binding site of FDH can be identified simply and specifically by examining T_4 binding at 4°C in serum diluted 1:100 in the presence of 1000-fold excess of unlabelled T_4, using dextran-charcoal separation (STOCKIGT et al. 1986). At an intermediate 50-fold excess of unlabelled T_4, the binding abnormality due to the [Thr^{109}]TTR variant can be distinguished from TBG excess and FDH (Fig. 3). Low temperature and immediate centrifugation after charcoal addition are important because of the rapid off-rate of lower affinity T_4-binding sites. A similar approach was used by REFETOFF et al. (1986) to compare the T_4 affinity of normal and variant TTR in diluted whole serum. By conventional Scatchard analysis, they were able to make comparisons of TTR affinity by considering only points with a bound/free ratio <1, which occurred with total T_4 > 150 n*M* at serum dilution 1:40, representing about a 50-fold excess over endogenous T_4.

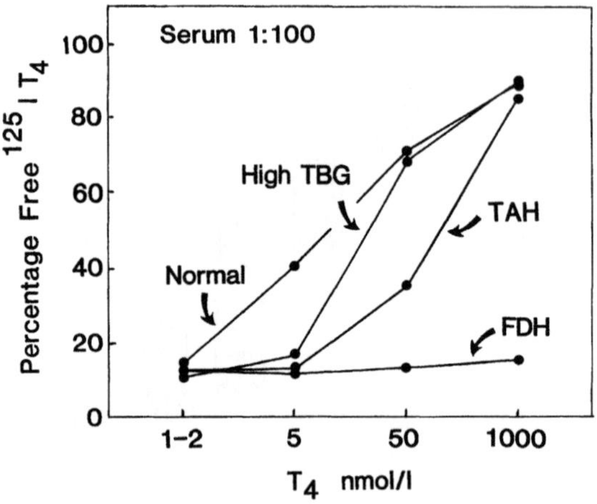

Fig. 3. Effect of progressive increase in the concentration of unlabelled T_4 on dextran-charcoal uptake of $[^{125}I]T_4$ in sera from normal subjects and those with TBG excess, transthyretin-associated hyperthyroxinaemia (*TAH*), and familial dysalbuminaemic hyperthyroxinaemia (*FDH*). The serum samples were diluted 1:100 in phosphate buffer, 0.04 mmol/l, pH 7.4, giving an endogenous T_4 concentration of 1–2 *nM*. When total T_4 is 1000-fold in excess, FDH serum shows a unique persistence in T_4 binding, consistent with an increased T_4 affinity for albumin. TAH was identified at an intermediate hormone load. Inhibition of binding is shown by an increase in the percentage of free $[^{125}I]T_4$

III. Specific Characterisation of TBG Binding

For studies of drug competition for T_4 binding to TBG, it was relevant to use a TBG-specific assay with the unmodified serum protein without the potential artefacts introduced by isolation and purification. Such a system required high serum dilution and very low ligand concentration. The TBG specificity of T_4 binding in serum diluted 1:10000 with a concentration of $[^{125}I]T_4$ of about $10^{-11} M$, with immediate dextran-charcoal separation at 4°C, was shown by: (1) lack of detectable T_4 binding in sera with total deficiency of TBG, (2) negligible binding after addition of $10^{-9} M$ unlabelled T_4 (300-fold excess at this dilution), and (3) Scatchard analysis of T_4 binding in normal sera, showing a single site with K_d $1.6 \times 10^{-11} M/l$ and capacity of about $3 \times 10^{-7} M/l$ (MOHR et al. 1987; MUNRO et al. 1989). Further, it could be shown that equivalent concentrations of TTR or albumin gave negligible binding in this system (Fig. 4).

IV. Assay of TBG

Using the principle described above, CROWE et al. (1995) were able to develop a TBG assay that could detect $<10^{-11} M$ protein, about 100-fold more sensitive than standard serum radioimmunoassays. The method gave precise measurement of the minute amounts of TBG secreted by cultured cells, and could

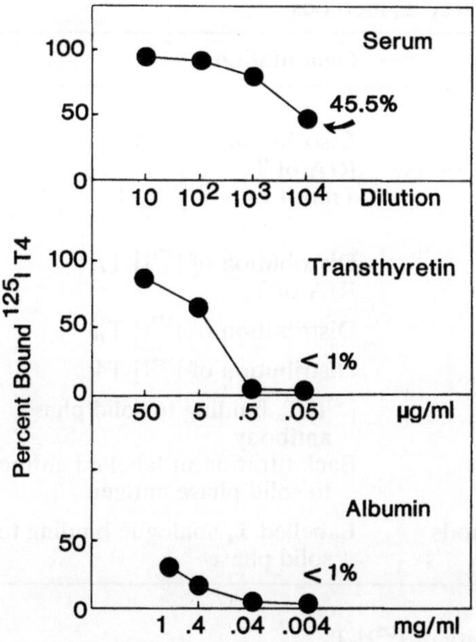

Fig. 4. Estimates of binding of $[^{125}I]T_4$ ($<10^{-11}$ *M*) using dextran-charcoal separation (4°C) at various dilutions of serum (*top*), and at equivalent concentrations of purified transthyretin (*middle*) or albumin (*lower*). At 1 : 10000 dilution of normal serum, 40%–50% of tracer T_4 is bound; transthyretin, 0.05 µg/ml, and albumin, 0.004 mg/ml, make a negligible contribution to binding

quantitate the downregulation of TBG secretion by physiological concentrations of T_3.

D. Free Hormone Measurement

There have been many approaches to the diagnostic measurement of the free, or active hormone concentration in serum, with much debate about the theoretical basis, practical utility, and validity of these methods (EKINS 1990). Although most free T_4 methods are a diagnostic improvement on total hormone values, which are influenced by the concentration of binding protein was well as by thyroid status, all are flawed in some respect. No current method directly measures the free hormone concentration in undisturbed, undiluted serum under physiological conditions. A classification of these methods is shown in Table 5. In view of the indirect nature of routine free T_4 methods, it is crucial that definitive measurements of total T_4 (and T_3) and of hormone-binding parameters be retained as reference methods that can be used to evaluate any free T_4 estimates that appear to be anomalous.

A distinction can be made between techniques that estimate the free hormone concentration in a fraction of serum, isolated by a procedure such as

Table 5. Summary of free T_4 methods

Method	Quantitation	Limitations
Dialysis		
Indirect	Distribution of $[^{125}I]$-T_4	1,2
Direct	RIA of T_4	2,3
Symmetric	Transit rate of $[^{125}I]$-T_4	1
Ultrafiltration		
Indirect	Distribution of $[^{125}I]$-T_4	1
Direct	RIA of T_4	3
Gelfitration	Distribution of $[^{125}I]$-T_4,	1,4
Adsorption	Distribution of $[^{125}I]$-T4,	1,4
Free hormone immunoassays	$[^{125}I]$-T_4 binding to solid phase antibody	3
	Back titration of labelled antibody to solid phase antigen	3,5
Analogue tracer methods	Labelled T_4 analogue binding to solid phase	6

Limitations:
1. Radiochemical purity of $[^{125}I]$-T_4.
2. Dilution of competitor into dialysate.
3. Sensitivity limited by antibody affinity.
4. Valid over limited range of dilutions only.
5. Shallow dose-response.
6. Variations in protein binding of labelled analogue tracer.

dialysis or ultrafiltration – the so-called direct methods – and the indirect methods that use the distribution of labelled hormone between bound and unbound phases to measure a free fraction, which is then used to calculate the free concentration from the total hormone value. Among the direct methods, those that isolate a fraction of the free T_4 pool (or some component directly related to it) from the binding proteins before the T_4 assay is performed tend to give valid T_4 estimates, while many one-step methods that attempt to measure free hormone in the presence of binding proteins are invalid if sample and standard differ in their binding of assay tracer (EKINS 1990). Although equilibrium dialysis is widely quoted as the "gold standard" for free T_4 measurement, this method is also subject to methodological errors, as summarised below.

To evaluate a free T_4 method critically, an assessment of serial dilutions of normal serum should be made. Many abbreviated methods show a rapid fall in apparent free T_4 concentration, suggesting that a component larger than true free T_4 is being measured (see below). Each method should also be tested in the full range of known binding protein abnormalities, in the presence of competitors of hormone binding, and in critically ill subjects who frequently show method-dependent anomalies of apparent free T_4 concentration. In general, two-step free T_4 methods that isolate a fraction of the T_4 pool from binding proteins tend to give high values in critical illness (possibly due to an in vitro effect of heparin – see below), while the one-step or analogue tracer methods generally tend to give falsely low free T_4 estimates (KAPTEIN 1994).

I. Factors Influencing Validity

1. Radiochemical Purity

Radiochemical purity is crucial whenever labelled hormone is used as a marker. In some systems, for example, equilibrium dialysis or ultrafiltration of undiluted serum, as little as 0.1% free [^{125}I] as iodide can lead to a 5- to 10-fold overestimate of the free hormone fraction. Hence, the radioactivity in each sample needs to be fractionated after separation by a procedure such as magnesium precipitation (STERLING and BRENNER 1966) or chromatography (SURKS et al. 1988) to separate authentic labelled hormone from contaminants.

2. Protein-Tracer Interactions

In some systems, such as the unbound analogue free T_4 assays (EKINS 1990), the labelled compound equilibrates with pools of T_4 other than the free hormone. Such assays depend on the assumption that a labelled T_4 analogue that binds to a T_4 antibody, but does not interact with serum T_4-binding proteins, will show antibody binding inversely proportional to free T_4. It is now clear that these labelled T_4 analogues do in fact interact with serum proteins, particularly albumin (EKINS 1990). If this interaction is identical in sample and standard, a useful free T_4 estimate can still be made. However, if the labelled analogue is protein bound to a greater extent in the sample than in the standard serum, less tracer is available to compete for the assay antibody, giving a falsely high free T_4 estimate, as in FDH (STOCKIGT et al. 1981b) and in the presence of iodothyronine-binding immunoglobulins (BECK PECCOZ et al. 1984). Conversely, if binding of labelled analogue is less in the sample than in the standard serum (e.g. lower sample albumin concentration, or occupancy of albumin by some other ligand, such as oleic acid), the results are falsely low (STOCKIGT et al. 1983).

3. Dilution Effects

Mass action dictates that dissociation of a bound ligand occurs with progressive sample dilution, so that its free concentration shows little decrease until the reservoir of bound ligand starts to become depleted. After dilution beyond the point where about 30% of bound ligand has dissociated, the free hormone concentration falls steeply; in human serum, this begins to occur at serum dilutions of greater than 1:100 for T_4. If, as is the case with many commercial assays, the free T_4 estimate decreases with dilution to a greater extent than is compatible with the mass action law, the method is in fact measuring a component larger than the true free fraction (i.e. the tracer is mixing with, interacting with, or "sampling from", a component other than free T_4). The correlation with true free T_4 may remain close if sample and standards show identical artefacts.

4. Other Factors

Few free T_4 assays properly reflect the effect of binding competitors (see below). The effect of competitors is generally underestimated, the error being greatest in the assays with the highest sample dilution.

Assay sensitivity may be the limiting factor in direct radioimmunoassays of free hormone that have been separated from undiluted serum by dialysis or ultrafiltration. Such assays require a specific antibody of extremely high affinity to achieve acceptable precision (Nelson and Tomei 1988).

While hormone binding in vivo relates to 37°C, many assays are equilibrated at room temperature. Results may then be biased in samples with anomalous TBG concentrations because of temperature-dependent differences in hormone dissociation between samples and the matrix used for assay standards (van der Sluis Veer 1992).

II. Non-isotopic Free T_4 Methods

Techniques that use non-radioactive detection systems do not overcome the problems inherent in isotopic free T_4 measurement. A detailed comparison of chemiluminometric and fluorometric free T_4 assays with radioimmunoassays in a large group of normal subjects and hyperthyroid, hypothyroid, pregnant, renal failure, intensive care, and heparin-treated patients showed that various non-isotopic and isotopic procedures had similar strengths and limitations (Perdrisot 1989). Problems of non-specific fluorescence have been identified in renal failure (Law et al. 1988).

III. Thyroid Hormone-Binding Ratio

A special example of a two-step method is the classical serum free T_4 index (Clark and Horn 1965), computed from the serum T_4 value and the thyroid hormone-binding ratio (THBR) (Larsen et al. 1987). The latter estimates the number of unoccupied serum-binding sites, based on distribution of tracer between diluted serum and a solid phase, such as resin, talc, or charcoal. This THBR value, relative to normal serum, is multiplied by the serum total T_4 (or T_3) concentration to yield the free T_4 (or free T_3) index. Proper use of the THBR requires that the calculation be made as matrix/serum, rather than as matrix/total counts, to improve the correction for very high and very low TBG concentrations (Larsen et al. 1987). This method is a useful correction for variations in TBG, but fails to correct for abnormalities of iodothyronine binding to transthyretin, albumin, or autoantibodies.

E. Interactions with Competitors

In contrast to binding proteins for corticosteroids, vitamin D, or sex hormones, which are highly specific for a single family of ligands, the iodothyronine-binding proteins show extensive cross-reactivity with unrelated hydrophobic ligands, such as non-esterified fatty acids (NEFA) and various drugs (Table 6). These effects can lead to diagnostically confusing test results and could also influence hormone delivery to tissues. Because each of these agents is itself highly bound to albumin, it is difficult to distinguish relevant from physiologically irrelevant competition in experimental systems where the albumin concentration is low, or where the sample has been diluted.

Hormone binding is often studied by examining displacement of labelled hormone from an isolated binding protein, using the unlabelled hormone as reference. Relative to T_4, the affinities of important drug competitors for TBG range from three orders of magnitude less (frusemide) to almost seven orders of magnitude less than T_4 itself, as in the case of aspirin (MUNRO et al. 1989). However, such direct studies do not reflect what happens in vivo, because they ignore the fact that competitor potency is a function of the free, rather than total, concentration of competitor; the free concentration of most competitors is determined by their binding to sites other than TBG, in particular to high-capacity sites such as albumin. Ultimately, the occupancy of albumin can influence the free competitor concentration.

Hence, binding needs to be studied in serum, as well as with isolated proteins. When working with a highly bound substance, such as T_4, it is technically much easier to study binding in diluted serum, and it is difficult to establish a diluted system in which the concentrations of free hormone, competitor(s), and unoccupied binding sites are maintained in the relationship that applies in vivo. Existing literature on competitor effects has become

Table 6. Drugs that can displace thyroid hormones from binding in normal human serum in vivo

Salicylates
Acetyl salicylic acid (aspirin)
Salicyl salicylic acid (salsalate)
Furosemide
Fenclofenac
Mefenamic acid
Naproxen
Diclofenac
Diflunisal
Phenytoin
Carbamazepine

Compiled from LARSEN (1972), STOCKIGT et al. (1985), LIM et al. (1988), MUNRO et al. (1989), BISHNOI et al. (1994), SURKS and DEFESI (1996).

confused because precise methodological details, particularly those related to dilution and albumin concentration, are often poorly defined. The terms "predilution" and "codilution" are useful in defining potential experimental artefacts.

I. Pre-dilution and Co-dilution

Pre-dilution occurs when the concentration of binding proteins is progressively decreased before particular concentrations of competitor are added (Fig. 5). The lower the concentration of albumin, the higher the occupancy of available binding sites for a given added concentration of competitor. If albumin is low, the free competitor concentration may increase disproportionately, thereby magnifying apparent competitor potency (Mendel et al. 1986). For example, in the case of a highly albumin bound competitor, the effect on T_4 binding of 5 *mM* oleic acid added to undiluted serum can be matched almost exactly by 0.5 *mM* oleic acid in serum diluted 1:10 (Lim et al. 1988).

Failure to consider such pre-dilution effects appears to have led to overestimates of the potency of long-chain NEFA, not only in T_4-binding interactions (Chopra et al. 1985), but in numerous other studies where direct biological activity has been attributed to them (e.g. Hwang et al. 1986; Ng and Hockaday 1986; Vallette et al. 1991). Where "physiological" concentrations of NEFA have been added to any albumin-free medium, their unbound concentrations are often unrealistically high by several orders of magnitude, leading to gross overassessment of inhibitor potency.

Co-dilution occurs when a competitor present in whole serum is serially diluted so that *total* concentrations of binding proteins, hormone, and competi-

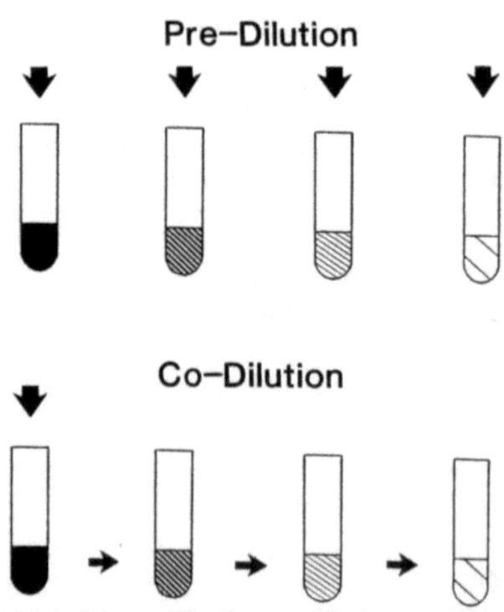

Fig. 5. *Pre-dilution*: the binding proteins are diluted, followed by addition of a particular concentration of competitor. *Co-dilution*: competitor is added to serum, followed by identical simultaneous dilution of binding proteins, total hormone, and total competitor concentrations

tors diminish in parallel. Notably, the free concentrations do not maintain this parallelism. Co-dilution effects lead to underestimation of the potency of competitors that are less highly protein bound than the hormone itself. The difference becomes clear if a hormone such as T_4 with a free fraction of about 1:4000 is compared with a drug that has a free fraction in serum of 1:50. Progressive dissociation will sustain the free T_4 concentration at 1:100 dilution while the free drug concentration decreases markedly after a dilution of only 1:10. As pointed out by EKINS (1990), a reverse effect, overestimation of potency with co-dilution, could occur with a competitor such as oleic acid that is more highly bound than T_4 itself. A co-dilution effect was the initial clue that led to the recognition of frusemide as an important inhibitor of T_4 binding in serum (STOCKIGT et al. 1984, 1985). When T_4 binding was studied in serial dilution in normal subjects and critically ill hypothyroxinaemic patients, some of them showed a marked increase in free T_4 fraction which became less obvious with progressive dilution; a threefold increase in T_4 free fraction was seen at 1:5 serum dilution, with almost no increase at 1:50 or 1:100. The effect of measured serum frusemide on T_4 binding was reproduced by addition of drug in vitro, evidence against the effect being due to a drug metabolite. Studies in serial dilution can be used to seek putative inhibitors; but such studies require highly sensitive methodology and meticulous attention to tracer purity (SURKS et al. 1988; WILCOX et al. 1994). SURKS and DEFESI (1996) have recently demonstrated that co-dilution effects have led to persistent underestimation of the importance of phenytoin and carbamazepine as inhibitors of T_4 binding.

II. Estimation of In Vivo Competitor Potency

Of the four factors that influence competition in vivo: kinetics of the competitor, total circulating concentration, free fraction, and affinity for the hormone-binding sites, only the latter can be determined by studying the binding protein in isolation. The precise free fractions of most highly albumin-bound drugs in serum at 37°C remain ill defined. Labelled drug preparations can be used to determine free fraction, but few are available.

A dialysis system can be devised to measure the drug free fraction without a labelled preparation, or a specific drug assay using a dialysis system (LIM et al. 1986). Unlabelled drug is added to a large dialysate volume; its serum binding is proportional to the measured decrease in this concentration after dialysis to equilibrium, as measured by spectrophotometry. Once the free fraction is known, drugs can be added to achieve the relevant free and total therapeutic concentrations at equilibrium in undiluted serum (LIM et al. 1988), allowing displacement of $[^{125}I]T_4$ from the serum compartment to be measured at equilibrium at predetermined total and free concentrations of competitor. For a drug with a millimolar total concentration such as aspirin, the free fraction will increase as its total concentration approaches that of albumin (TOZER 1984).

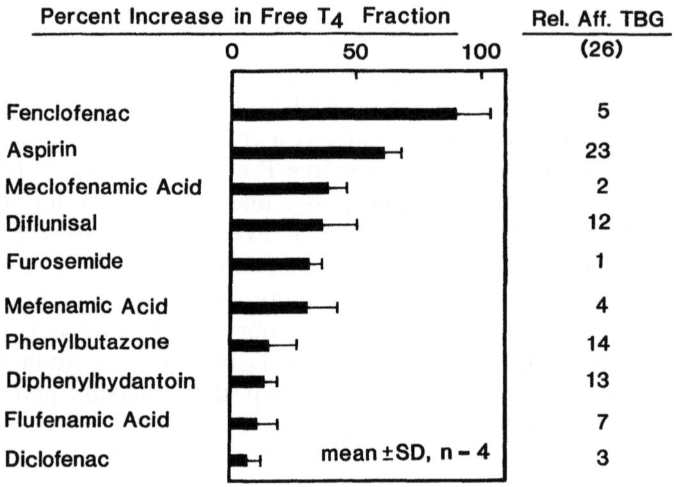

Fig. 6. Relationship between the potency of drugs in increasing the free T_4 fraction in whole serum at 37°C at their relevant therapeutic concentrations (LIM et al. 1988) and their rank order (from 1 to 26) as inhibitors of T_4 binding to TBG alone at 4°C (MUNRO et al. 1989). Frusemide (furosemide), the most potent drug on a molar basis in isolation, was only fifth most potent at its relevant serum concentration. Aspirin, ranked 23rd on a molar basis, ranked second in whole serum because of its high therapeutic concentration and relatively high unbound fraction

The main drugs that can displace thyroid hormones in human serum are shown in Table 6. Figure 6 shows the hierarchy of drug inhibitor potency for T_4 binding at relevant therapeutic concentrations in undiluted serum. Of the drugs evaluated by LIM et al. (1988), fenclofenac was the most potent in serum, followed by aspirin, meclofenamic acid, diflunisal, and frusemide. These estimates differed markedly from the hierarchy of drug affinities for TBG or TTR in isolation (MUNRO et al. 1989). Although few drugs have been tested directly for T_3 displacement, it is presumed that proportional changes in free T_3 and free T_4 are comparable.

SURKS and DEFESI (1996) recently demonstrated that therapeutic concentrations of phenytoin and carbamazepine increased the free fraction of T_4 by 40%–50% using ultrafiltration of undiluted serum. During continuing drug therapy, total T_4 was lowered by 25%–50%, resulting in calculated free concentrations within the normal range. In contrast, a commercial single-step free T_4 assay after 1:5 serum dilution gave subnormal free T_4 levels, attributable to a co-dilution effect, as described above.

III. In Vivo Kinetics of Competitors

The kinetics of the competitor itself will influence the way it affects hormone binding in vivo, as reflected by comparison of a short half-life competitor, such as frusemide ($t_{1/2}$ ~2 h) with fenclofenac ($t_{1/2}$ ~20–40 h). As a competitor of long half-life approaches its steady state concentration, the free hormone concentration will tend to rise. Increased clearance and feedback inhibition of TSH secretion then tend to decrease the total hormone concentration to a new steady state with little change in free concentration for the period of drug administration (KURTZ et al. 1981). In contrast, a competitor of short half-life such as frusemide will show fluctuating effects on hormone binding. The total T_4 concentration may show only transient changes in response to frusemide, except in situations where the feedback relationships is disrupted, as for example when this drug is used in combination with dopamine (STOCKIGT et al. 1984), which inhibits the TSH response to hypothyroxinaemia (VAN DEN BERGHE et al. 1994).

When thyroid status is assessed in patients receiving repeated high oral doses of frusemide, the time interval between drug dosage and blood sampling needs to be taken into account. Thyroid hormone levels measured at various times in patients treated with frusemide 80, 120, and 250 mg twice daily showed time-dependent changes in total T_4, binding index, and free thyroxine index; changes were maximal 3–4 h after each dose (NEWNHAM et al. 1987), with a tendency for total T_4 to fall, associated with inhibition of binding and a rise in the free thyroxine index. Although it is not yet known whether intermittent competitor-induced increases in free hormone concentration can augment hormone action in man, it has been shown that a T_3 and T_4-displacing synthetic flavonoid has a transient thyromimetic effect in rats (LUEPRASITSAKUL et al. 1990).

IV. Interaction Between Competitors

From the outline given above, it follows that increasing concentrations of any substance that shares albumin sites with a competitor could increase the free concentration of that competitor. Two substances with the potential to exert such a "cascade effect" on T_4 binding in serum are oleic acid (LIM et al. 1991) and 3-carboxy-4-methyl-5-propyl-2-furanpropanoic acid (CMPF) (LIM et al. 1993), a naturally occurring furanoid acid that accumulates in renal failure (MABUCHI and NAKAHASHI 1987). At concentrations that had only a minimal direct effect on the binding of T_4 in undiluted normal serum, CMPF (Fig. 7) and oleic acid augmented the T_4-displacing effect of numerous drug competitors for T_4 binding to TBG (LIM et al. 1991, 1993).

V. Spurious Competition

The effect of heparin to increase the apparent free T_4 concentration in vitro is potentially misleading because it does not reflect true changes in circulating free T_4 (MENDEL et al. 1987b). It appears that increases in free T_4 as a result of heparin treatment are due to in vitro generation of NEFA during assay incubation as a result of heparin-induced lipase activity (MENDEL et al. 1987b). The studies of ZAMBON et al. (1993) demonstrated that in vitro generation of nonesterified fatty acids also occurs during room temperature storage of samples from heparin-treated subjects. This phenomenon may account for the fre-

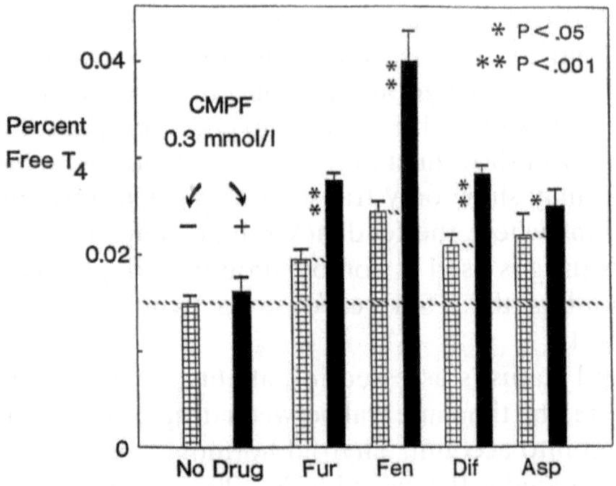

Fig. 7. Influence of 3-carboxy-4-methyl-5-propyl-2-furanpropanoic acid (*CMPF*) on the T_4-displacing effects of therapeutic concentrations of frusemide (*Fur*), fenclofenac (*Fen*), diflunisal (*Dif*) and aspirin (*Asp*) in undiluted serum at 37°C (equilibrium dialysis). Percentage free T_4 is shown in the presence (*solid columns*) and absence (*hatched columns*) of 0.3 m*M* CMPF. Each drug together with CMPF increased free T_4 more than the sum of drug alone and CMPF alone (**$P < 0.001$). (From LIM et al. 1993)

quent reports of apparent increases in free T_4 in critically ill subjects, when measurements are done by analytically correct two-step free T_4 methods (KAPTEIN 1994).

VI. Drug Competition at Other Sites

While studied less extensively than in serum, it is clear that many drugs can compete for tissue binding of thyroid hormones, as reviewed in Chap. 13, this volume, on potential thyroid hormone antagonists (see Table 7). Nuclear T_3 binding to the β_1 thyroid hormone receptor can be inhibited by desethylamiodarone (Chap. 10, this volume; BAKKER et al. 1994). Phenytoin (SMITH and SURKS 1984) and several non-steroidal anti-inflammatory agents (TOPLISS et al. 1988; BARLOW et al. 1994) also bind weakly to nuclear T_3 receptors, although the class of receptor has not been defined.

Cell uptake of T_3 by hepatic and pituitary cells in culture is subject to competition by a variety of drugs (TOPLISS et al. 1989; LIM et al. 1995), including calcium channel blockers (TOPLISS et al. 1993). CHALMERS et al. (1993) investigated the ability of 26 phenylanthranilic acid analogues related to mefenamic and flufenamic acids to inhibit T_3 uptake by cultured hepatocytes and found that inhibitory activity was highly dependent on hydrophobicity of the compounds, suggesting that competition may depend on physicochemical rather than specific structural properties. Cytoplasmic T_3 binding in mammalian liver can also be displaced by some anti-inflammatory agents and non-bile acid cholephils (BARLOW et al. 1994).

Table 7. Inhibitors of cellular T_3 or T_4 binding

A Plasma membrane
- Non-steroidal anti-inflammatory drugs (NSAID) (Topliss et al. 1989)
  - diclofenac, fenclofenac
  - flufenamic acid, meclofenamic acid
  - mefenamic acid
- Non-bile acid cholephils (Topliss et al. 1989)
  - bromosulfophthalein, indocyanine green
  - bilirubin
- Calmodulin antagonists (Topliss et al. 1993)
  - naphthalene sulfonamides (W7, W12, W13)
  - calmidazolium, trifluoperazine
- Calcium channel blockers (Topliss et al. 1993)
  - nifedipine, verapamil, diltiazem
- Anticonvulsants (Topliss et al. 1989)
  - diphenylhydantoin
- Sedatives
  - benzodiazepines (Kragie and Doyle 1992)
- Cholecystographic agents (Topliss et al. 1989)
  - iopanoic acid
- Others
  - phloretin (Topliss et al. 1989)
  - EMD21388 (synthetic flavanoid) (Lim et al. 1996)
  - phenylanthranilic acid analogues (Chalmers et al. 1993)

B Cytoplasm
- NSAIDs (Barlow et al. 1994)
  - acetylsalicylic acid, diclofenac, diflunisal
  - fenclofenac, fenoprofen, flufenamic acid
  - indomethacin, meclofenamic acid, mefenamic acid
- Non-bile acid cholephils (Barlow et al. 1994)
  - bromosulfophthalein
- Cholecystographic agents (Barlow et al. 1994)
  - iopanoic acid
- Others (Barlow et al. 1991)
  - SKF 94901

C Nuclear
- NSAIDs (Topliss et al. 1988)
  - diclofenac, fenclofenac
  - meclofenamic acid, mefenamic acid
- Diuretics (Topliss et al. 1988)
  - furosemide
- Anti-convulsants (Smith and Surks 1984; Topliss et al. 1988)
  - diphenylhydantoin
- Anti-arrhythmic agents
  - desethylamiodarone (Bakker et al. 1994)
- Others
  - SKF 94901 (Barlow et al. 1991)

Studies of competition for cellular binding sites are prone to the artefacts of pre-dilution described above (i.e. the relevant free concentrations of competitor at the specific binding site are not known), so that the physiological or pharmacological importance of these competitive effects remains uncertain.

References

Ain KB, Mori Y, Refetoff S (1987) Reduced clearance rate of thyroxine-binding globulin (TBG) with increased sialylation: a mechanism for estrogen-induced elevation of serum TBG concentration. J Clin Endocrinol Metab 65:689–696

Ain KB, Refetoff S (1988) Relationship of oligosaccharide modification to the cause of serum thyroxine-binding globulin excess. J Clin Endocrinol Metab 66:1037–1043

Andrea TA, Cavalieri RR, Golfine ID, Jorgensen EC (1980) Binding of thyroid hormones and analogues to the human plasma protein prealbumin. Biochemistry 19:55–63

Bakker O, van Beeren HC, Wiersinga WM (1994) Desethylamiodarone is a noncompetitive inhibitor of the binding of thyroid hormone to the thyroid hormone β_1-receptor protein. Endocrinology 134:1665–1670

Barlow JW, Csicsmann JM, White EL, Funder JW, Stockigt JR (1982) Familial euthyroid thyroxine excess: characterization of abnormal intermediate affinity thyroxine binding to albumin. J Clin Endocrinol Metab 55:244–250

Barlow JW, Raggatt LE, Lim C-F, Kolliniatis E, Topliss DJ, Stockigt JR (1991) The thyroid hormone analogue SKF-94901 and iodothyronine binding sites in mammalian tissues: differences in cytoplasmic binding between liver and heart. Acta Endocrinologica (Copenh) 124:37–44

Barlow JW, Curtis AJ, Raggatt LE, Loidl NM, Topliss DJ, Stockigt JR (1994) Drug competition for intracellular triiodothyronine-binding sites. Eur J Endocrinol 130:417–421

Bartalena L, Tata JR, Robbins J (1984) Characterization of nascent and secreted thyroxine-binding globulin in cultured human hepatoma (Hep G2) cells. J Biol Chem 259:13605–13609

Bartalena L (1990) Recent achievements in studies of thyroid hormone binding proteins. Endocr Rev 11:47–64

Bartalena L (1994) Thyroid hormone-binding proteins: update 1994. In: Braverman LE, Refetoff S (eds) Clinical and molecular aspects of diseases of the thyroid. Endocrine review monographs, vol 3. The Endocrine Society, pp 140–142

Beck-Peccoz P, Romelli PB, Cattaneo MG, Faglia G, White EL, Barlow JW, Stockigt JR (1984) Evaluation of free T_4 methods in the presence of iodothyronine autoantibodies. J Clin Endocrinol Metab 58:736–739

Benvenga S, Trimarchi F, Robbins J (1987) Circulating thyroid hormone antibodies. J Endocrinol Invest 10:605–619

Benvenga S, Gregg RE, Robbins J (1988) Binding of thyroid hormones to human plasma lipoproteins. J Clin Endocrinol Metab 67:6–16

Benvenga S, Cahnmann HJ, Robbins J (1993) Characterization of thyroid hormone binding to apolipoprotein-E: localization of the binding site in the exon 3-coded domain. Endocrinology 133:1300–1305

Bishnoi A, Carlson HE, Gruber BL, Kaufman LD, Bock JL, Lidonnici K (1994) Effects of commonly prescribed nonsteroidal anti-inflammatory drugs on thyroid hormone measurements. Am J Med 96:235–238

Chalmers DK, Scholz GH, Topliss DJ, Kolliniatis E, Munro SLA, Craik DJ, Iskander MN, Stockigt JR (1993) Thyroid hormone uptake by hepatocytes: structure-activity relationships of phenylanthranilic acids with inhibitory activity. J Med Chem 36:1272–1277

Chopra IJ, Chua Teco GN, Mead JF, Huang T-S, Beredo A, Solomon DH (1985) Relationship between serum free fatty acids and thyroid hormone binding inhibitor in nonthyroid illnesses. J Clin Endocrinol Metab 60:980–984

Clark F, Horn DB (1965) Assessment of thyroid function by the combined use of the serum protein-bound iodine and resin uptake of ^{131}I-triiodothyronine. J Clin Endocr 25:39–45

Crowe TC, Cowen NL, Loidl NM, Topliss DJ, Stockigt JR, Barlow JW (1995) Down-regulation of thyroxine-binding globulin messenger ribonucleic acid by 3,5,3′-

triiodothyronine in human hepatoblastoma cells. J Clin Endocrinol Metab 80:-2233–2237

Curtis AJ, Scrimshaw BJ, Topliss DJ, Stockigt JR, George PM, Barlow JW (1994) Thyroxine binding by human transthyretin variants: mutations at position 119, but not position 54, increase thyroxine binding affinity. J Clin Endocrinol Metab 78:459–462

Dickson PW, Howlett GJ, Schreiber G (1982) Metabolism of prealbumin in rats and changes induced by acute inflammation. Eur J Biochem 129:289–293

Divino CM, Schussler GC (1990) Receptor-mediated uptake and internalization of transthyretin. J Biol Chem 265:1425–1429

Docter R, Bos G, Krenning EP, Fekkes D, Visser TJ, Hennemann G (1981) Inherited thyroxine excess. A serum abnormality due to an increased affinity for modified albumin. Clin Endocrinol (Oxf) 15:363–371

Docter R, Bos G, Krenning EP, Hennemann G (1984) Specific thyroxine binding albumin is a constituent of normal human serum. Lancet 1:50

Ekins R (1990) Measurement of free hormones in blood. Endocr Rev 11:5–46

Emerson CH, Seiler CM, Alex S, Fang SL, Mori Y, DeVito WJ (1993) Gene expression and serum thyroxine-binding globulin are regulated by adrenal status and corticosterone in the rat. Endocrinology 133:1192–1196

Ferguson RN, Edelhoch H, Saroff HA, Robbins J (1975) Negative co-operativity in the binding of thyroxine to human serum prealbumin. Biochemistry 14:282–289

Flink IL, Bailey TJ, Gustafson TA, Markham BE, Morkin E (1986) Complete amino acid sequence of human thyroxine-binding globulin deduced from cloned DNA: close homology to the serine antiproteases. Proc Natl Acad Sci 83:7708–7712

Glinoer D, McGuire R, Dubois A, Cogan J, Robbins J, Berman M (1979) Thyroxine-binding globulin metabolism in rhesus monkeys: effects of hyper- and hypothyroidism. Endocrinology 104:175–183

Hammond GL, Smith CL, Goping IS, Underhill DA, Harley MJ, Reventos J, Musto NA, Gunsalus GL, Bardin CW (1987) Primary structure of human corticosteroid binding globulin, deduced from hepatic and pulmonary cDNAs, exhibits homology with serine protease inhibitors. Proc Natl Acad Sci USA 84:5153–5157

Heller J, Horowitz J (1974) The binding stoichiometry of human retinol binding protein to prealbumin. J Biol Chem 249:5933–5938

Hennemann G, Docter R, Krenning EP, Bos G, Otten M, Visser TJ (1979) Raised total thyroxine and free thyroxine index but normal free thyroxine. Lancet 1:639–642

Hillier AP (1971) Human thyroxine-binding globulin and thyroxine-binding prealbumin: dissociation rates. J Physiol 217: 625–634

Hillier AP (1975) Thyroxine dissociation in human plasma: measurement of its rate by a continuous-flow dialysis method. Acta Endocrinologica 78:32–38

Hwang PLH (1986) Unsaturated fatty acids as endogenous inhibitors of tamoxifen binding to anti-oestrogen-binding sites. Biochem J 237:749–755

Ingbar SH (1963) Observations concerning the binding of thyroid hormones by human serum prealbumin. J Clin Invest 42:143–160

Jacobsson B, Carlstrom A, Plotz A, Collins VP (1990) Transthyretin messenger ribonucleic acid expression in the pancreas and in endocrine tumors of the pancreas and gut. J Clin Endocrinol Metab 71:875–880

Janssen OE, Büttner C, Treske B, Wagner SS, Gunn SK, Refetoff S (1994) The new variant thyroxine-binding globulin-Houston has reduced thyroxine-binding affinity but normal concentration in serum. Program of the 76th Annual Meeting of The Endocrine Society, Anaheim CA, p 478 (Abstract)

Jornvall H, Carlstrom A, Pettersson T, Jacobsson B, Persson M, Mutt V (1981) Structural homologies between prealbumin, gastrointestinal prohormones and other proteins. Nature 291:261–263

Kallee E (1996) Bennhold's analbuminemia: a follow-up study of the first two cases (1953–1992). J Lab Clin Med 127:470–480

Kaptein EM (1994) Thyroid in vitro testing in non-thyroidal illness. Exp Clin Endocrinol 102 [Suppl 2]:92–101
Konno N, Kakinoki K, Hagiwara K, Taguchi H, Minami R (1985) Serum concentrations of unsaturated thyroxine-binding globulin in hyper- and hypothyroidism. Clin Endocrinol 22:249–255
Korcek L, Tabachnick M (1976) Thyroxine-protein interactions. Interaction of thyroxine and triiodothyronine with human TBG. J Biol Chem 251:3558–3562
Kragh-Hansen U (1981) Molecular aspects of ligand binding to serum albumin. Pharmacol Rev 33:17–53
Kragie L, Doyle D (1992) Benzodiazepines inhibit temperature-dependent L-[^{125}I] triiodothyronine accumulation into human liver, human neuroblast, and rat pituitary cell lines. Endocrinology 130:1211–1216
Kurtz AB, Capper SJ, Clifford J, Humphrey MJ, Lukinac L (1981) The effect of fenclofenac on thyroid function. Clin Endocrinol (Oxf) 15:117–124
Lalloz MRA, Byfield PGH, Himsworth RL (1984) A prealbumin variant with an increased affinity for T_4 and reverse-T_3. Clin Endocrinol 21:331–338
Larsen PR (1972) Salicylate-induced increases in free triiodothyronine in human serum. J Clin Invest 51:1125–1134
Larsen PR, Alexander NM, Chopra IJ et al (1987) Revised nomenclature for tests of thyroid hormones and thyroid-related proteins in serum. J Clin Endocrinol Metab 64:1089–1092
Larsson M, Pettersson T, Carlström A (1985) Thyroid hormone binding in serum of 15 vertebrate species: isolation of thyroxine-binding globulin and prealbumin analogs. Gen Comp Endocrinol 58:360–375
Law LK, Cheung CK, Swaminathan R (1988) Falsely high thyroxine results by fluorescence polarization in sera with high background fluorescence. Clin Chem 34:1918
Lim C-F, Wynne KN, Barned JM, Topliss DJ, Stockigt JR (1986) Non-isotopic spectrophotometric determination of the unbound fraction of drugs in serum. J Pharm Pharmacol 38:795–800
Lim C-F, Bai Y, Topliss DJ, Barlow JW, Stockigt JR (1988) Drug and fatty acid effects on serum thyroid hormone binding. J Clin Endocrinol Metab 67:682–688
Lim C-F, Curtis AJ, Barlow JW, Topliss DJ, Stockigt JR (1991) Interactions between oleic acid and drug competitors influence specific binding of thyroxine in serum. J Clin Endocrinol Metab 73:1106–1110
Lim C-F, Stockigt JR, Curtis AJ, Wynne KN, Barlow JW, Topliss DJ (1993) Influence of a naturally-occurring furanoid acid on the potency of drug competitors for specific thyroxine binding in serum. Metabolism 42:1468–1474
Lim C-F, Stockigt JR, Hennemann G (1995) Alterations in hepatocyte uptake and plasma binding of thyroxine in nonthyroidal illness and caloric deprivation. Trends Endocrinol Metab 6:17–20
Lim C-F, Loidl NM, Kennedy JA, Topliss DJ, Stockigt JR (1996) Drug effects on triiodothyronine uptake by rat anterior pituitary cells in vitro. Exp Clin Endocrinol Diabetes 104:151–157
Lueprasitsakul W, Alex S, Fang SL, Pino S, Irmscher K, Köhrle J, Braverman LE (1990) Flavonoid administration immediately displaces thyroxine (T_4) from serum transthyretin, increases serum free T_4 and decreases serum thyrotropin in the rat. Endocrinology 126:2890–2895
Mabuchi H, Nakahashi H (1987) Determination of 3-carboxy-4-methyl-5-propyl-2-furanpropanoic acid, a major endogenous ligand substance in uremic serum, by high-performance liquid chromatography with ultraviolet detection. J Chromatogr 415:110–117
Mendel CM, Frost PH, Cavalieri RR (1986) Effect of free fatty acids on the concentration of free thyroxine in human serum: the role of albumin. J Clin Endocrinol Metab 63:1394–1399
Mendel CM, Weisiger RA, Jones AL, Cavalieri RR (1987a) Thyroid hormone-binding proteins in plasma facilitate uniform distribution of thyroxine within tissues: a perfused rat liver study. Endocrinology 120:1742–1749

Mendel CM, Frost PH, Kunitake ST, Cavilieri RR (1987b) Mechanism of the heparin-induced increase in the concentration of free thyroxine in plasma. J Clin Endocrinol Metab 65:1259–1264
Mendel CM (1989a) The free hormone hypothesis: a physiologically based mathematical model. Endocr Rev 10:232–274
Mendel CM, Cavalieri RR, Gavin LA, Pettersson T, Inoue M (1989b) Thyroxine transport and distribution in Nagase analbuminemic rats. J Clin Invest 83:143–148
Mendel CM, Weisiger RA (1990) Thyroxine uptake by perfused rat liver. J Clin Invest 86:1840–1847
Mohr VS, Barlow JW, Topliss DJT, O'Dea K, Stockigt JR (1987) Evaluation of T_4 and T_3 binding kinetics in the thyroxine binding globulin abnormality of Australian aborigines. Clin Endocrinol 26:531–540
Mori Y, Miura Y, Takeuchi H, Igarashi Y, Sugiura J, Saito H, Oiso Y (1995) Gene amplification as a cause of inherited thyroxine-binding globulin excess in two Japanese families. J Clin Endocrinol Metab 80:3758–3762
Moses AC, Lawlor J, Haddow J, Jackson IMD (1982) Familial euthyroid hyperthyroxinemia resulting from increased thyroxine binding to thyroxine-binding prealbumin. N Engl J Med 306:966–969
Moses AC, Rosen HN, Moller DE, Tsuzaki S, Haddow JE, Lawlor J, Liepieks JJ, Nichols WC, Benson MD (1990) A point mutation in transthyretin increases affinity for thyroxine and produces euthyroid hyperthyroxinaemia. J Clin Invest 86:2025–2033
Munro SL, Lim C-F, Hall JG, Barlow JW, Craik DJ, Topliss DJ, Stockigt JR (1989) Drug competition for thyroxine binding to transthyretin (prealbumin): comparison with effects on thyroxine-binding globulin. J Clin Endocrinol Metab 68:1141–1147
Murata Y, Refetoff S, Sarne DH, Dick M, Watson F (1985) Variant thyroxine-binding globulin in serum of Australian aborigines: its physical, chemical and biological properties. J Endocrinol Invest 8:225–232
Nelson JC, Tomei RT (1988) Direct determination of free thyroxine in undiluted serum by equilibrium dialysis/radioimmunoassay. Clin Chem 34:1737–1744
Newnham HH, Hamblin PS, Long F, Lim C-F, Topliss DJ, Stockigt JR (1987) Effect of oral furosemide on diagnostic indices of thyroid function. Clin Endocrinol (Oxf) 26:423–431
Ng LL, Hockaday TDR (1986) Non-esterified fatty acids may regulate human leucocyte sodium pump activity. Clin Sci 71:737–742
Oppenheimer J, Werner S (1966) Effect of prednisone on thyroxine-binding proteins. J Clin Endocrinol Metab 26:715–721
Palha JA, Episkopou V, Maede S, Shimada K, Gottesman ME, Saraiva MJM (1994) Thyroid hormone metabolism in a transthyretin-null mouse strain. J Biol Chem 269:33135–33139
Pardridge WM (1981) Transport of protein-bound hormones into tissue in vivo. Endocr Rev 2:103–123
Perdrisot R, Bounaud M-P, Bounaud J-Y, Jallet P (1989) Four nonisotopic immunoassays of free thyroxine evaluated. Clin Chem 35:115–120
Peters T Jr (1985) Serum albumin. Adv Protein Chem 37:161–245
Petersen CE, Scottolini AG, Cody LR, Mandel M, Reimer N, Bhagavan NV (1994) A point mutation in the human serum albumin gene results in familial dysalbuminaemic hyperthyroxinaemia. J Med Genet 31:355–359
Petersen CE, Ha CE, Mandel M, Bhagavan NV (1995) Expression of a human serum albumin variant with high affinity for thyroxine. Biochem Biophys Res Comm 214:1121–1129
Prince HP, Ramsden DB (1977) A new theoretical description of the binding of thyroid hormones by serum proteins. Clin Endocrinol 7:307–324
Refetoff S, Robin NI, Fang VS (1970) Parameters of thyroid function in serum of 16 selected vertebrate species: a study of PBI, serum T_4, free T_4, and the pattern of T_4 and T_3 binding to serum proteins. Endocrinology 86:793–805

Refetoff S, Dwulet FE, Benson MD (1986) Reduced affinity for thyroxine in two of three structural thyroxine-binding prealbumin variants associated with familial amyloidotic polyneuropathy. J Clin Endocrinol Metab 63:1432–1437
Refetoff S (1989) Inherited thyroxine-binding globulin abnormalities in man. Endocr Rev 10:275–293
Refetoff S (1994) Inherited thyroxine-binding globulin abnormalities in man: Update 1994. In: Barverman LE, Refetoff S (eds) Clinical and molecular aspects of diseases of the thyroid. Endocr reviews monographs, vol 3. The Endocrine Society pp 162–164
Richardson SJ, Bradley AJ, Duan W, Wettenhall REH, Harms PJ, Babon JJ, Southwell BR, Nicol S, Donnellan SC, Schreiber G (1994) Evolution of marsupial and other vertebrate thyroxine-binding plasma proteins. Am J Physiol 266:R1359-R1370
Robbins J, Cheng S-Y, Gershengorn MC, Glinoer D, Cahnmann HJ, Edelnoch H (1978) Thyroxine transport proteins of plasma, molecular properties and biosynthesis. Rec Prog Horm Res 34:477–519
Robbins J, Johnson ML (1979) Theoretical considerations in the transport of thyroid hormones in blood. In: Ekins RP, Faglia G, Pennisi T, Pinchera A (eds) International symposium of free thyroid hormones. Excerpta Medica, Amsterdam, pp 1–14
Rosen HN, Moses AC, Murrell JR, Liepnieks JJ, Benson MD (1993) Thyroxine interactions with transthyretin: a comparison of 10 different naturally occurring human transthyretin variants. J Clin Endocrinol Metab 77:370–374
Rosner W (1990) The functions of corticosteroid-binding globulin and sex hormone-binding globulin: recent advances. Endocr Rev 11:80–91
Rouaze-Romet M, Savu L, Vranckx R, Bleiberg-Daniel F, Le Moullac B, Gouache P, Nunez EA (1992) Re-expression of thyroxine-binding globulin in post-weaning rats during protein or energy malnutrition. Acta Endocrinologica 127:441–448
Sakata SO, Nakamura S, Miura K (1985) Autoantibodies against thyroid hormone or iodothyronine: implications in diagnosis, thyroid function, treatment and pathogenesis. Ann Intern Med 103:579–589
Saraiva MJM (1995) Transthyretin mutations in health and disease. Hum Mutat 5:191–196
Savu L, Vranckx R, Maya M, Nunez EA (1987) A thyroxine-binding globulin (TBG)-like protein in the sera of developing and adult rats. Biochem Biophys Res Comm 148:1165–1173
Savu L, Vranchx R, Rouaze-Romet M, Maya M, Nunez EA, Tréton J, Flink IL (1991) A senescence up-regulated protein: the rat thyroxine-binding globulin (TBG). Biochim Biophys Acta 1097:19–22
Schreiber G (1987) Synthesis, processing and secretion of plasma proteins by the liver and other organs and their regulation. In: Putnam PW (ed) The plasma proteins: structure, function and genetic control, 2nd edn, vol V. Acadmic, Orlando, pp 293–363
Schreiber G, Aldred AR, Jaworowski A, Milsson C, Achen MG, Segal MB (1990) Thyroxine transport from blood to brain via transthyretin synthesis in choroid plexus. Am J Physiol 258:R338–R345
Smith PJ, Surks MI (1984) Multiple effects of diphenylhydantoin on the thyroid hormone system. Endocr Rev 5:514–524
Smith TJ, Davis FB, Deziel MR, Davis PJ, Ramsden DB, Schoenl M (1994) Retinoic acid inhibition of thyroxine binding to human transthyretin. Biochim Biophys Acta 1199:76–80
Snyder SM, Cavalieri RR, Goldfine ID, Ingbar SH, Jorgenson EC (1976) Binding of thyroid hormones and their analogues to thyroxine-binding globulin in human serum. J Biol Chem 251:6489–6494
Sterling K, Brenner MA (1966) Free thyroxine in human serum: simplified measurement with aid of magnesium precipitation. J Clin Invest 45:153–163

Stockigt JR, Topliss DJ, Barlow JW, White EL, Hurley DM, Taft P (1981a) Familial euthyroid thyroxine excess: an appropriate response to abnormal thyroxine binding associated with albumin. J Clin Endocrinol Metab 53:353–359

Stockigt JR, DeGaris M, Csicsmann J, Barlow JW, White EL, Hurley DM (1981b) Limitations of a new free thyroxine assay (AmerlexR free T_4). Clin Endocrinol (Oxf) 15:313–318

Stockigt JR, Stevens V, White EL, Barlow JW (1983) "Unbound analog" radioimmunoassays for free thyroxin measure the albumin-bound hormone fraction. Clin Chem 29:1408–1410

Stockigt JR, Lim C-F, Barlow JW, Stevens V, Topliss DJ, Wynne FN (1984) High concentrations of furosemide inhibit plasma binding of thyroxine. J Clin Endocrinol Metab 59:62–66

Stockigt JR, Lim C-F, Barlow JW, Wynne KN, Mohr VS, Topliss DJ, Hamblin PS, Sabto J (1985) Interaction of furosemide with serum thyroxine-binding sites: in vivo and in vitro studies and comparison with other inhibitors. J Clin Endocrinol Metab 60:1025–1031

Stockigt JR, Dyer SA, Mohr VS, White EL, Barlow JW (1986) Specific methods to identify plasma binding abnormalities in euthyroid hyperthyroxinemia. J Clin Endocrinol Metab 62:230–233

Surks MI, Hupart KH, Chao P, Shapiro LE (1988) Normal free thyroxine in critical nonthyroidal illnesses measured by ultrafiltration of undiluted serum and equilibrium dialysis. J Clin Endocrinol Metab 67:1031–1039

Surks MI, Sievert R (1995) Drugs and thyroid function. N Engl J Med 1688–1694

Surks MI, Defesi CR (1996) Normal serum free thyroid hormone concentrations in patients treated with phenytoin or carbamazepine: a paradox resolved. JAMA 275:1495–1498

Topliss DJ, Hamblin PS, Kolliniatis E, Lim C-F, Stockigt JR (1988) Furosemide, fenclofenac, diclofenac, mefenamic acid and meclofenamic acid inhibit specific T_3 binding in isolated rat hepatic nuclei. J Endocrinol Invest 11:355–360

Topliss DJ, Kolliniatis E, Barlow JW, Lim C-F, Stockigt JR (1989) Uptake of T_3 cultured rat hepatoma cells is inhibitable by non-bile acid cholephils, diphenylhydantoin and non-steroidal anti-inflammatory drugs. Endocrinology 124:980–986

Topliss DJ, Scholz GH, Kolliniatis E, Barlow JW, Stockigt JR (1993) Influence of calmodulin antagonists and calcium channel blockers on triiodothyronine uptake by rat hepatoma and myoblast cell lines. Metabolism 42:376–380

Tozer TN (1984) Implications of altered plasma protein binding in disease states. In: Benet LZ, Massoud N, Gambertoglio JG (eds) Pharmacokinetic basis for drug treatment. Raven, New York, pp 173–193

Trevorrow V (1939) Studies on the nature of the iodine in blood. J Biol Chem 127:737–750

Vallette G, Vanet A, Sumida C, Nunez EA (1991) Modulatory effects of unsaturated fatty acids on the binding of glucocorticoids to rat liver glucocorticoid receptors. Endocrinology 129:1363–1369

van den Berghe G, de Zegher F, Lauwers P (1994) Dopamine and the sick euthyroid syndrome in critical illness. Clin Endocrinol 41:731–737

van der Sluijs Veer G, Vermes I, Bonte HA, Hoorn RKJ (1992) Temperature effects on free-thyroxine measurements: analytical and clinical consequences. Clin Chem 38:1327–1331

Vranckx R, Rouaze M, Savu L, Nunez EA, Beaumont C, Flink IL (1990) The hepatic biosynthesis of rat thyroxine binding globulin (TBG): demonstration, ontogenesis and up-regulation in experimental hypothyroidism. Biochem Biophys Res Comm 167:317–322

Vranckx R, Rouaze-Romet M, Savu L, Mechighel P, Maya M, Nunez EA (1994) Regulation of rat thyroxine-binding globulin and transthyretin: studies in

thyroidectomized and hypophysectomized rats given tri-iodothyronine or/and growth hormone. J Endocrinol 142:77–84
Vyas SK, Wilkin TJ (1994) Thyroid hormone autoantibodies and their implications for free thyroid hormone measurement. J Endocrinol Invest 17:15–21
Wilcox RB, Nelson JC, Tomei RT (1994) Heterogeneity in affinities of serum proteins for thyroxine among patients with nonthyroidal illness as indicated by the serum free thyroxine response to serum dilution. Eur J Endocrinol 131:9–13
Zambon A, Hashimoto SI, Brunzell JD (1993) Analysis of techniques to obtain plasma for measurement of levels of free fatty acids. J Lipid Res 34:1021–1028

CHAPTER 6

Molecular Biology of Thyroid Hormone Action

J.A. FRANKLYN and V.K.K. CHATTERJEE

A. Introduction

The major biologically active thyroid hormone 3,5,3′-triiodothyronine (T_3) exerts effects upon almost every cell and tissue of the body influencing function, as well as in many cases the growth and development of that tissue. T_3 is known to regulate the level of expression of a large number of specific genes expressed in a variety of tissues, often by stimulating or inhibiting the rate of transcription of those genes; much of this chapter concentrates upon the mechanisms of regulation of transcription by T_3. Nonetheless, there are a number of steps which precede the binding of T_3 to its receptor within the nucleus and which therefore have the potential to modulate the actions of T_3 and these will be considered briefly first.

B. Extranuclear Mechanisms of Thyroid Hormone Action

I. Plasma Membrane and Intracellular Transport of Thyroid Hormones

Chapter 5 has discussed the transport of thyroid hormones in the circulation. While it is clear that the principle mechanism determining the intracellular supply of the "prohormone" thyroxine (T_4) and the biologically active hormone T_3 is the concentration of non-protein-bound or "free" hormone outside the cell and hence the amount of passive diffusion into the cell, it is also clear that there exists an energy-dependent, high-affinity, low-capacity system which contributes to the cellular uptake of thyroid hormones (KRENNING et al. 1981). Furthermore, an active energy-dependent system may modulate transport inside the cell and uptake of T_3 into the nucleus (OPPENHEIMER and SCHWARTZ 1985). It is postulated that modulation of these energy-dependent systems may play a part in ultimately determining thyroid hormone action, especially in the context of "non-thyroidal" illnesses in which marked abnormalities of circulating concentrations of thyroid hormones are frequent and in which there are often discrepancies between thyroid hormone concentrations in serum and clinical thyroid state.

The metabolism of thyroid hormones has been discussed in Chap. 4, this volume, and emphasises that while the major determinant of T_3 supply to the cell is the circulating concentration of that hormone, local deiodination of T_4 to T_3, through the action of the enzyme 5′-monodeiodinase, is an important regulator of T_3 supply. This is especially pertinent to tissues such as the brain and anterior pituitary, where intracellular deiodination accounts for at least 50% of available T_3 (LARSEN et al. 1982). Modulation of deiodination itself, in situations such as "non-thyroidal" illness and during therapy with a variety of drugs, thus represents a further potential level of control of thyroid hormone action.

II. Extranuclear Sites of Thyroid Hormone Action

It has been proposed for some years that T_3 may act, at least in part, through extranuclear mechanisms (STERLING et al. 1977). High-affinity, limited-capacity binding sites for T_3 have been described in mitochondria and studies, indicating increased oxygen consumption by isolated mitochondria after T_3 treatment in vitro lends support for a role for these intracellular organelles in T_3 action. Direct effects of T_3 upon plasma membrane uptake of amino acids have also been reported.

The contribution of these extranuclear systems to thyroid hormone action remains unclear and the subject of considerable debate. Nonetheless, overwhelming evidence suggests that the major actions of T_3 are mediated via binding to specific nuclear thyroid hormone receptor proteins (TRs), as discussed below.

C. Identification of High-Affinity Nuclear-Binding Sites for Thyroid Hormones

The concept that the first step in the initiation of thyroid hormone action results from a direct effect upon the nucleus arose from the work of TATA and WIDNELL (1966). They reported stimulation of RNA polymerase activity in rat liver cell nuclei after administration of T_3 or T_4 to the hypothyroid animal. The presence of high-affinity, limited-capacity binding sites or receptors in the nuclei of rat hepatocytes was later demonstrated by OPPENHEIMER et al. (1972). Nuclear binding sites for T_3 with similar high affinity (K_d 10^{-10}–10^{-11} M) and specificity were subsequently described in a number of other rat tissues and a variety of cell lines.

A large number of studies using radioactively labelled thyroid hormones as receptor-binding ligands were carried out; these studies demonstrated that the affinity of binding sites for T_3, T_4 and a variety of other thyroid hormones and their analogues paralleled their biological potency. In addition, there appeared to be a close correlation between the number of high-affinity binding sites for T_3 present in the nuclei of a given tissue and the apparent responsiveness of that tissue to thyroid hormones. Liver and anterior pituitary cells were calculated to have 8000–10000 TRs per cell nucleus, while tissues considered unresponsive to thyroid hormones, such as testis and spleen, were found to have little or no demonstrable ligand binding. These findings from ligand-binding studies were consistent with an important role of nuclear receptors in the initiation of thyroid hormone effects, evidence pointing to the presence of a single class of such receptors in all the tissues of a given organism (OPPENHEIMER et al. 1972; SAMUELS et al. 1983).

Further biochemical characterization of TRs was hindered by the intrinsic instability of receptor proteins. Considerable efforts were made to purify such proteins, the results of such efforts indicating that TRs were heterogeneous in nature, ranging in molecular weight from 47 to 57 kDa, heterogeneity being thought at the time to represent protein degradation or post-translational modification. Furthermore, it became clear that these nuclear receptor proteins were able to bind with high affinity to nuclear chromatin, providing early insight into their mechanism of action.

D. Cloning of cDNAs Encoding Nuclear Receptors for T_3

Although purification of receptors for T_3 using standard biochemical approaches proved largely unsuccessful, this was not the case for receptors for steroid hormones which were purified using radiolabelled high-affinity binding steroid hormone analogues. Isolation of glucocorticoid and oestrogen receptor proteins allowed the production of antibodies against these receptors, tools which led ultimately to cloning and sequencing of receptor cDNAs and deduction of receptor structure. Investigation of the role of the oestrogen receptor in the growth of breast tumours led to recognition of marked structural homology between the human oestrogen receptor and the v-erbA gene of the transforming avian erythroblastosis virus (GREEN et al. 1986). It was postulated that the normal cellular counterpart of this gene, the c-erbA proto-oncogene, might encode a receptor for a steroid hormone other than oestrogen but two reports published simultaneously demonstrated that the in vitro translation products of both a chicken and a human c-erbA cDNA bound thyroid hormones, rather than steroid hormones, with high affinity (SAP et al. 1986; WEINBERGER et al. 1986). The molecular weights of these c-erbA gene products were similar to those described previously for T_3 receptors and the products were shown to bind T_3, T_4 and their analogues with similar relative affinities to those derived from studies of ligand binding to cell nuclei and nuclear extracts.

The deduced amino acid sequences of the chicken and human cDNAs revealed that they encoded proteins which are members of a larger and ever expanding "superfamily" of structurally related proteins which includes receptors for glucocorticoids, mineralocorticoids, gonadal steroids, vitamin D_3, all-*trans* retinoic acid and 9-*cis* retinoic acid (termed retinoic acid and retinoid X receptors, respectively), as well as further molecules whose ligands have yet to be identified but which are likely to act as independent transcription factors (GREEN and CHAMBON 1988). Each of the receptor molecules within the family has a region near its N-terminal end which has the potential to form "zinc finger" structures capable of binding to DNA, while the carboxy-terminal region of each molecule corresponds to the ligand-binding domain; the function of these specific domains is discussed in detail below.

E. Recognition of Two Genes Encoding Two Major Classes of TR

Hybridisation of the human c-erbA cDNA to digested placental DNA revealed the presence of multiple c-erbA genes which were located on more than one chromosome (WEINBERGER et al. 1986), implying the existence of more than one gene encoding the T_3 receptor. THOMPSON et al. (1987) proceeded to isolate from a rat brain cDNA library a putative "neuronal" form of T_3 receptor cDNA. The rat protein encoded by this cDNA was shown to be more closely related structurally to the chicken than the human receptor already described; the rat and chicken receptors were therefore designated α forms and the human receptor was designated β. It was confirmed that the α form represented a distinct gene product, since Southern blotting revealed hybridization to chromosome 17, while the human β receptor gene was mapped to chromosome 3.

The view, arising from the initial cloning of distinct α- and β-receptor cDNAs, that there existed more than one form of T_3 receptor protein was soon supported by cloning and expression of further rat and human receptor cDNAs. BENBROOK and PFAHL (1987) cloned, from a human testis cDNA library, a cDNA with a product of 55 kDa demonstrating characteristic DNA-binding and ligand-binding domains. The human α-type receptor cDNA demonstrated incomplete homology with the previously described human β-receptor, with only 87% similarity in their DNA-binding regions. This report was followed by description of another human T_3 receptor cDNA cloned from a kidney cDNA library (NAKAI et al. 1987). These human α-receptor cDNAs were shown to be similar to, but not identical with, the previously described rat α_1 receptor cDNA and were designated α_2 forms. It soon became clear that, unlike their α_1 counterparts, the products of α_2 genes are unable to bind T_3 with high affinity but retain some ability to bind to DNA (LAZAR et al. 1988). It is known that the T_3 receptor α gene transcript is alternatively spliced to produce α_1 or α_2 mRNAs. Further multiple splice variants of the rat c-erbA α_2 product have also been described (IZUMO and MAHDAVI 1988). The picture has been further complicated by evidence that there exists, on both the rat and human T_3 receptor α gene, a transcript on the opposite DNA strand which encodes a further member of the thyroid/steroid hormone receptor superfamily with a function which is as yet unclear (LAZAR et al. 1989). The product of this gene, termed rev-erbA α, does not bind T_3 but may act through an "antisense" mechanism to inhibit translation of the α_1 and α_2 gene transcripts or may itself bind to regulatory DNA sequences of T_3 target genes (SPANJAARD et al. 1994).

The T_3 receptor β gene also utilises the mechanisms of alternate promoter sites or RNA splicing in order to produce β_1 and β_2 mRNAs. It is of interest that the product of the β_2 gene is expressed most abundantly in the anterior pituitary (HODIN et al. 1989), in contrast to the β_1 product, which demonstrates widespread expression. However, the presence of β_2 transcripts or protein detected by reverse transcriptase polymerase chain reaction amplification or immunocytochemistry, respectively, has been reported in other tissues, especially within the central nervous system (COOK et al. 1992; LECHAN et al. 1993).

F. Thyroid Hormone Response Elements

Considerable attention has focused on definition of the sequences of DNA termed thyroid hormone response elements (TREs) to which T_3 receptor isoforms bind in order to regulate gene transcription. Definition of the sequences that mediate thyroid hormone responsiveness has involved analysis of the promoter regions of target genes through synthesis of chimaeric constructs, comprising varying lengths of promoter DNA linked to reporter genes (genes with easily measured products), such as that encoding the bacterial enzyme chloramphenicol acetyl transferase, and transiently expressed in mammalian cells in culture. Parallel studies defining the specific site of binding of receptor proteins to regulatory sequences within target gene promoters have utilised methods for analysis of protein-DNA binding including DNAse 1 footprinting, gel mobility shift assays and methylation interference.

Initial transfection studies of promoter deletion constructs upstream of reporter genes investigated the rat growth hormone gene and indicated that the DNA elements which mediated T_3 stimulation of transcription of this gene resided within 235 base pairs of its transcriptional start site (CREW and SPINDLER 1986). Similar transfection studies led to localisation within 5′-flanking DNA of the TRE of other thyroid hormone responsive genes such as those encoding malic enzyme, the α-myosin heavy chain and the TSH α- and β-subunits (Fig. 1; GUSTAFSON et al. 1987; CARR et al. 1989; CHATTERJEE et al. 1989).

There is no evidence from such studies that there exists a single "consensus" sequence of DNA to which T_3 receptors bind in order to mediate T_3 effects upon every T_3 responsive gene. Nonetheless there exists up to 80% homology between the TREs of various genes and this homology has led to description of an ideal "consensus half-site" with the structure AGGT(C/A)A (BRENT et al. 1989) (Fig. 1). Three such half sites similar in structure to this idealised TRE have been shown to exist within the 5′-flanking DNA of the rat growth hormone gene (between −188 and −165 bases relative to the transcriptional start site) and it has been reported that each is required for full T_3

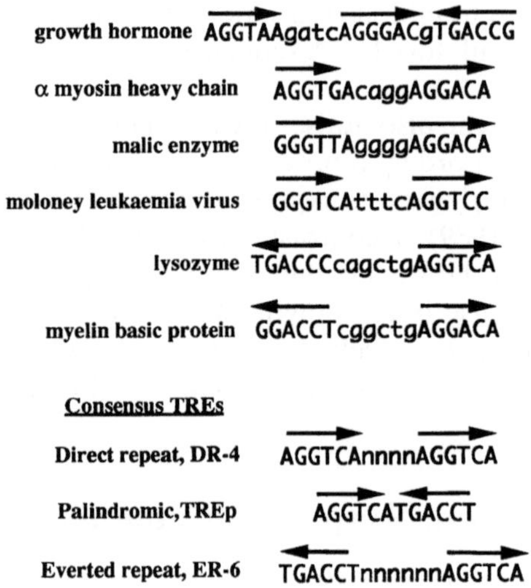

Fig. 1. Nucleotide sequences from the promoter regions of different target genes that are induced by thyroid hormone are shown. From these, three major types of consensus thyroid response element (*TRE*) can be derived, consisting of the hexameric sequence AGGTCA arranged either as a direct repeat with a four-nucleotide spacing (*DR-4*), palindromically (*TREp*) or as an everted repeat with a six-nucleotide spacing (*ER-6*). TREs from negatively regulated genes are quite variable in configuration such that no clear consensus can be derived

stimulation of transcription, the nature and relative position of the TREs influencing their activity (BRENT et al. 1991). Three similar half sites are observed in the promoter of the rat α-myosin heavy-chain gene.

It is notable that consensus binding sequences for glucocorticoid receptors and oestrogen receptors are identical or very similar to the "consensus" TRE, the consensus glucocorticoid RE comprising two GGTACA hexamers in a palindromic arrangement separated by three base pairs, while a consensus oestrogen RE comprises two AGGTCA hexamers also arranged as a symmetrical palindrome with a three base pair gap (CARSON-JURICA et al. 1990). The situation for TREs is, however, more complicated than that which applies to the response elements mediating glucocorticoid and oestrogen effects, since analysis of wild-type promoters of T_3 target genes demonstrates that T_3 receptors do not bind to consensus palindromic sequences in nature. Furthermore, T_3 receptors can recognise DNA-binding sites containing between one and four hexamers, often of degenerate sequence, which can be arranged in combinations of any relative orientation (WILLIAMS and BRENT 1992; WILLIAMS et al. 1992). Despite this, T_3 receptors usually bind to direct repeat response elements containing two hexamers homologous to the AGGTCA sequence.

At the present time, controversy exists over the precise nature and position of response elements mediating T_3 receptor actions. The complexity of structure of TREs, as well as the structural and functional complexity of T_3

receptor isoforms, which is discussed below, determines that receptors can bind to dually regulated elements (GLASS et al. 1989; YARWOOD et al. 1993), as well as to overlapping binding sites for other receptors or transcription factors (DIAMOND et al. 1990), and are able to heterodimerise with several potential functional partners (YU et al. 1991; FORMAN et al. 1992; KLIEWER et al. 1992a,b; YEN et al. 1995). These observations determine that the regulation of specific target genes by T_3 is highly complex and cannot be explained by a simple model of receptor binding to DNA.

G. Structural Characteristics of TRs and Identification of Functional Domains

Following the cloning of TRs, inspection of their primary amino acid sequence indicated high homology with steroid receptors (e.g. glucocorticoid,

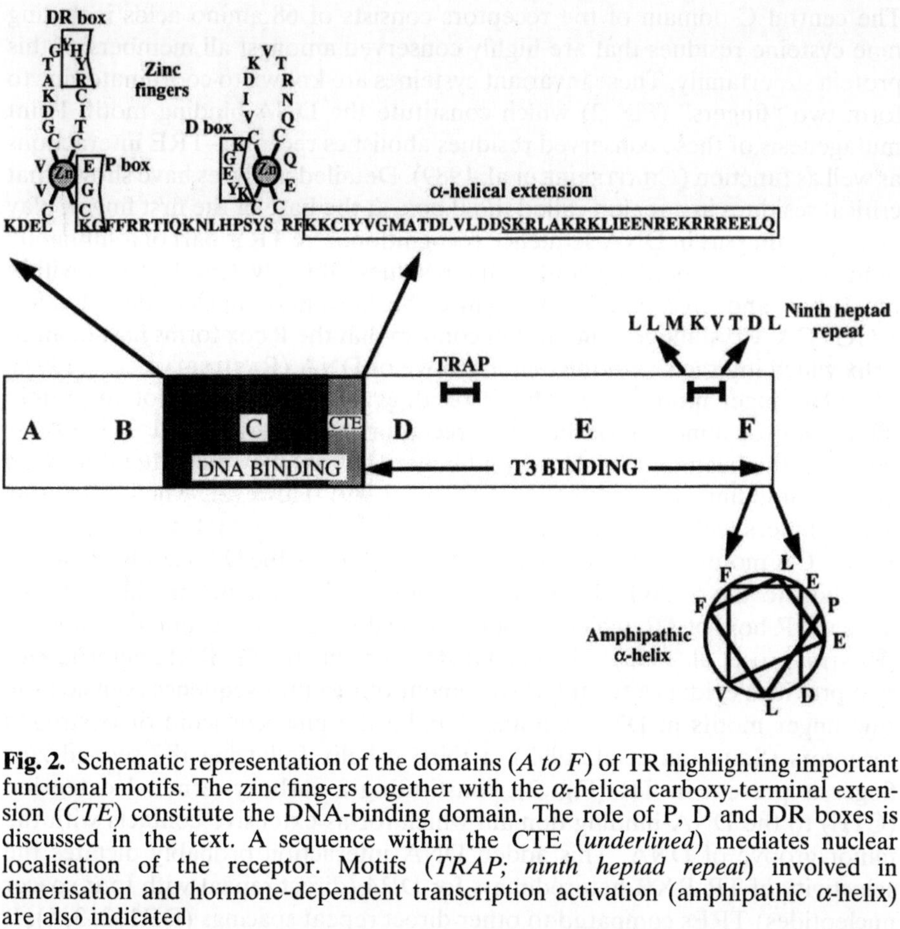

Fig. 2. Schematic representation of the domains (*A to F*) of TR highlighting important functional motifs. The zinc fingers together with the α-helical carboxy-terminal extension (*CTE*) constitute the DNA-binding domain. The role of P, D and DR boxes is discussed in the text. A sequence within the CTE (*underlined*) mediates nuclear localisation of the receptor. Motifs (*TRAP; ninth heptad repeat*) involved in dimerisation and hormone-dependent transcription activation (amphipathic α-helix) are also indicated

oestrogen), suggesting that they were part of this family of proteins (EVANS 1988). When aligned by sequence similarity, the receptors can be subdivided into distinct domains (A to F) (Fig. 2) which mediate specific functions. A central C domain is the most highly conserved region and is organised into zinc finger motifs which mediate binding to DNA and the carboxy-terminal (D/E/F) domains encode ligand binding and dimerisation functions. The role of amino-terminal (A/B) domains is less well understood, but they have a transcription activation function which manifests variably depending on cell type and gene promoter context (GREEN and CHAMBON 1988). In common with other members of the steroid/nuclear receptor family, the TR acts as a ligand-inducible transcription factor to activate or repress target gene transcription in a hormone-dependent manner. The structural features within each domain which mediate specific functions will now be considered in more detail.

I. DNA-Binding Domain

The central C domain of the receptors consists of 68 amino acids including nine cysteine residues that are highly conserved amongst all members of this protein superfamily. These invariant cysteines are known to coordinate zinc to form two "fingers" (Fig. 2) which constitute the DNA-binding motif. Point mutagenesis of these conserved residues abolishes receptor–TRE interactions as well as function (CHATTERJEE et al. 1989). Detailed analyses have shown that critical residues in a region called the P box, at the base of the first finger, play an important part in DNA sequence recognition. The TR is part of a subfamily of nuclear receptors which contain the residues Glu, Gly, Cys, Lys, Gly within the P box and preferentially recognise the hexameric nucleotide sequence AGGTCA. Crystallographic studies confirm that the P box forms part of an α-helix which interacts with the major groove of DNA (RASTINEJAD et al. 1995). The zinc finger motifs also contain residues which mediate protein-protein interaction or dimerisation between receptor monomers bound to DNA. A region at the beginning of the second finger (D box) may mediate interaction in TR homodimers (UMESONO and EVANS 1989). However, when TR forms heterodimers with the retinoid X receptor (RXR) on a TRE containing two AGGTCA motifs arranged as a direct repeat (Fig. 1), the D box of RXR which is bound to the 5′ AGGTCA motif interacts with residues in the first zinc finger (DR box) of TR, which is bound to the downstream hexameric sequence (RASTINEJAD et al. 1995). The crystal structure of the TR-RXR heterodimer also provides evidence for the involvement of receptor sequences outside the zinc finger motifs in DNA binding. Unlike the glucocorticoid or oestrogen receptors (SCHWABE et al. 1993), a third α-helix following the second zinc finger is present in TR (Fig. 2), constituting a carboxy-terminal extension (CTE) to the DNA-binding domain which forms extensive contacts with the minor groove of DNA. This added DNA interaction probably dictates the selectivity of TR-RXR heterodimers for DR4 (direct repeat with four spacer nucleotides) TREs compared to other direct repeat spacings (DR1, 2, 3, 5). It may also explain why the TR, uniquely, can bind moderately well as a monomer to a slightly extended half-site recognition sequence (TAAGGTCA) (KATZ and KOENIG 1993).

II. Hormone-Binding Domain

Experiments in which various domains of the TR were coupled to a heterologous DNA-binding domain indicate that the hormone-binding and transactivation functions of TRs are encompassed within the D/E/F domains (THOMPSON and EVANS 1989). However, further deletions extending either from the D domain (LIN et al. 1991) or from truncation of amino acids at the carboxy terminus (CHATTERJEE et al. 1991) lead to a dramatic loss of ligand-binding capacity. Single point mutations within this region are equally deleterious (ADAMS et al. 1994), suggesting that the ability to bind ligand is distributed widely across this region of the receptor. Most recently, the crystal of the hormone-binding domain of the TRα has been elucidated. The domain consists of 11 α-helices arranged as a three-layered antiparallel sandwich, harbouring an internal hydrophobic core which contains the ligand (WAGNER et al. 1995). As suggested by mutational analyses, the buried ligand makes extensive contacts with at least eight different structural elements throughout the length of the hormone-binding domain.

III. Nuclear Localisation

Immunocytochemical studies show that, unlike other members of the steroid receptor superfamily, the TR is constitutively located in the cell nucleus (MACCHIA et al. 1990), probably reflecting the fact that it is not associated with cytosolic heat shock proteins (DALMAN et al. 1990). Nevertheless, the entry of receptor into the nucleus is thought to be mediated by a specific sequence of amino acids resembling those identified in other proteins such as the SV40 large T antigen or progesterone receptor (GUICHON-MANTEL et al. 1989). When coupled to a heterologous cytoplasmic protein, a short basic peptide sequence within the α-helical extension to the DNA-binding domain (Fig. 2) is indeed capable of targeting it to the nucleus (DANG and LEE 1989) and mutations within this motif impair nuclear localisation (LEE and MADHAVI 1993).

IV. Dimerisation

As has been discussed previously, the TR can bind to DNA as a monomer or homodimer or as a heterodimer with RXR. TR homodimers are particularly evident on everted repeat and palindromic configurations of TRE, whereas TR-RXR heterodimers are formed preferentially on direct repeat response elements (Fig. 1). Furthermore, the addition of ligand disrupts the homodimer complex, whereas the heterodimer remains stable (Fig. 3) (YEN et al. 1992). In

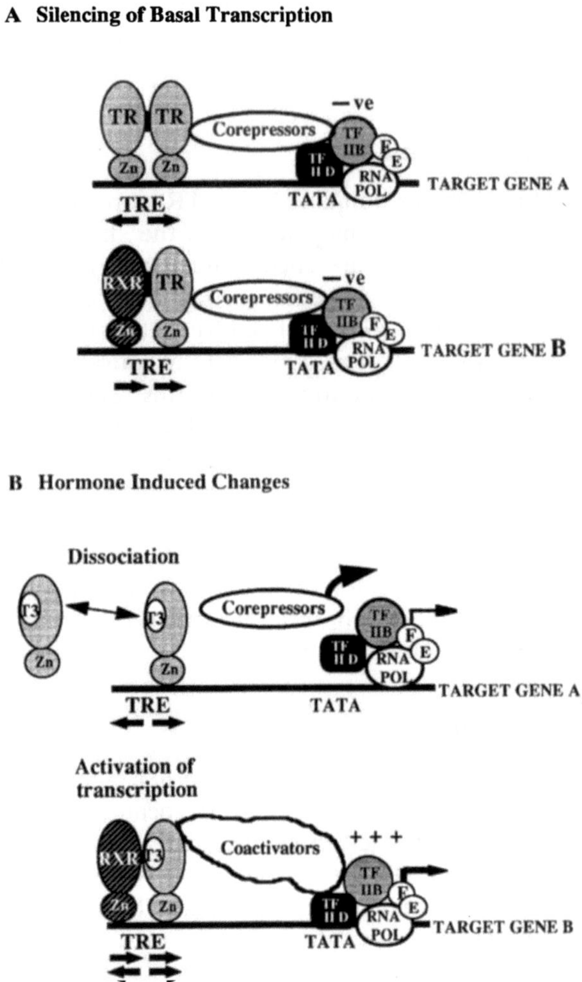

Fig. 3. A In the absence of ligand, the thyroid hormone receptor binds to response elements as either a homodimer or a heterodimer with RXR. Basal gene transcription is inhibited via intermediary corepressors. **B** Following T_3 binding, TR homodimers dissociate and release of corepressor leads to derepression. The TR-RXR heterodimer remains stable and recruits coactivators to enhance target gene transcription

addition to sequences within the DNA-binding domain, regions within the hormone-binding domain have also been implicated in dimerisation. FORMAN and SAMUELS (1989) inspected the primary amino acid sequence of this domain and delineated a series of nine repeats consisting of conserved hydrophobic residues at the first, fifth and eighth positions. These heptad repeats were analogous to the "leucine zipper" motif which forms a coiled-coil helical structure in transcription factors such as Fos and Jun and mediates dimerisation. Mutagenesis experiments have confirmed that the ninth heptad repeat (Fig. 2) is important for both homo- and heterodimerisation (AUFLIEGNER et al. 1993). However, naturally occurring receptor mutations, identified in the syndrome of resistance to thyroid hormone (RTH), overlap the first and second heptad repeats and dimerise normally, arguing against their importance for this function (COLLINGWOOD et al. 1994). Interestingly, some natural mutant receptors in RTH (e.g. R316H, R338W, R429Q) exhibit a failure to form homodimers yet heterodimerise normally, suggesting that different regions of the hormone-binding domain are involved in the two types of interaction.

A second region which lies further upstream in the hormone-binding domain (Fig. 2) was first shown to be important for the interaction of TR with auxiliary factors (TRAPs) from nuclear extracts and designated the TRAP domain (O'DONNELL et al. 1990). It is now believed that the TRAP activity in many cell types is synonymous with RXR and the TRAP domain has indeed been shown to be involved in TR interaction with RXR (ROSEN et al. 1993).

The hormone-binding domain of TRa crystallises as a monomer, such that only limited inferences about the nature of the dimer interface can be drawn. Nevertheless, the hydrophobic residues of the ninth heptad are found on the surface of helix 11, with the potential to participate in protein-protein interaction. However, elucidation of the exact nature of homo- and heterodimeric interfaces awaits crystallisation of full-length receptors bound to DNA.

V. Silencing of Basal Gene Transcription by Unliganded TR

v-erbA, the oncogenic counterpart of TR, was first shown to act as a transcriptional repressor (DAMM et al. 1989), but many groups have since made the observation that when hormone-inducible reporter genes (containing positive TREs) are cotransfected with TR, the basal level of transcription is inhibited (Fig. 3). This was best exemplified by studies of the chicken lysozyme gene (BANIAHMAD et al. 1990), where an everted repeat TRE in the promoter was shown to mediate transcriptional "silencing" by recruiting TR in the absence of ligand. The subsequent addition of hormone relieved this repression.

Further studies have shown that silencing is mediated by the carboxy-terminal hormone-binding domain of TR (BANIAHMAD et al. 1992). One hypothesis for this effect was that the receptor might directly inhibit components of the basal transcriptional machinery. This was supported by experiments which showed that TR could indeed interact with factors such as TF-IIB (BANIAHMAD et al. 1993; FONDELL et al. 1993) or TATA-binding protein (TBP) (TONE et al. 1994) and that these interactions were disrupted by ligand. An alternative hypothesis suggested the existence of an additional cellular factor containing an intrinsic repression function, which could be recruited by unliganded TR but dissociated from the receptor in the presence of hormone (CASANOVA et al. 1994).

Two groups have now isolated cellular factors, called N-CoR and SMRT, respectively, that are candidate corepressors which interact with TR and related nuclear receptors in the absence of hormone (HORLEIN et al. 1995; CHEN and EVANS 1995). N-CoR is a 270-kDa protein which interacts optimally with TR/RXR heterodimers bound to DNA and dissociates following the addition of T_3.

VI. Transcription Activation

In keeping with other nuclear receptors, TRs have been shown to contain two types of transcription activation function: their amino-terminal A/B regions may encode a weak activation function (AF-1), which is constitutive and manifests even with unliganded receptor bound to a TRE; in contrast, the carboxy-terminal D/E/F regions contain a powerful activation function (AF-2) which is strictly hormone dependent.

1. Hormone-Dependent Activation of Transcription (AF-2)

Previous studies of the oncogene v-erbA had shown that it was unable to regulate transcription in a hormone-dependent manner. Comparisons of TR and v-erbA indicated that this function mapped to nine amino acids at the carboxy terminus of the receptor (ZENKE et al. 1990). A helical wheel plot indicated that the carboxy-terminal motif, made up of hydrophobic and acidic residues, could form an amphipathic helix (Fig. 2), analogous to transcription activation domains present in factors such as GAL4 and VP16. Further studies supported this hypothesis, showing that mutation of leucine and glutamic acid residues, which are highly conserved amongst nuclear receptors, abrogated AF-2 function with preservation of hormone and DNA binding (TONE et al. 1994; BARETTINO et al. 1994).

The crystal structure of TRa confirmed the presence of an amphipathic α-helix (helix 12) at the carboxy terminus of the receptor, which is also present in the crystal structures of the retinoic acid (RARγ) and RXRα. Interestingly, the position of this helix in unliganded RXRα versus liganded RARγ differs markedly (RENAUD et al. 1995), suggesting that hormone-binding induces a marked conformational change in the D/E/F domains. Although similar direct comparisons cannot be made for TR, other evidence (e.g. measurements of secondary structure by circular dichroism) suggests a similar hormone-dependent alteration of conformation (TONEY et al. 1993).

The conformational change is known to be accompanied by a relief of repression or silencing by TR due to dissociation of corepressor. By analogy, this led to the hypothesis that transcription activation involved the recruitment of coactivators by the receptor. Using either the yeast two-hybrid system or Far Western blotting, several groups have identified a number of different cellular cofactors which interact with TR and other nuclear receptors in a strictly hormone dependent manner. Such putative coactivators include SUG1/TIF1 (LEE et al. 1995), RIP140 (CAVAILLES et al. 1995), SRC-1 (ONATE et al. 1995) and CBP (KAMEI et al. 1996). In each case it appears that the C-terminal amphipathic α-helix is important for receptor interaction with the cofactor. The relative importance and functional role of these different proteins in mediating transcription activation remains to be elucidated.

2. Constitutive Transcription Activation (AF-1)

In contrast to the high homology (~80%) between TRα_1 and TRβ_1 receptor isoforms in their DNA- and hormone-binding domains, the amino-terminal A/B regions of these receptors and TRβ_2 are quite dissimilar (<15% homology) (Fig. 4), suggesting divergent functions for this domain. As the tissue distribution of these receptor isoforms differs markedly, one hypothesis is that the A/B regions mediate cell-type or promoter-specific differences in target gene regulation by the different receptors. For example, cotransfection of TRα_1 with the Rous sarcoma virus promoter enhances basal transcription (Saatcioglu et al. 1993). This ligand-independent activation (AF-1) function mapped to the A/B domain of TRα_1 and the β_1 receptor did not exhibit a similar effect. The chick TRα_1 can be phosphorylated on serine residues at positions 12 and 28 by protein kinase A or casein kinase II, respectively (Goldberg et al. 1988; Glineur et al. 1989). However, the contribution of such post-translational modification to AF-1 activity is not known. In another study (Sjoberg and Vennstrom 1995), the amino-terminal domain of TRβ_2 was also found to contain strong AF-1 activity which was markedly attenuated by mutating conserved tyrosine residues. Whether these residues modulate receptor interaction with cofactors (corepressors/coactivators) remains to be elucidated.

The amino-terminal A/B domains of TRs have also been shown to augment the hormone-dependent activation function (AF-2) of the carboxy-terminal region. For example, TRα_1 is more transcriptionally active than TRβ_1

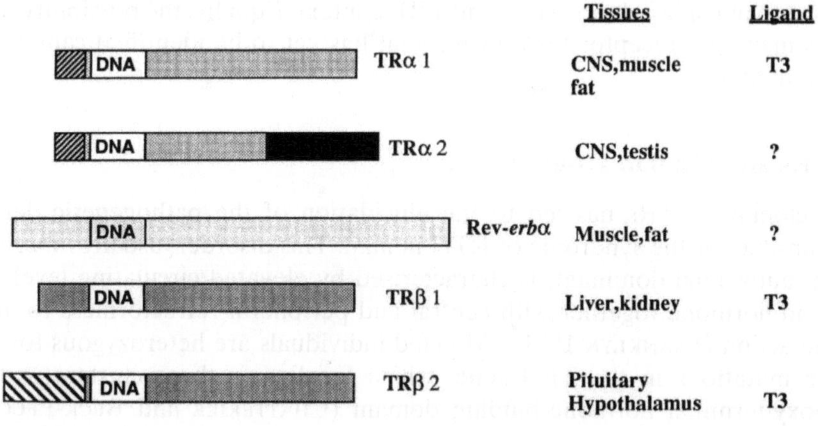

Fig. 4. Organisation and tissue distribution of thyroid hormone receptor isoforms (TRα_1, TRβ_1, TRβ_2) and related proteins (TRα_2, Rev-erbα). The proteins are aligned via their DNA-binding domains, which are most homologous. TRα_2 is identical to TRα_1 except at the carboxy terminus (*black*), and the amino terminus of TRβ_2 (*bars*) diverges from TRβ_1

when compared using synthetic TREs in JEG-3 choriocarcinoma cells (HOLLENBERG et al. 1995) and TRβ_1 is more potent than TRβ_2 when tested with TREs from the myelin basic protein and malic enzyme genes in NIH 3T$_3$ cells (TOMURA et al. 1995). In both cases, these differences were abolished by A/B domain deletions. Possible explanations include the interaction of TRα_1 and β_1, but not TRβ_2, with the basal transcription factor TF-IIB (TOMURA et al. 1995), or that TRβ_2 exhibits stronger homodimeric binding to some TREs which fail to dissociate with ligand to allow the formation of transcriptionally active heterodimers (NG et al. 1995).

H. Role of the TR Splice Variant TRα_2

As a result of alternate splicing of the TRα gene, the receptor variant TRα_2 (Fig. 4) has a divergent carboxy terminus and does not bind thyroid hormone (LAZAR et al. 1988). As it is distributed ubiquitously, often with TRα_1 or TRβ_1, this raised the possibility that the α_2 variant might act as an endogenous modulator of thyroid hormone action. Initial experiments using a direct repeat type of TRE suggested that TRα_2 could indeed inhibit the action of coexpressed TRα_1 or TRβ_1 (KOENIG et al. 1989), but a subsequent study with a palindromic TRE (RENTOUMIS et al. 1990) could not reproduce this effect. These differences were reconciled by the later observation that TRα_2 forms heterodimers with RXR more efficiently on direct repeat versus palindromic TREs to mediate its inhibitory effects (NAGAYA and JAMESON 1993). Most recently, KATZ et al. (1995) have shown that the DNA-binding and inhibitory activities of TRα_2 can also be inhibited by casein kinase II dependent phosphorylation of a serine within the unique divergent carboxy terminus. Overall, these studies suggest that TRα_2 may be a natural inhibitor of TR action, subject to phosphorylation state and TRE context. Equally, the possibility that TRα_2 may be a receptor for a ligand that has yet to be identified cannot be discounted.

I. TRs and Human Disease

The cloning of TRs has led to the elucidation of the pathogenetic defect responsible for the syndrome of RTH in man. This disorder, usually inherited as an autosomal dominant, is characterised by elevated circulating levels of thyroid hormone together with central and peripheral refractoriness to hormone action (FRANKLYN 1991). Affected individuals are heterozygous for diverse mutations in the TRβ gene, which localise to three clusters in the carboxy-terminal hormone-binding domain (CHATTERJEE and BECK-PECCOZ 1994). The clinical manifestations of RTH are highly variable, ranging from asymptomatic individuals deemed to have generalised resistance (GRTH), to thyrotoxic features such as failure to thrive, low body mass index, tachycardia or dysrhythmia, suggesting predominant pituitary resistance (PRTH). Both

GRTH and PRTH are associated with TRβ mutations, indicating that the two disorders represent phenotypic variants of a single genetic entity (ADAMS et al. 1994). In keeping with their location, mutant receptors in RTH exhibit impaired hormone-binding and transcriptional activity. In addition, the mutant receptors are capable of inhibiting the action of their wild-type counterparts when coexpressed (CHATTERJEE et al. 1991). Clinical observations from two other unusual cases of RTH provide evidence in support of a "dominant negative" inhibitory effect of mutant receptors in vivo. In a unique family with recessively inherited RTH (REFETOFF et al. 1967), individuals who were heterozygous for a deletion of one allele of the TRβ gene were clinically and biochemically normal and this has also been confirmed in heterozygote TRβ knockout mice (FORREST et al. 1996); conversely, another child who was homozygous for two "dominant negative" mutant TRβ alleles showed severe growth and mental retardation together with biochemical evidence of extreme resistance to thyroid hormone action (ONO et al. 1991). To date, no naturally occurring defects in human TRα_1 have been described, although based on its tissue distribution (Fig. 4) this would be unlikely to manifest as classical thyroid hormone resistance.

References

Adams M, Matthews C, Collingwood TN, Tone Y, Beck-Peccoz P, Chatterjee VKK (1994) Genetic analysis of 29 kindreds with generalised and pituitary resistance to thyroid hormone. J Clin Invest 94:506–515

Au-Fliegner M, Helmer E, Casanova J, Raaka BM, Samuels HH (1993) The conserved ninth C-terminal heptad in thyroid hormone and retinoic acid receptors mediates diverse responses by affecting heterodimer but not homodimer formation. Mol Cell Biol 13:5725–5737

Baniahmad A, Ha I, Reinberg D, Tsai S, Tsai M-J, O'Malley BW (1993) Interaction of human thyroid hormone receptor β with transcription factor TFIIB may mediate target gene derepression and activation by thyroid hormone. Proc Natl Acad Sci USA 90:8832–8836

Baniahmad A, Kohne AC, Renkawitz R (1992) A transferable silencing domain is present in the thyroid hormone receptor, in the v-erbA oncogene product and in the retinoic acid receptor. EMBO J 11:1015–1023

Baniahmad A, Steiner C, Kohne AC, Renkawitz R (1990) Modular structure of a chicken lysozyme silencer: involvement of an unusual thyroid hormone receptor binding site. Cell 61:505–514

Barettino D, Vivanco Ruiz MM, Stunnenberg HG (1994) Characterization of the ligand-dependent transactivation domain of thyroid hormone receptor. EMBO J 13:3039–3049

Benbrook D, Pfahl M (1987) A novel thyroid hormone receptor encoded by a cDNA clone from a human testis library. Science 238:788–791

Brent GA, Harney JW, Chen Y, Warne RL, Moore DD, Larsen PR (1989) Mutations of the rat growth hormone promoter which increase and decrease response to thyroid hormone define a consensus thyroid hormone response element. Mol Endocrinol 3:1996–2004

Brent GA, Williams GR, Harney JW, Forman BM, Samuels HH, Moore DD, Larsen PR (1991) Mol Endocrinol 5:542–548

Carr FE, Burnside J, Chin WW (1989) Thyroid hormones regulate rat thyrotropin-β gene promoter activity expressed in GH3 cells. Mol Endocrinol 3:709–716

Carson-Jurica MA, Schrader WT, O'Malley BW (1990) Steroid receptor family: structure and functions. Endoc Rev 11:201–220
Casanova J, Helmer E, Selmi-Ruby S, Qi J-S, Au-Fliegner M, Desai-Yajnik V, Koudinova N, Yarm F, Raaka BM, Samuels HH (1994) Functional evidence for ligand-dependent dissociation of thyroid hormone and retinoic acid receptors from an inhibitory cellular factor. Mol Cell Biol 14:5756–5765
Cavailles V, Dauvois S, L'Horset F, Lopez G, Hoare S, Kushner PJ, Parker MG (1995) Nuclear factor RIP140 modulates transcriptional activation by the estrogen receptor. EMBO J 14:3741–3751
Chatterjee VKK, Beck-Pecoz (1994) Thyroid hormone resistance. In: Sheppard MC, Stewart PM (eds) Ballieres clinical endocrinology and metabolism, vol 8. Hormones, enzymes and receptors, pp 267–283
Chatterjee VKK, Lee JK, Rentoumis A, Jameson JL (1989) Negative regulation of the thyroid stimulating hormone a gene by thyroid hormone: receptor interaction adjacent to the TATA box. Proc Natl Acad Sci USA 86:9114–9118
Chatterjee VKK, Nagaya T, Madison LD, Datta S, Rentoumis A, Jameson JL (1991) Thyroid hormone resistance syndrome: inhibition of normal receptor function by mutant thyroid hormone receptors. J Clin Invest 87:1977–1984
Chen JD, Evans RM (1995) A transcriptional co-repressor that interacts with nuclear hormone receptors. Nature 377:454–457
Collingwood TN, Adams M, Tone Y, Chatterjee VKK (1994) Spectrum of transcriptional dimerization and dominant negative properties of twenty different mutant thyroid hormone β receptors in thyroid hormone resistance syndrome. Mol Endocrinol 8:1262–1277
Cook CB, Kakucska I, Lechan RM, Koenig RA (1992) Expression of thyroid hormone receptor β_2 in rat hypothalamus. Endocrinology 130:1077–1079
Crew MD, Spindler SR (1986) Thyroid hormone regulation of the transfected rat growth hormone promoter. J Biol Chem 261:5018–5022
Dalman FC, Koenig RJ, Perdew GH, Massa E, Pratt WB (1990) In contrast to the glucocorticoid receptor the thyroid hormone receptor is translated in the DNA binding state and is not associated with hsp90. J Biol Chem 265:3615–3618
Damm K, Thompson CC, Evans RM (1989) Protein encoded by v-erbA functions as a thyroid hormone receptor antagonist. Nature 339:593–597
Dang CV, Lee WMF (1989) Nuclear and nucleolar targeting sequences of c-erbA, c-myb, N-myc, p53, hsp70 and HIV tat proteins. J Biol Chem 264:18019–18023
Diamond MI, Miner JN, Yoshinaga SK, Yamamoto KR (1990) Transcription factor interactions: selectors of positive and negative regulation from a single DNA element. Science 249:1266–1272
Evans RM (1988) The steroid and thyroid hormone receptor superfamily. Science 240:889–895
Fondell JD, Roy AL, Roeder RG (1993) Unliganded thyroid hormone receptor inhibits its formation of a functional preinitiation complex: implications for active repression. Genes Develop 7:1400–1410
Forman BM, Casanova J, Raaka BM, Ghysdael J, Samuels HH (1992) Half-site spacing and orientation determines whether thyroid hormone and retinoic acid receptors and related factors bind to DNA response elements as monomers, homodimers, or heterodimers. Mol Endocrinol 6:429–442
Forman BM, Samuels HH (1990) Interactions among a subfamily of nuclear hormone receptor: the regulatory zipper model. Mol Endocrinol 9:1293–1301
Forrest D, Hanebuth E, Smeyne RJ, Everds N, Stewart CL, Wehner JM, Curran T (1996) Recessive resistance to thyroid hormone in mice lacking thyroid hormone receptor β: evidence for tissue-specific modulation of receptor function. EMBO J 15:3006–3015
Franklyn JA (1991) Syndromes of thyroid hormone resistance. Clin Endocrinol 34: 237–245

Glass CK, Lipkin SM, Devary OV, Rosenfeld MG (1989) Positive and negative regulation of gene transcription by a retinoic acid-thyroid hormone receptor heterodimer. Cell 59:697–708

Glineur C, Bailly M, Ghysdael J (1989) The c-erbAa encoded thyroid hormone receptor is phosphorylated in its amino terminal domain by casein kinase II. Oncogene 4:1247–1254

Goldberg Y, Glineur C, Gesquiere JC, Ricouart A, Sap J, Veenstrom B, Ghysdael J (1988) EMBO J 7:2425–2433

Green S, Chambon P (1987) Oestradiol induction of a glucocorticoid responsive gene by a chimaeric receptor. Nature 325:75–78

Green S, Chambon P (1988) Nuclear receptors enhance our understanding of transcription regulation. Trends Gen 4:309–314

Green S, Walter P, Kumar VJ et al (1986) Human oestrogen receptor cDNA: sequence, expression and homology to v-erbA. Nature 320:134–139

Guichon-Mantel A, Loosfelt H, Lescop P et al (1989) Mechanisms of nuclear localization of the progesterone receptor: evidence for interaction between monomers. Cell 57:1147–1154

Gustafson TA, Markham BE, Bahl JJ, Morkin E (1987) Thyroid hormone regulates expression of a transfected α myosin heavy chain fusion gene in fetal heart cells. Proc Natl Acad Sci USA 84:3122–3126

Hodin RA, Lazar MA,Wintman BI, et al (1989) Identification of a thyroid hormone receptor that is pituitary specific. Science 244:76–79

Hollenberg AN, Monden T, Wondisford FE (1995) Ligand-independent and -dependent functions of thyroid hormone receptor isoforms depend on their distinct amino termini. J Biol Chem 270:14274–14280

Horlein AJ, Naar AM, Heinzel T, Torchia J, Gloss B, Kurokawa R, Ryan A, Kamei Y, Soderstrom M, Glass CK, Rosenfeld MG (1995) Ligand-independent repression by the thyroid hormone receptor mediated by a nuclear receptor co-repressor. Nature 377:397–404

Izumo S, Mahdavi V (1988) Thyroid hormone receptor α isoforms generated by alternative splicing differentially activate myosin heavy chain gene transcription. Nature 334:539–542

Kamei Y, Xu L, Heinzel T, Torchia J, Kurokawa R, Gloss B, Lin S-C, Heyman RA, Rose DW, Glass CK, Rosenfeld MG (1996) A CBP integrator complex mediates transcriptional activation and AP-1 inhibition by nuclear receptors. Cell 85:403–414

Katz D, Reginato MJ, Lazar MA (1995) Functional regulation of thyroid hormone receptor variant TRα_2 by phosphorylation. Mol Cell Biol 15:2341–2348

Katz RW, Koenig RJ (1993) Nonbiased identification of DNA sequences that bind thyroid hormone receptor α_1 with high affinity. J Biol Chem 268:19392–19397

Kliewer SA, Umesono K, Heyman RA et al (1992a) Retinoid X receptor-COUP-TF interactions modulate retinoic acid signalling. Proc Natl Acad Sci USA 89:1448–1452

Kliewer SA, Umesono K, Mangelsdorf DJ, Evans RM (1992b) Retinoid X receptor interacts with nuclear receptors in retinoic acid, thyroid hormone and vitamin D3 signalling. Nature 355:446–449

Koenig RJ, Lazar MA, Hodin RA, Brent GA, Larsen PR, Chin WW, Moore DD (1989) Inhibition of thyroid hormone action by a non-hormone binding c-erbA protein generated by alternative mRNA splicing. Nature 337:659–661

Krenning EP, Docter R, Bernhard HL et al (1981) Characteristics of active transport of thyroid hormone into rat hepatocyte. Biochim Biophys Acta 676:314–316

Larsen PR (1982) Thyroid pituitary interaction. Feedback regular of thyrotrophin secretion by thyroid hormones. N Engl J Med 306:26–32

Lazar MA, Hodin RA, Darling DS, Chin WW (1988) Identification of a rat c-erbAa-related protein which binds DNA but does not bind thyroid hormone. Mol Endocrinol 2:893–901

Lazar MA, Hodin RA, Darling DS, Chin WW (1989) A novel member of the thyroid/steroid hormone receptor family is encoded by the opposite strand of the rat c-erbAα transcriptional unit. Mol Cell Biol 9:1128–1136
Lechan RM, Qi Y, Berrodin TJ, Davis KD, Schwartz HL, Strait KA, Oppenheimer JH, Lazar MA (1993) Immunocytochemical delineation of thyroid hormone receptor β_2-like immunoreactivity in the rat central nervous system. Endocrinology 132:2461–2469
Lee JW, Ryan F, Swaffield JC, Johnston SA, Moore DD (1995) Interaction of thyroid-hormone receptor with a conserved transcriptional mediator. Nature 374:91–94
Lee Y, Mahdavi V (1993) The D domain of the thyroid hormone receptor α_1 specifies positive and negative transcriptional regulation functions. J Biol Chem 268:2021–2028
Lin KH, Parkison C, McPhie P, Cheng S-Y (1991) An essential role of domain D in the thyroid hormone binding activity of human β_1 thyroid hormone nuclear receptor. Mol Endocrinol 5:485–492
Macchia E, Nakai A, Janiga et al (1990) Characterization of site-specific polyclonal antibodies to c-erbA peptides recognising the human thyroid hormone receptors α_1, α_2 and β and native 3,5,3′-triiodothyronine receptor and a study of tissue distribution of the antigen. Endocrinology 126:3232–3239
Nagaya T, Jameson JL (1993) Distinct dimerization domains provide antagonist pathways for thyroid hormone receptor action. J Biol Chem 268:24278–24282
Nakai A, Seino S, Sakurai A et al (1987) Characterization of a thyroid hormone receptor expressed in human kidney and other tissues. Proc Natl Acad Sci USA 85:2781–2785
Ng L, Forrest D, Haugen BR, Wood WM, Curran T (1995) N-terminal variants of thyroid hormone receptor β: differential function and potential contribution to syndrome of resistance to thyroid hormone. Mol Endocrinol 9:1202–1213
O'Donnell AL, Koenig RJ (1990) Mutational analysis identifies a new functional domain of the thyroid hormone receptor. Mol Endocrinol 4:715–720
Onate SA, Tsai SY, Tsai M-J, O'Malley BW (1995) Sequence and characterization of a coactivator for the steroid hormone receptor superfamily. Nature 270:1354–1357
Ono S, Schwartz ID, Mueller OT, Root AW, Usala SJ, Bercu BB (1991) Homozygosity for a dominant negative thyroid hormone receptor gene responsible for generalized resistance to thyroid hormone. J Clin Endocrinol Metab 73:990–994
Oppenheimer JH, Koerner D, Schwartz AL, Surks MI (1972) Specific nuclear triiodothyronine binding sites in liver and kidney. J Clin Endocrinol Metab 35:330–333
Oppenheimer JH, Schwartz HL (1985) Stereospecific transport of T_3 from plasma to cytosol and from cytosol to nucleus in rat liver, kidney, brain and heart. J Clin Invest 75:147–151
Rastinejad F, Perlmann T, Evans RM, Sigler PB (1995) Structural determinants of nuclear receptor assembly on DNA direct repeats. Nature 375:203–211
Refetoff S, DeWind LT, DeGroot LJ (1967) Familial syndrome combining deaf-mutism, stippled epiphyses, goiter and abnormally high PBI: possible target organ refractoriness to thyroid hormone. J Clin Endocrinol Metab 27:279–294
Renaud J-P, Rochel N, Ruff M, Vivat V, Chambon P, Gronemeyer H, Moras D (1995) Crystal structure of the RARγ ligand-binding domain bound to all-trans retinoic acid. Nature 378:681–689
Rentoumis A, Chatterjee VKK, Madison LD, Datta S, Gallagher GD, DeGroot LJ, Jameson JL (1990) Negative and positive transcriptional regulation by thyroid hormone receptor isoforms. Mol Endocrinol 4:1522–1531
Rosen ED, Beninghof EG, Koenig RJ (1993) Dimerization interfaces of thyroid hormone, retinoic acid, vitamin D and retinoid X receptors. J Biol Chem 268:11534–11541

Saatcioglu F, Deng T, Karin M (1993) A novel cis element mediating ligand-independent activation by c-erbA: implications for hormonal regulation. Cell 75:1095–1105
Samuels HH (1983) Identification and characterization of thyroid hormone receptors and action using cell culture techniques. In: Oppenheimer JH, Samuels JH (eds) Molecular basis of thyroid hormone action. Academic Press, New York, pp 36–66
Sap J, Munoz A, Damm K et al (1986) The c-erbA protein is a high affinity receptor for thyroid hormone. Nature 324:635–640
Schwabe JWR, Chapman L, Finch JT, Rhodes D (1993) The crystal structure of the estrogen receptor DNA-binding domain bound to DNA: how receptors discriminate between their response elements. Cell 75:567–578
Sjoberg M, Vennstrom B (1995) Ligand-dependent and -independent transactivation by thyroid hormone receptor β_2 is determined by the structure of the hormone response element. Mol Cell Biol 15:4718–4726
Spanjaard RA, Nguyen VP, Chin WW (1994) Rat rev-erbAα, an orphan receptor related to thyroid hormone receptor, binds to specific thyroid hormone response elements. Mol Endocrinol 8:286–295
Sterling K, Mitch PO, Lazarus JH (1977) Thyroid hormone action: the mitochondrial pathway. Science 197:996–999
Tata J, Widnell CC (1966) Ribonucleic acid synthesis during the early action of thyroid hormones. Biochem J 98:604–620
Thompson CC, Evans RM (1989) Trans-activation by thyroid hormone receptors: functional parallels with steroid hormone receptors. Proc Natl Acad Sci USA 86:3494–3498
Thompson CC, Weinberger C, Lebo L, Evans RM (1987) Identification of a novel thyroid hormone receptor expressed in the mammalian central nervous system. Science 237:1610–1614
Tomura H, Lazar J, Phyillaier M, Nikodem VM (1995) The N-terminal region (A/B) of rat thyroid hormone receptors α_1, β_1 but not β_2 contains a strong thyroid hormone-dependent transactivation function. Proc Natl Acad Sci USA 92:5600–5604
Tone Y, Collingwood TN, Adams M, Chatterjee VKK (1994) Functional analysis of a transactivation domain in the thyroid hormone β receptor. J Biol Chem 269:31157–31161
Toney JH, Wu L, Summerfield AE, Sanyal G, Forman BM, Zhu J, Samuels HH (1993) Conformational changes in chicken thyroid hormone receptor α_1 induced by binding to ligand or to DNA. Biochemistry 32:2–6
Umesono K, Evans RM (1989) Determinants of target gene specificity for steroid/thyroid hormone receptors. Cell 57:1139–1146
Wagner RL, Apriletti JW, McGrath ME, West BL, Baxter JD, Fletterick RJ (1995) A structural role for hormone in the thyroid hormone receptor. Nature 378:690–697
Weinberger C, Thompson CC, Ong ES et al (1986) The c-erbA gene encodes a thyroid hormone receptor. Nature 324:641–646
Williams GR, Brent GA (1992) Specificity of nuclear hormone receptor action: who conducts the orchestra? J Endocrinol 135:191–194
Williams GR, Harney JW, Moore DD, Larsen PR, Brent GA (1992) Differential capacity of wild type promoter elements for binding and transactivation by retinoic acid and thyroid hormone receptors. Mol Endocrinol 6:1527–1537
Yarwood NJ, Gurr J, Sheppard MC, Franklyn JA (1993) Estradiol modulates thyroid hormone regulation of the human glycoprotein hormone α subunit gene. J Biol Chem 268:21984–21989
Yen PM, Darling DS, Carter RL, Forgione M, Umeda PK, Chin WW (1992) Triiodothyronine (T_3) decreases binding to DNA by T_3-receptor homodimers but not receptor-auxiliary protein heterodimers. J Biol Chem 267:3565–3568
Yen PM, Wilcox EC, Chin WW (1995) Steroid hormone receptors selectively affect transcriptional activation but not basal repression by thyroid hormone receptors. Endocrinology 136:440–445

Yu VC, Delsert C, Andersen B et al (1991) RXR beta: a coregulator that enhances binding of retinoic acid, thyroid hormone and vitamin D receptors to their cognate response elements. Cell 67:1251–1266
Zenke M, Munoz A, Sap J, Vennstrom B, Beug H (1990) v-erbA oncogene activation entails the loss of hormone-dependent regulator activity of c-erbA. Cell 61:1035–1049

CHAPTER 7

Iodine: Metabolism and Pharmacology

S. NAGATAKI and N. YOKOYAMA

A. Introduction

The synthesis of normal quantities of thyroid hormones containing iodine in the molecules depends on the availability of adequate quantities of exogenous iodine. Iodine participates not only in an essential substrate for thyroid hormone biosynthesis, but also in many pharmacological actions. Therefore, the effect of iodine on the thyroid is a combination of the effects of pharmacological action and the effects of iodine as a substrate for thyroid hormone.

In the 1940s, it was proposed that iodine might have a direct influence on thyroid structure. In comparisons of thyroids from hypophysectomized rats given high and low iodine diets, thyroids in animals receiving low iodine diets were heavier and more vascular, and had a greater mean acinar cell height than those in iodine-rich diets (CHAPMAN 1941). In comparisons of the growth response of thyroid glands to thyroid-stimulating hormone (TSH) in hypophysectomized rats, thyroids with mild iodine deficiency displayed a smaller response to both a standard dose and a higher threshold dose of TSH for thyroid growth than thyroids with severe iodine deficiency (BRAY 1968).

There exists a mechanism whereby iodine directly influences thyroid growth with or without trophic stimulations. The possible effects of such autoregulation of thyroid function are manifold., including the involuting action of iodine on the diffuse goitre of Graves' disease. The same mechanism operating in reverse may facilitate the development on maintenance of simple goitre, in which thyroid organic iodine is decreased (RAPOPORT et al. 1972). In this matter, it has traditionally been postulated that enhanced TSH secretion to impaired hormone synthesis is the primary cause of goitre. Nevertheless, patients with simple goitre do not necessarily have elevated serum TSH levels (YOUNG et al. 1975). There may be another mechanism that permits the development and maintenance of goitre via an enhanced growth response to normal TSH levels.

It is clear that the thyroid itself is an unfilled reservoir of both iodine and thyroid hormone, that the extracellular fluid and tissues are themselves reservoirs of hormones, and that these reservoirs provide a strong factor of physiological stability. It would be desirable that the mechanisms for maintenance of thyroid homeostasis not only respond to various concentrations of thyroid hormone in the blood, but also respond to the glandular content of hormone. The thyroid indeed contains intrinsic mechanisms responsive to variations in the quantity of iodine available and often to the resulting changes in thyroidal organic iodine contents (see also Chap. 4, this volume).

B. Iodide Transport and Organification

Iodine is actively transported against the electrical gradient at the basal membrane of the thyroid follicular cell and diffuses with a specialized channel from the thyroid cell to the follicular lumen at the apical membrane. Iodide transport into the thyroid is the first step in the biosynthesis of thyroid hormones. TSH stimulates all aspects of thyroid function, including iodide transport. The Na^+/I^- symporter is an intrinsic membrane protein located in the follicular cells and is responsible for the active Na^+-dependent accumulation of iodide (CARRASCO 1993; DUMONT and VASSART 1995; VILIJIN and CARRASCO 1989). The identification, solubilization, purification and reconstitution in a functional state of the Na^+/I^- symporter have been characterized to elucidate the molecular mechanisms involved in iodide accumulation and its regulation (CARRASCO 1993; DUMONT and VASSART 1995; VILIJIN and CARRASCO 1989; GERARD et al. 1994; KAMINSKY et al. 1994). After considerable progress in iodine transport research over the last few decades, the cloning and characterization of the thyroid Na^+/I^- symporter has just been reported (DAI et al. 1996). A cDNA clone that encodes this symporter was isolated as a result of functional screening of a cDNA library from a rat thyroid-derived cell line (FRTL-5) in *Xenopus laervis* oocytes. Oocyte microinjection of an RNA transcript made in vitro from this cDNA clone elicited a more than 700-fold increase in perchlorate-sensitive Na^+/I^- symport activity. The Na^+/I^- symporter cDNA expresses 3.1 kb with 12 trans-membrane regions and is composed of 680 amino acids.

The responses of iodine organification and coupling mechanisms to the administration of additional iodine are complex in thyroid glands, which depend on the dosage and duration of administered iodide. Under normal circumstances, the quantity of iodide delivered into the thyroid gland by the iodide transport mechanism does not exceed the capacity of peroxidatic mechanisms to carry out oxidation and organic binding to yield monoiodotyrosine (MIT) and diiodotyrosine (DIT). Similarly, the coupling mechanism proceeds to synthesize hormonally active iodotyronines from a portion of the iodotyrosine precursors. Hence, when radioiodine is administered, only a small proportion of radioiodine in the thyroid is present as inorganic iodide. The remainder is present in organic forms, principally MIT and DIT, with lesser proportions of the active hormones (T_3 and T_4).

C. Thyroid Autoregulation

Iodine is central to any consideration of thyroid physiology, and the concept of thyroid autoregulation was established several decades ago. Autoregulation was originally defined as regulation of thyroidal iodine metabolism independent of TSH or other external stimulators, and the major autoregulatory factor was considered to be excess iodide (NAGATAKI 1974; PISAREV 1985).

In humans, autoregulation results in the maintenance of normal thyroid secretion despite wide variations in dietary iodide intake. Although the intake of iodide varies from 50 μg to several milligrams per day in iodine-sufficient areas, serum thyroid hormone concentrations as well as TSH concentrations are remarkably constant in these areas. Even in mildly iodine deficient areas, many people are euthyroid with normal serum thyroid hormone and TSH concentrations. In patients with hyperthyroidism, excess iodide ameliorates the symptoms and signs of thyrotoxicosis and decreases serum thyroid hormone concentrations. This antithyroid effect of excess iodide disappears, however, during continuous administration of iodide, and thyrotoxicosis reappears (escape or adaptation).

In animal thyroid, acute inhibition of thyroidal organification of iodine by excess iodide, escape from the acute inhibitory effect of excess iodide, and changes of thyroid radioiodine uptake in hypophysectomized animals in response to variations in dietary iodide intake are representative examples of autoregulation. The acute inhibitory effect of excess iodide (Wolff-Chaikoff effect) is temporary and escape occurs despite continuous administration of iodide. Escape also occurs in hypophysectomized animals, indicating that it is not dependent on changes in TSH secretion. When hypophysectomized rats are fed a low iodine diet, thyroidal radioactive iodine uptake increases, and the increase is abolished by excess iodide.

Organic iodine content and iodide-transport activity are inversely related even in hypophysectomized rats (HALMI 1961). In hypophysectomized rats, the weight of the thyroid gland and uptake of radioactive iodine were higher if the rats had been iodine depleted before hypophysectomy, and administration of TSH produces a greater effect in the iodine-depleted rats (HALMI and SPIRTOS 1955).

I. Autoregulation in Animals

1. Wolff-Chaikoff Effect and Escape

The acute inhibitory effects of excess iodide were first demonstrated in the 1940s (MORTON et al. 1944; WOLFF and CHAIKOFF 1948). In rats injected with 100 μg iodide containing a tracer quantity of radioiodine, serum iodide concentrations decreased rapidly with time, and thyroidal iodine organification was inhibited as long as serum iodide concentrations were above 20–30 μg/dl. When serum iodide concentration decreased below this range, organification of newly accumulated iodide began. This inhibition of thyroidal iodine organification in response to the acute increase of serum iodide is commonly called the Wolff-Chaikoff effect.

When a high concentration of serum iodide (100–200 μg/dl) is maintained by repeated administration of iodide, the inhibitory effect disappears and thyroidal iodine organification increases (WOLFF et al. 1949). This is the so-called escape from the Wolff-Chaikoff effect. Studies of the mechanism of escape suggested that it occurs because of impairment in the ability of the thyroid to concentrate sufficient iodide to inhibit thyroidal iodine organification (BRAVERMAN and INGBAR 1963; RABEN 1949). Escape from the acute inhibitory effect of iodide explains why hypothyroidism or goitre formation do not occur in humans or animals maintained on high doses of iodide for a long time; however, the exact mechanism for the decrease in iodide transport activity in response to chronic excess iodide remains unresolved.

2. Effects of Graded Doses of Iodide

Even during the acute Wolff-Chaikoff effect, a small amount of organic iodine is formed in thyroid gland, but the newly formed organic iodine consists mostly of MIT and DIT, and very little thyroxine (T_4) or triiodothyronine (T_3) can be detected. The thyroid, however, concentrates substantial proportions of iodide when plasma iodide concentrations are only moderately increased (NAGATAKI and INGBAR 1964). Figure 1 shows the results of studies in which rats were given graded doses of iodide (2.5–250 μg) and a tracer dose of radioiodine (^{131}I) 30 min before killing, to determine the incorporation of radioiodine into several thyroidal components. Two phases of response could be distinguished. The percentage of thyroidal radioiodine as inorganic iodide increased and the percentage of ^{131}I amino acids as T_4 and T_4 decreased, with increasing iodide dose above 50 μg. The ratio of labelled MIT/DIT also increased. As for the total quantity of newly formed organic iodine, the changes in total organification were biphasic, increasing as the iodide dose increased to 50 μg and then decreasing T_4 and T_3 formation more abruptly than did total organification.

The effects of excess iodide can be divided into four categories (NAGATAKI 1974). Firstly, with relatively low doses of iodide, which do not change the proportionate metabolism of iodine, the percentage uptake and incorporation of radioactive iodine into iodinated amino acids is unaltered. The total accumulation and incorporation of stable iodide into T_4 and T_3 increases with and remains proportional to the dose of stable iodide administered. Secondly, moderate doses of iodide decrease the percentage uptake of administered iodide, the proportion of newly formed organic iodine and the proportion of T_4 and T_3 among the newly formed iodinated amino acids, but increase the absolute rate of organic iodination and T_4 and T_3 synthesis. Thirdly, large doses of iodide decrease both the percentage incorporation of administered iodine and the absolute rate of organic iodine formation (Wolff-Chaikoff

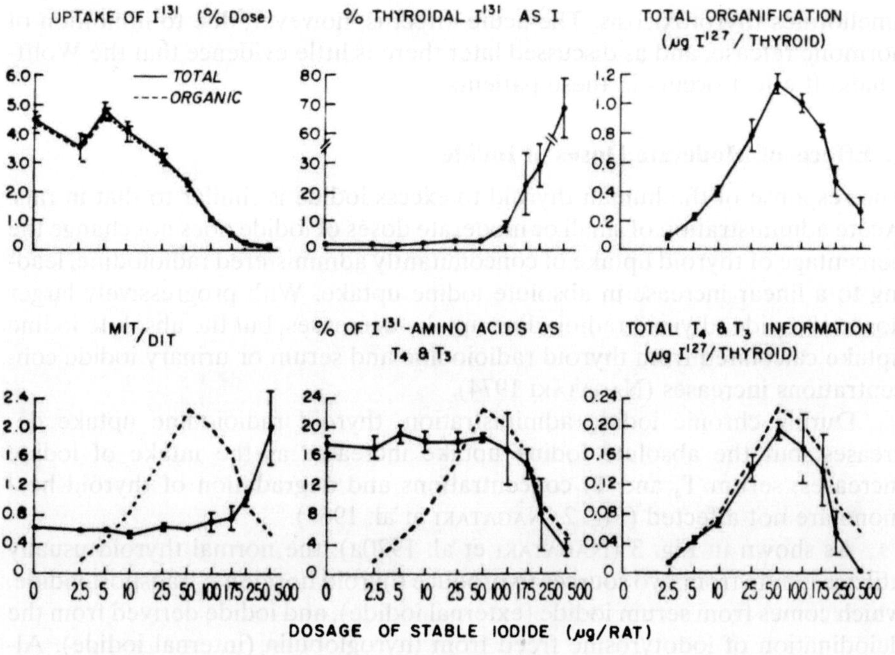

Fig. 1. Effects of graded doses of iodide administered 30 min before killing on the thyroidal metabolism of iodine in rats. The results shown are the means ± SE (*bars*) of values obtained from five rats. For reference purposes, the curve of total organic iodination is shown as *a dashed line in the lower three panels*. (Adapted from NAGATAKI and INGBAR 1964)

effect). Finally, very large doses of iodide acutely saturate the mechanism for iodide transport.

II. Autoregulation in Humans

When the iodide dose reaches a certain level (more than 1 mg/day) in man, the thyroidal uptake of tracer doses of radioiodine decreases, and the administration of perchlorate or thiocyanate results in discharge of radioiodine from the thyroid, indicating a proportionate decrease in organification of thyroidal iodide. There is no evidence, however, that overall organification is actually decreased by excess iodide; that is, there is no evidence for an acute Wolff-Chaikoff effect in man. The discharge of iodide means only that it has accumulated in excess of the thyroid's ability to organify iodide. If a large dose is given, the thyroid radioiodine uptake is so low that the absolute iodine uptake cannot be calculated. Hence, it is not possible to demonstrate either a Wolff-Chaikoff effect or escape from it.

In contrast, in patients with hyperthyroidism caused by Graves' disease, acute administration of iodide decreases serum T_4 and T_3 concentrations and ameliorates thyrotoxicosis. The acute effect is, however, due to inhibition of hormone release, and as discussed later there is little evidence that the Wolff-Chaikoff effect occurs in these patients.

1. Effects of Moderate Doses of Iodide

The response of the human thyroid to excess iodide is similar to that in rats. Acute administration of small or moderate doses of iodide does not change the percentage of thyroid uptake of concomitantly administered radioiodine, leading to a linear increase in absolute iodine uptake. With progressively larger doses of iodide, thyroid radioiodine uptake decreases, but the absolute iodine uptake calculated from thyroid radioiodine and serum or urinary iodide concentrations increases (NAGATAKI 1974).

During chronic iodide administration, thyroid radioiodine uptake decreases, but the absolute iodine uptake increases as the intake of iodide increases; serum T_4 and T_3 concentrations and degradation of thyroid hormone are not affected (Fig. 2, NAGATAKI et al. 1967).

As shown in Fig. 3 (NAGATAKI et al. 1970a), the normal thyroid usually utilizes iodide from two sources to produce thyroid hormone: transport iodide, which comes from serum iodide (external iodide), and iodide derived from the deiodination of iodotyrosine freed from thyroglobulin (internal iodide). Al-

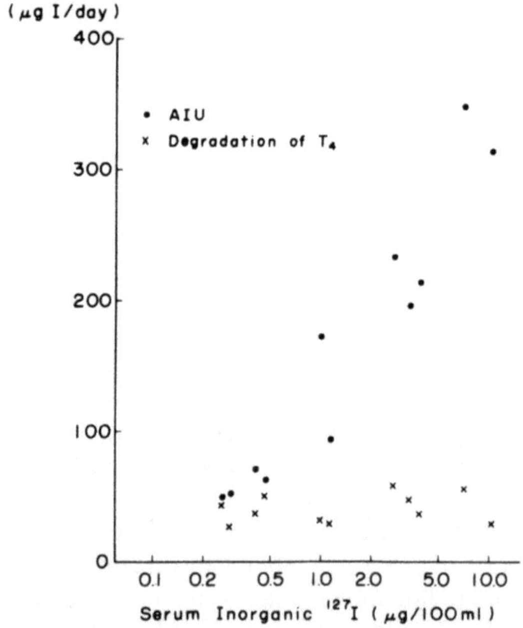

Fig. 2. Thyroidal absolute iodine uptake and degradation of thyroxine measured in the same subjects. Values for both are expressed as micrograms iodine per day. *Circles*, AIU calculated from thyroid clearance and serum inorganic ^{127}I. *Crosses*, degradation of thyroxine. (Adapted from NAGATAKI et al. 1967)

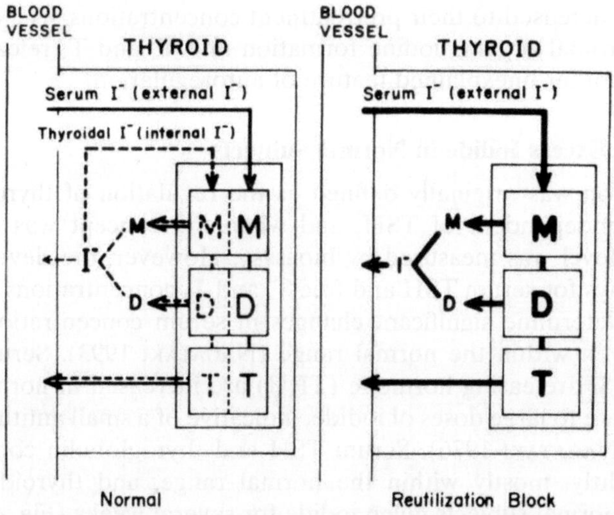

Fig. 3. Scheme of iodine metabolism in the normal thyroid and in the thyroid in which the reutilization of iodide is blocked. This blocking of the reutilization of iodide is the postulated result of iodide in excess given over a relatively long time. *M*, monoiodotyrosine; *D*, diiodotyrosine; *T*, triiodothyronine plus thyroxine. (Adapted from NAGATAKI et al. 1970a)

though these two iodide pools are reported to mix nearly completely, absolute iodine uptake, or thyroidal organic iodine formation, which is calculated from the incorporation of serum radioactive iodide into thyroidal organic iodine, represents only the organification of external iodide. If internal iodide is reutilized completely, the organification of internal iodide should be two to four times greater than the organification of external iodide, because the amount of iodotyrosine iodine freed from thyroglobulin is from two to four times greater than that transported from the blood and the release of iodotyrosine iodine should be roughly equal to the organification of external iodide in the steady state. If the organification of internal iodide could be decreased when that of external iodide is increased, then the organification of external iodide could be increased from two to four times without changing the total thyroidal iodination and hormone production.

In patients with Graves' hyperthyroidism, the absolute iodine uptake increases severalfold during iodide treatment. In one study, thyroid radioiodine uptake 24 h after injection averaged 20% of the dose, despite daily administration of 10 mg of iodide, and the proportion of inorganic radioiodine was only about 14% of total thyroidal content of radioiodine (NAGATAKI et al. 1970b). Thus, thyroidal organic iodine formation in Graves' hyperthyroidism is increased by iodide treatment despite a significant decrease in T_4 and T_3 secretion. Furthermore, thyroidal organic iodine formation did not change after escape from inhibition of hormone release when serum T_4 and T_3 concentrations had increased to their pretreatment concentrations. The dissociation between thyroidal organic iodine formation and T_4 and T_3 release in these patients is another unexplained feature of autoregulation.

2. Effects of Excess Iodide in Normal Subjects

Autoregulation was originally defined as the regulation of thyroidal iodine metabolism independent of TSH, and when the concept was established, serum TSH level was measured by bioassay. However, the development of sensitive assays for serum TSH and free T_4 and T_3 concentrations has made it possible to determine significant changes in serum concentrations of these hormones even within the normal range (NAGATAKI 1993). Serum TSH responses to TSH-releasing hormone (TRH) are increased in normal subjects given moderate to large doses of iodide, indicative of a small antithyroid effect (IKEDA and NAGATAKI 1976). Serum TSH and thyroglobulin concentrations increase slightly, mostly within the normal range, and thyroid gland size increases in normal subjects given iodide for several weeks (Fig. 4, NAMBA et al. 1993). In addition, the administration of as little as 0.75–1.5 mg iodide daily to normal subjects leads to unsustained increases in serum TSH concentrations and TSH responses to TRH (GARDNER et al. 1988; CHOW et al. 1991) (Table 1).

These results indicate that moderate doses of iodide have antithyroid actions, even if the action is sufficient to decrease serum free T_4 concentrations by only about 25%. Thus, many phenomena of autoregulation may in fact be dependent on TSH, and the definition of autoregulation may have to be reconsidered, because serum TSH concentrations are significantly increased by excess iodide, at least in normal human subjects.

Table 1. Effects of iodide on serum TSH levels (adapted from NAGATAKI 1993)

	Iodide dose	T_4	T_3	FT_4	TRH test	Basal TSH	
1974	190 mg/day 10 days	↓	↓		↑	↑	VAGENAKIS et al. (1974)
1975	50 mg/day 250 mg/day 13 days	→ ↑	↓ ↓		↑ ↑	↑ ↑	SABERI and UTIGER (1975)
1976	10 mg/day 1 week	→	→		↑	↑	IKEDA and NAGATAKI (1976)
1988	(0.5) 1.5, 4.5 mg/day 14 days	↓		↓	↑	↑	GARDNER et al. (1988)
1991	0.75 mg/day 28 days			↓		↑	CHOW et al. (1991)
1993	27 mg/day 28 days	→	→	↓		↑	NAMBA et al. (1993)

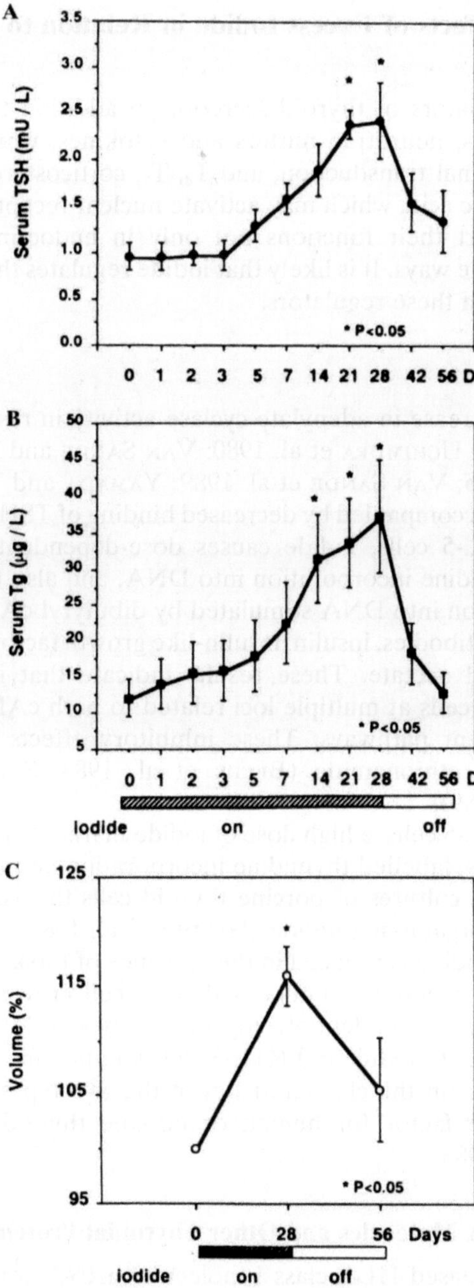

Fig. 4. Serum TSH (**A**), and Tg (**B**) concentrations and thyroid volume (**C**) measured by ultrasonography before, during and after administration of 27 mg iodine daily in ten normal subjects. *, $P < 0.05$ vs. value before iodide administration. (Adapted from NAMBA et al. 1993)

III. Intracellular Effects of Excess Iodide in Relation to Other Regulators

There are other regulators of thyroid secretion in addition to TSH. These include growth factors, neurotransmitters and cytokines, which may affect thyroid membrane signal transduction, and T_4, T_3, corticosteroids, estrogen, vitamin D_3 and retinoic acid, which may activate nuclear receptors in thyroid. These regulators exert their functions not only in endocrine but also in paracrine and autocrine ways. It is likely that iodide regulates thyroid function at least in part through these regulators.

1. Signal Transduction

Iodide inhibits the increase in adenylate cyclase activity in response to TSH (RAPOPORT et al. 1975; UCHIMURA et al. 1980; VAN SANDE and DUMONT 1973; VAN SANDE et al. 1975; VAN SANDE et al. 1989; YAMADA and TAKASU 1985). This inhibition is not accompanied by decreased binding of TSH to thyroid cell membranes. In FRTL-5 cells, iodide causes dose-dependent inhibition of TSH-stimulated thymidine incorporation into DNA, and also the increase in thymidine incorporation into DNA stimulated by dibutyryl cAMP, forskolin, thyroid-stimulating antibodies, insulin, insulin-like growth factor I (IGF-I) and tetradecanoyl phorbol acetate. These results indicate that iodide inhibits the growth of thyroid cells at multiple loci related to both cAMP-dependent and cAMP-independent pathways. These inhibitory effects are abolished by methimazole and ethionamide (BECKS et al. 1988; SAJI et al. 1988; TRAMONTANO et al. 1989).

In contrast to FRTL-5 cells, a high dose of iodide markedly increases c-*myc* mRNA concentrations, labelled thymidine incorporation and mitotic activity in primary suspension cultures of porcine thyroid cells that, unlike FRTL-5 cells, are capable of organifying iodide (HELDIN et al. 1987). Moreover, the stimulatory effect of iodide is reduced in the presence of forskolin, suggesting that an organic form of iodide stimulates thyroid cell growth and that the stimulatory pathway is independent of exogenous polypeptide growth factors. The different responses to iodide in FRTL-5 cells and porcine cells are probably due to differences in the characteristics of the two types of cells, since TSH is not a growth factor for human or porcine thyroid cells in vitro (WESTERMARK et al. 1983).

2. Expression of HLA Molecules and Other Thyroidal Proteins

Iodide markedly decreased HLA class I molecule mRNA concentrations in both TSH-treated and untreated FRTL-5 cells. The effect of iodide on class I gene expression reflects iodide autoregulation, and does not require TSH-induced iodide transport. Understanding the basis for iodide regulation of class I gene expression and the relationship of the action of iodide to the inhibitory effect of methimazole on class I gene transcription may contribute to understanding of the mechanism of iodide autoregulation as well as methimazole action (SAJI et al. 1992). The increase in thyroglobulin mRNA induced by methimazole is inhibited by iodide in FRTL-5 rat thyroid cells (ISOZAKI et al. 1991). Incubation with iodide decreases the cellular content of thyroid peroxidase (TPO) and TPO gene expression in primary cultures of human thyroid cells (YOKOYAMA et al. 1991) and TPO activity in porcine thyroid cells in primary culture (KASAI et al. 1992).

3. Protein Synthesis

Iodide-induced suppression of iodide transport in cat thyroid slices is inhibited by the addition of cycloheximide or puromycin. Two-dimensional column chromatography of iodoproteins of control and cycloheximide-treated tissue suggest that the iodide-induced effects are associated with reduced iodination of an 8- to 10-kDa soluble component of the thyroid gland (SHERWIN and PRINCE 1986). Iodide decreases amino acid transport in dog thyroid cells in primary culture. The effect is abolished by methimazole, and iodide does not inhibit amino acid transport in cells lacking a mechanism for iodide organification (FILETTI and RAPOPORT 1984).

4. Organic Iodinated Lipids

Iodinated lipids, including iodinated derivatives of arachidonic acid or purified iodolactone, inhibit radioactive uptake, basal and TSH-induced organification of radioiodine, and uridine incorporation into total RNA in calf thyroid slices (CHAZENBALK et al. 1984, 1988). These iodinated lipids decrease the action of iodide on thyroid growth and cAMP production in rat thyroid tissue in vitro. They also inhibit growth of FRTL-5 cells, which is not abolished by methimazole (PISAREV et al. 1992). In isolated porcine thyroid follicles, iodolactone inhibits, dose dependently, epidermal growth factor-induced thyroid cell growth, which is also not abolished by methimazole. Basal as well as TSH-induced cAMP formation, however, is not changed by iodolactone (DUGRILLION et al. 1990). Iodotyrosines (MIT or DIT) inhibit iodide transport and cAMP generation in the presence of TSH in porcine thyroid cell cultures, suggesting that iodotyrosines can serve as a negative control factor for thyroid hormone formation (NASU and SUGAWARA 1994).

5. Growth Factors

IGF-I and transforming growth factor-β (TGF-β) are both produced by thyroid follicular cells, and the inhibitory action of TGF-β on cell growth may involve a decrease in the thyroidal production of IGF-I. Furthermore, the attenuating action of iodide on cell growth may in part reflect increased production of TGF-β (BEERE et al. 1991; COWIN et al. 1992). Iodide induces TGF-β1 mRNA in sheep thyroid cells (YUASA et al. 1992), and TGF-β inhibits TSH-induced DNA synthesis and iodide uptake and DNA synthesis induced by IGF-I in FRTL-5 rat thyroid cells (PANG et al. 1992).

In human thyroid cells, iodide increases thyroidal TGF-β1 mRNA expression, and TGF-β1 almost completely abolishes cAMP-induced stimulation of iodide uptake and TPO synthesis (COWIN and BIDEY 1994; TATON et al. 1993). These results emphasize the potentially major role of TGF-β1 as a local modulator of thyroid functions.

Endothelin (ET)-1 is a potent vasoconstrictive substance and immunoreactive ET-1 and ET-1 mRNA are expressed in porcine thyroid cells. Iodide increases ET-1 mRNA expression and the effect of iodide is attenuated by methimazole, indicating that ET-1 gene expression is induced by organified iodine compounds in thyroid cells in a manner very similar to the inhibitory actions of iodide on thyroid cell function. ET-1 produced by thyroid cells may be involved in autoregulation including thyroid blood flow (ISOZAKI et al. 1993). Iodine levels in the thyroid are inversely related to blood flow.

IV. Mechanism of Autoregulation

1. Acute Inhibitory Effect (Wolff-Chaikoff Effect)

Despite the numerous reports on the effects of excess iodide on thyroid gland, little is known about the mechanism of autoregulation. Various effects of excess iodide are abolished by thiocyanate or by methimazole (RABEN 1949; HELDIN et al. 1987). For example, methimazole inhibits the effects of excess iodide on expression of the mRNAs for c-*myc* and TGF-β1 (FILETTI and RAPOPORT 1984; COWIN et al. 1992). It also inhibits the effects of iodide on amino acid transport, cell toxicity (MANY et al. 1992) and inhibition of H_2O_2 production (CORVILAIN et al. 1991), but not the expression of HLA class I molecules by excess iodide (SAJI et al. 1992). Hence, production of one or more organic iodine compounds has been proposed to be important in autoregulation (BECKS et al. 1987; BURKE 1970; CORVILAIN et al. 1988; GROLLMAN et al. 1986; PRICE and SHERWIN 1986).

In the acute inhibitory effect of excess iodide, inhibition of organification of intrathyroidal iodide is a fundamental phenomenon. TPO-catalysed iodination requires the peroxidase, an acceptor (protein or free tyrosine), iodide, and H_2O_2.

It was originally proposed that the acute inhibitory effect of excess iodide was due to formation of I_2 preference to iodination of protein (TAUROG 1970).

In dog thyroid slices, H_2O_2 generation is stimulated by TSH and by carbamylcholine. The action of carbamylcholine is mimicked by ionomycin and by phorbol myristate ester, suggesting that the action is mediated by signals generated by the Ca^{2+}/phosphatidyl-inositol cascade. Preincubation of dog thyroid slices with excess iodide greatly inhibits iodide organification and H_2O_2 generation stimulated by TSH and by carbamylcholine. While inhibition of H_2O_2 generation may be the cause of the acute inhibitory effect, the nature of the organic iodine compound that inhibits H_2O_2 generation is unknown (CORVILAIN et al. 1988). Monoamine oxidase (MAO) in the thyroid has been postulated to play a role in the biosynthesis of thyroid hormone because of its ability to generate hydrogen peroxide, but MAO inhibitor was found to inhibit thyroid iodide transport in rats (CABANILLAS et al. 1994).

Iodinated phospholipids and iodinated derivatives of arachidonic acid or iodolactone inhibit organification of iodide in both calf thyroid slices and homogenates, whereas arachidonic acid has no such effect (CHAZENBALK et al. 1984, 1988). It is possible that iodinated arachidonic acid plays an important role in the acute inhibitory effect of excess iodide.

2. Mechanism of Adaptation

Decreased iodide transport is an important mechanism in the adaptation to or escape from the acute inhibitory effect of iodide. Iodinated arachidonic acid or iodolactone is one of the iodinated compounds that is proposed to reduce iodide transport. Iodinated arachidonic acid may decrease iodide transport, but it is hard to see how the same substance could inhibit organification of iodide on the one hand and mediate the adaptation by which organification of iodide increases in response to chronic iodide administration on the other. However, the changes in iodide transport in response to excess iodide could be due mainly to changes in sodium transport and not to the production of an organic iodine compound (SAITO et al. 1989).

The amounts of iodide taken up by the thyroid and incorporated into iodoamino acids and iodothyronines differ greatly according to dietary iodide intake, but the amount of T_4 and T_3 released from the thyroid is remarkably constant in both humans and animals. Inhibition of hormone release by iodide is a well-known phenomenon in Graves' disease and other forms of hyperthyroidism, and the inhibitory effect of excess iodide on thyroid hormone secretion has been demonstrated in sheep thyroid cell cultures (NAGATAKI 1974). Preferential inhibition of hormone secretion, however, cannot explain the balance between hormone formation and hormone release unless thyroid gland has an almost infinite capacity to store thyroid hormones.

The acute Wolff-Chaikoff effect, the escape from this effect, and the increased thyroidal iodide uptake in hypophysectomized rats fed a low iodine diet are the typical autoregulations in animals. In contrast, constant hormone release regardless of the amount of iodide taken up by the thyroid and inhibition of hormone release from the thyroid by iodide are the important autoregulatory effects in humans. It is still, however, not clear whether these types of autoregulation share the same mechanism or are due to different mechanisms.

Most recent studies of autoregulation have been performed in vitro using thyroid slices, primary cell cultures and cell lines from different species. Although they clearly showed the effects of iodine on certain functions, the results are not compatible with the mechanism of autoregulation defined from in vivo studies (PRICE and SHERWIN 1986; PENEL et al. 1987; TAKASU et al. 1985).

3. Species Differences in Autoregulation

Species differences in thyroid sensitivity to the acute inhibitory effect of iodide and escape from the inhibitory effect of iodide have been demonstrated in many studies. The rarity of hypothyroidism and goitre formation in humans despite exposure of many patients to excess iodide suggests that the human thyroid can easily escape from the inhibitory effect of iodide. This also explains the difficulty in producing iodide goitre in rats. In contrast to humans and rats, long-term iodide feeding leads to colloid goitre in mice despite functional adaptation to iodide excess. Iodide feeding to hens leads to colloid goitre in their chicks, and guinea pigs treated with excess iodide show signs of histological activation of the thyroid. These variations in iodide effects in different species make it difficult to propose a uniform mechanism for autoregulation.

4. Role of TSH in Autoregulation

Although serum or medium TSH levels are constant, responses of iodine metabolism to TSH can be regulated by iodide through many other regulators. Furthermore, serum TSH levels are significantly changed by excess iodide, at least in normal human subjects. Many phenomena of autoregulation may be dependent on TSH and the definition of autoregulation may have to be reconsidered.

References

Becks GP, Eggo MC, Burrow GN (1988) Organic iodine inhibits deoxyribonucleic acid synthesis and growth in FRTL-5 thyroid cells. Endocrinology 123:545–551

Becks GP, Eggo MC, Burrow GN (1987) Regulation of differentiated thyroid function by iodide: preferential inhibitory effect of excess iodide on thyroid hormone secretion in sheep thyroid cell cultures. Endocrinology 120:2569–2575

Beere HM, Soden J, Tomlinson S, Bidey SP (1991) Insulin-like growth factor-I production and action in porcine thyroid follicular cells in monolayer: regulation by transforming growth factor-β. J Endocrinol 130:3–9

Braverman LE, Ingbar SH (1963) Changes in thyroidal function during adaptation to large doses of iodide. J Clin Invest 42:1216–1231

Bray GA (1968) Increased sensitivity of the thyroid in iodine-depleted rats to the goitrogenic effect of thyrotropin. J Clin Invest 47:1640–1647

Burke G (1970) Effects of iodide on thyroid stimulation. J Clin Endocrinol 30:76–84

Cabanillas AM, Masini-Repiso AM, Costamagna ME (1994) Thyroid iodide transport is reduced by administration of monoamine oxidase A inhibitors to rats. J Endocrinol 143:303–308

Carrasco N (1993) Iodine transport in the thyroid gland. Biochem Biophys Acta 1154:65–82

Chapman A (1941) The relation of the thyroid and pituitary glands to iodine metabolism. J Endocrinol 29:680–685

Chazenbalk GD, Valsecchi RM, Krawiec L, Burton G, Juvenal GJ, Monteagudo E, Chester HA, Pisalev MA (1988) Thyroid autoregulation: inhibitory effects of iodinated derivatives of arachidonic acid on iodine metabolism. Prostaglandins 36:163

Chazenbalk GD, Pisarev MA, Krawiec L, Juvenal GJ, Burton G, Vulsecchi RM (1984) In vitro inhibitory effects of an iodinated derivative of arachidonic acid on calf thyroid. Acta Physiol Pharmacol Latinoam 34:367
Chow CC, Phillips DIW, Lazarus JH, Parkes AB (1991) Effect of low dose iodide supplementation on thyroid function in potentially susceptible subjects: are dietary iodide levels in Britain acceptable? Clin Endocrinol 34:413–416
Corvilain B, Van Sande J, Laurent E, Dumont JE (1991) The H_2O_2-generating system modulates protein iodination and the activity of the pentose phosphate pathway in dog thyroid. Endocrinology 128:779–785
Corvilain B, Van Sande J, Dumont JE (1988) Inhibition by iodide of iodide binding to proteins: the "Wolff-Chaikoff" effect is caused by inhibition of H_2O_2 generation. Biochem Biophys Res Commun 154:1287–1292
Cowin AJ, Bidey SP (1994) Transforming growth factor-β1 synthesis in human thyroid follicular cells: differential effects of iodide and plasminogen on the production of latent and active peptide forms. J Endocrinol 141:183–190
Cowin AJ, Davis JRE, Bidey SP (1992) Transforming growth factor-β1 production in porcine thyroid follicular cells: regulation by intrathyroidal organic iodine. J Mol Endocrinol 9:197–205
Dai G, Levy O, Carrasco N (1996) Cloning and characterization of the thyroid iodide transporter. Nature 379:458–460
Dugrillion A, Bechtner G, Uedelhoven WM, Weber PC, Gärtner R (1990) Evidence that an iodolactone mediates the inhibitory effect of iodide on thyroid cell proliferation but not on adenosine 3′, 5′-monophosphate formation. Endocrinology 127:337–343
Dumont JE, Vassart G (1995) Thyroid regulation. In: DeGroot LJ (ed) Endocrinology, 3rd edn. Saunders, Philadelphia, p 543
Filetti S, Rapoport B (1984) Autoregulation by iodine of thyroid protein synthesis: influence of iodine on amino acid transport in cultured thyroid cells. Endocrinology 114:1379–1385
Galton VA, Pitt-Rivers R (1959) The effect of excessive iodine on the thyroid of the rat. Endocrinology 64:835–839
Gardner DF, Centor RM, Utiger RD (1988) Effects of low dose oral iodide supplementation on thyroid function in normal men. Clin Endocrinol 28:283–288
Gerard C, Rigot V, Penel C (1994) Chloride channel blockers inhibit the Na^+/I^- symporter in thyroid follicles in culture. Biochem Biophys Res Comm 204:1265–1271
Grollman E, Smolar A, Ommaya A, Tombaccini D, Santisteban P (1986) Iodine suppression of iodine uptake in FRTL-5 thyroid cells. Endocrinology 118:2477–2482
Halmi NS (1961) Thyroidal iodide transport. Vitam Horm 19:133–163
Halmi NS, Spirtos BN (1955) Analysis of the modifying effect of dietary iodine levels on the thyroidal response of hypophysectomized rats to thyrotropin. Endocrinology 56:157–160
Heldin NE, Karlsson FA, Westermark B (1987) A growth stimulatory effect of iodide is suggested by its effect on c-myc messenger ribonucleic acid levels, [^{3}H]thymidine incorporation, and mitotic activity of porcine follicular cells in suspension culture. Endocrinology 121:757–764
Ikeda H, Nagataki S (1976) Augmentation of thyrotropin responses to thyrotropin-releasing hormone following inorganic iodide. Endocrinol Jpn 23:431–436
Isozaki O, Tsushima T, Emoto N, Saji M, Tsuchiya Y, Demura H, Sato Y, Shizume K, Kimura S, Kohn LN (1991) Methimazole regulation of thyroglobulin biosynthesis and gene transcription in rat FRTL-5 thyroid cells. Endocrinology 128:3113–3121
Isozaki O, Tsushima T, Miyakawa M, Emoto N, Demura H, Sato Y, Shizume K, Arai M (1993) Iodine regulation of endothelin-1 gene expression in cultured porcine thyroid cells: possible involvement in autoregulation of the thyroid. Thyroid 3:239–244

Kaminsky SM, Levy O, Salvador C, Dai G, Carrasco N (1994) Na^+/I^- symport activity is present in membrane vesicles from thyrotropin-deprived non-I^--transporting cultured thyroid cells. Proc Natl Acad Sci USA 91:3789–3793

Kasai K, Yamaguchi F, Hosoya T, Ichimura K, Banba N, Emoto T, Hiraiwa M, Hishinuma A, Hattori Y, Shimoda S (1992) Effects of inorganic iodide, epidermal growth factor and phorbol ester on hormone synthesis by porcine thyroid follicles cultured in suspension. Life Sci 51:1095–1103

Many MC, Mestdagh C, Van Den Hove MF, Denef JF (1992) In vitro study of acute toxic effects of high iodide doses in human thyroid follicles. Endocrinology 131:621–630

Morton ME, Chaikoff IL, Rosenfeld S (1944) Inhibiting effect of inorganic iodide on the formation in vitro of thyroxine and diiodotyrosine by surviving thyroid tissue. J Biol Chem 154:381–387

Nagataki S (1974) Effect of excess quantities of iodide. In: Greer MA, Solomon DH (eds) Handbook of physiology, Sect 7. Endocrinology 3. American Physiological Society, Washington DC, p 329

Nagataki S (1993) Autoregulation of thyroid function by iodide. In: Delange F, Dunn JT, Glinoer D (eds) Iodine deficiency in Europe: a continuing concern. Plenum, New York, p 43

Nagataki S, Ingbar SH (1964) Relation between qualitative and quantitative alterations in thyroid hormone synthesis induced by varying doses of iodide. Endocrinology 74:731–736

Nagataki S, Shizume K, Nakao K (1970a) Alternations in intrathyroidal iodine metabolism in response to chronic iodine administration. Endocrinology 87:1218–1227

Nagataki S, Shizume K, Nakao K (1970b) Effect of iodide on thyroidal iodine turnover in hyperthyroid subjects. J Clin Endocrinol Metab 30:469–478

Nagataki S, Shizume K, Nakao K (1967) Thyroid function in chronic excess iodide ingestion: comparison of thyroidal absolute iodine uptake and degradation of thyroxine in euthyroid Japanese subjects. J Clin Endocrinol Metab 27:638–647

Namba H, Yamashita S, Kimura H, Yokoyama N, Usa T, Otsuru A, Izumi M, Nagataki S (1993) Evidence of thyroid volume increase in normal subjects receiving excess iodide. J Clin Endocrinol Metab 76:605–608

Nasu M, Sugawara M (1994) Exogenous free iodotyrosine inhibits iodide transport through the sequential intracellular events. Eur J Endocrinol 130:601–607

Pang X-P, Park M, Hershman JM (1992) Transforming growth factor-β blocks protein kinase-A-mediated iodide transport and protein kinase-C-mediated DNA synthesis in FRTL-5 rat thyroid cells. Endocrinology 131:45–50

Penel C, Rognoni JB, Bastiani P (1987) Thyroid autoregulation: impact on thyroid structure and function in rats. Am J Physiol 253:165–172

Pisarev MA (1985) Thyroid autoregulation. J Endocrinol Invest 8:475–484

Pisarev MA, Bocanera LV, Chester HA, Kleiman DL, Juvenal GJ, Pregliasco LB, Krawiec L (1992) Effect of iodoarachidonates on thyroid FRTL-5 cell growth. Horm Metab Res 24:558–561

Price DJ, Sherwin JR (1986) Autoregulation of iodide transport in the rabbit: absence of autoregulation in fetal tissue and comparison of maternal and fetal thyroid iodination products. Endocrinology 119:2547–2552

Raben MS (1949) The paradoxical effects of thiocyanate and of thyrotropin on the organic binding of iodine by the thyroid in the presence of large amounts of iodide. Endocrinology 45:296–304

Rapoport B, Niepomniszcze H, Bigazze M, Hati R, DeGroot LJ (1972) Studies on the pathogenesis of poor thyroglobulin iodination in non-toxic multinodular goiter. J Clin Endocrinol Metab 34:822–830

Rapoport B, West MN, Ingbar SH (1975) Inhibitory effect of dietary iodine on the thyroid adenylate cyclase response to thyrotropin in the hypophysectomized rat. J Clin Invest 56:516–519

Saberi M, Utiger RD (1975) Augmentation of thyrotropin response to thyrotropin-releasing hormone following small decreases in serum thyroid hormone concentrations. J Clin Endocrinol Metab 46:435–441

Saito K, Yamamoto K, Nagayama I, Uemura J, Kuzuya T (1989) Effect of internally loaded iodide, thiocyanate, and perchlorate on sodium-dependent iodide uptake by phospholipid vesicles reconstituted with thyroid plasma membranes: iodide counterflow mediated by the iodide transport carrier. J Biochem 105:790–793

Saji M, Isozaki O, Tsushima T, Arai M, Miyakawa M, Ohba Y, Tsuchiya Y, Sano T, Shizume K (1988) The inhibitory effect of iodide on growth of rat thyroid (FRTL-5) cells. Acta Endocrinol (Copenh) 119:145–151

Saji M, Moriarty J, Ban T, Singer DS, Kohn LD (1992) Major histocompatibility complex class I gene expression in rat thyroid cells is regulated by hormones, methimazole, and iodide as well as interferon. J Clin Endocrinol Metab 75: 871–878

Sherwin JR, Prince DJ (1986) Autoregulation of thyroid iodide transport: evidence for the mediation of protein synthesis in iodide-induced suppression of iodide transport. Endocrinology 119:2553–2559

Takasu N, Honda Y, Kawaoi A, Shimizu Y, Yamada T (1985) Effects of iodide on thyroid follicle structure and electrophysiological potentials of culture thyroid cells. Endocrinology 117:71–76

Taton M, Lamy F, Roger PP, Dumont JE (1993) General inhibition by transforming growth factor β1 of thyrotropin and cAMP responses in human thyroid cells in primary culture. Mol Cel Endocrinol 95:13–21

Taurog A (1970) Thyroid peroxidase and thyroxine biosynthesis. Recent Prog Horm Res 26:189–247

Tramontano D, Veneziani BM, Lombardi A, Villone G, Ingbar SH (1989) Iodine inhibits the proliferation of rat thyroid cells in culture. Endocrinology 125:984–992

Uchimura H, Chiu SC, Kuzuya N, Ikeda H, Ito K, Nagataki S (1980) Effect of iodine enrichment in vitro on the adenylate cyclase-adenosine 3′, 5′ monophosphate system in thyroid glands from normal subjects and patients with Graves' disease. J Clin Endocrinol Metab 50:1066–1070

Vagenakis AG, Rapoport B, Azizi F, Portnay GI, Braverman LE, Ingbar SH (1974) Hyperresponse to thyrotropin-releasing hormone accompanying small decreases in serum thyroid hormone concentrations. J Clin Invest 54:913–918

Van Sande J, Dumont JE (1973) Effects of thyrotropin, prostaglandin E_1 and iodide on cyclic 3′, 5′-AMP concentration in dog thyroid slices. Biochim Biophys Acta 313:320–326

Van Sande J, Lefort A, Beebe S, Roger P, Parret J, Corbin J, Dumont JE (1989) Pairs of cyclic AMP analogs, that are specifically synergistic for type I and type II cAMP-dependent protein kinase, mimic thyrotropin effects on the function, differentiation expression and mitogenesis of dog thyroid cells. Eur J Biochem 183:699–708

Van Sande J, Grenier G, Willems C, Dumont JE (1975) Inhibition by iodide of the activation of the thyroid cyclic 3′, 5′-AMP system. Endocrinology 96:781–786

Vilijin F, Carrasco N (1989) Expression of the thyroid sodium/iodine symporter in Xenopus laevis oocytes. J Biol Chem 264:11901–11903

Westermark K, Karlsson FA, Westermark B (1983) Epidermal growth factor modulates thyroid growth and function in culture. Endocrinology 112:1680–1686

Wolff J, Chaikoff IL (1948) Plasma inorganic iodide as a homeostatic regulator of thyroid function. J Biol Chem 174:555–564

Wolff J, Chaikoff IL, Goldberg RC, Meier JR (1949) The temporary nature of the inhibitory action of excess iodide on organic iodine synthesis in the normal thyroid. Endocrinology 45:504–513

Yamada T, Takasu N (1985) Effects of excess iodide on thyroid hormone synthesis and release. In: Hall R, Kobberling J (eds) Thyroid disorders associated with iodine deficiencies and excess. Raven, New York, p 319

Yokoyama N, Tominaga T, Eishima K, Izumi M (1991) Effect of iodide on human thyroid peroxidase in thyroid cells. In: Gordon A, Gross J, Hennemann G (eds) Progress in thyroid research. Balkema, Rotterdam, p 483
Young RL, Harvey WC, Mazzaferri EL, Reynolds JC, Hamilton CR Jr. (1975) Thyroid-stimulating hormone levels in idiopathic euthyroid goiter. J Clin Endocrinol Metab 41:21–26
Yuasa R, Eggo MC, Meinkoth J, Dillmann WH, Burrow GN (1992) Iodide induces transforming growth factor beta$_1$ (TGF-β_1) mRNA in sheep thyroid cells. Thyroid 2:141–145

CHAPTER 8

Antithyroid Drugs: Their Mechanism of Action and Clinical Use

M. EL SHEIKH and A.M. MCGREGOR

A. Introduction

The treatment of hyperthyroidism is directed towards reducing thyroid hormone production and release from thyroid follicular cells. The mainstay of treatment is the use of antithyroid drugs (COOPER 1984), though cure of the disease often relies on either surgical treatment by partial thyroidectomy or the use of radioactive iodine (FRANKLYN 1994). Studies in the early 1940s demonstrated that the treatment of rats with thiourea or sulphaguanidine led to goitre formation, with subsequent studies demonstrating that these goitres resulted from the inhibition of thyroid hormone production, and the consequent stimulation of thyroid gland growth by the rise in thyroid-stimulating hormone (TSH) secretion. Based on these initial observations, Astwood conducted clinical trials with these agents which demonstrated that they were effective in controlling hyperthyroidism in man (ASTWOOD 1943). The two main groups of antithyroid drugs (known collectively as thionamides) (Fig. 1) can be divided into the thiouracils, which have a six-membered ring, with propylthiouracil (6-propyl-2-thiouracil, PTU) being the only compound of this group in current clinical use, and the imidazoles, which have five-membered rings; the drugs in current clinical use from this group are methimazole (1-methyl-2-mercaptoimidazole, MMI) and carbimazole (1-methyl-2-thio-3-carbethoxy-imidazole, CBZ). CBZ is rapidly metabolised to MMI following ingestion.

B. Hyperthyroidism

A number of different situations lead to the development of hyperthyroidism. In areas of the world where iodine intake is adequate, over 75% of the patients presenting with hyperthyroidism to endocrine clinics do so because of underlying Graves' disease. In the majority of the remaining patients, hyperthyroidism is usually attributable to a toxic multinodular goitre or to a solitary toxic adenoma (hot nodules). The remaining causes of hyperthyroidism are exceedingly rare. Since the cause of the hyperthyroidism does influence the subsequent course of management, correct diagnosis is important. Clinical assessment of the thyroid with the demonstration of diffuse enlargement coupled with extrathyroidal manifestations, most commonly in women and

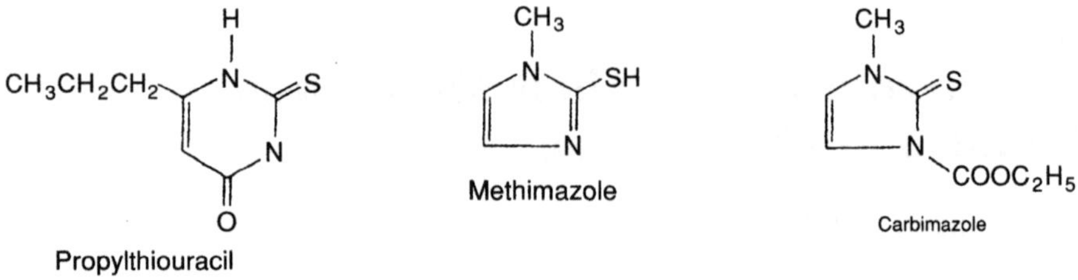

Fig. 1. The thioureylenes; structures of the commonly used antithyroid drugs. The six-membered ring thiouracils (e.g. propylthiouracil) and the five-membered ring imidazoles (e.g. methimazole and carbimazole) both contain the thioureylene moiety within the ring structure and are known collectively as thionamides

often with a family history of autoimmune thyroid disease, makes the diagnosis of Graves' disease exceedingly likely. This can be confirmed by diffuse uptake of isotope on a thyroid scan and by the presence of thyroid autoantibodies. If on clinical grounds the diagnosis of a multinodular or solitary nodule cannot be confidently made, then again an isotope scan will demonstrate the presence of a multinodular goitre or a solitary toxic nodule. In patients with solitary toxic adenomata the treatment of choice is radioactive iodine and there is no role for antithyroid drugs. In patients with a toxic multinodular goitre, our own preference again is to use radioactive iodine except in situations where (1) the size of the goitre is a cause for concern, in which case antithyroid medication is used to establish euthyroidism prior to partial thyroidectomy, or (2) in patients with severe disease in whom drugs may be indicated prior to radioiodine. In our own clinic, therefore, the main role for antithyroid drugs is in the treatment of hyperthyroid Graves' disease, and it is in this context that these drugs are considered in this chapter.

C. Pharmacokinetics

Propylthiouracil (PTU) is well absorbed after oral administration, with peak serum levels being achieved about 60 min after ingestion (Table 1). Its serum half-life is approximately 60–120 min, and is not affected by hyperthyroidism, or by hepatic or renal disease. The majority of the drug is bound to albumin. After its breakdown into its native metabolites by the liver it is excreted by the kidneys. The duration of action is between 12 and 24 h and this depends largely on its intrathyroidal concentration rather than on serum levels.

MMI and CBZ are also completely absorbed from the gut, with peak serum levels being achieved approximately 60–120 min after ingestion (Table 1). Their serum half-life ranges between 6 and 8 h and these are again not influenced by hyperthyroidism or renal disease, but, in contrast to PTU, the half-life of these drugs is increased by severe liver disease. Negligible amounts of MMI are protein bound and its inactive metabolites are excreted by the kidneys. The duration of action of MMI depends on the intrathyroidal drug

Table 1. Pharmacology of antithyroid drugs

	Propylthiouracil	Methimazole
Absorption	Rapid	Rapid
Bioavailability	≈100%	≈100%
Peak serum level (dose related)	60 min	60–120 min
Serum protein binding	>75%	Nil
Serum half-life	60–120 min	6–8 h
Intrathyroidal concentrations	Unknown	5×10^{-5} mol/l (in hyperthyroid phase)
Intrathyroidal turnover	Moderate	Slow
Metabolism in illness (influence on drug half-life)		
Hyperthyroidism	Nil	Nil
Renal	Nil	Nil
Liver	Nil	Prolonged
Excretion	Renal	Renal
Crosses placenta and breast epithelium	Minimal	Yes (not protein bound)
Potency	1	>10 (more potent inhibitor of thyroid peroxidase)
Duration of action	12–24 h	>24 h (can be given once daily)

levels achieved and these are much higher than in serum with a much slower turnover and, therefore, a duration of action which is greater than 24 h.

D. Mechanism of Action

In restoring euthyroidism and inducing remission in patients with hyperthyroid Graves' disease, the antithyroid drugs act predominantly to inhibit the crucial thyroid follicular cell enzyme thyroid peroxidase (TPO), thus interfering with thyroid hormone biosynthesis (Taurog 1991). In addition, in patients with Graves' disease, they may influence the autoimmune response and in so doing may contribute to controlling the disease by immunosuppression (Ratanachaiyavong and McGregor 1985).

I. Inhibition of TPO

1. Thyroid Hormone Synthesis

Thyroglobulin (TG), the precursor of thyroid hormones, is a large, tyrosine-containing glycoprotein. Following transcription and mRNA translation, the TG is glycosylated and thence packaged in the Golgi apparatus of the thyroid follicular cell into exocytotic vesicles. These vesicles fuse with the follicular cell apical membrane and so release TG into the follicular lumen. Iodination of the tyrosine residues of TG takes place at this apical surface. Iodide is actively transported (trapped) from the extracellular fluid into the follicular cell. Within the cell this inorganic iodide is incorporated into the tyrosine residues of TG (organified). This process is mediated by TPO – a membrane-bound haemoprotein, in the presence of hydrogen peroxide (H_2O_2). The iodinated tyrosine residues of TG combine (couple) to form iodothyronines so that two diiodotyrosines (DIT) combine to form thyroxine (T_4), and a DIT molecule coupled with a monoiodotyrosine (MIT) forms triiodothyronine (T_3). As well as being important in the initial formation of iodotyrosines, TPO is essential for the coupling process. Thyroid peroxidase therefore catalyses all steps in the synthesis of T_3 and T_4.

2. Drug Action

The antithyroid drugs do not inhibit iodide transport (nor do they block the release of preformed, stored thyroid hormone). Instead, like iodide, they are actively trapped by the thyroid follicular cell. Their roles in inhibiting thyroid hormone synthesis depend on their ability to influence TPO-mediated iodine oxidation and organification and iodothyronine coupling (Taurog 1991). In the presence of iodine, the drugs compete with tyrosyl residues of TG for oxidised iodine, thus diverting oxidised iodine away from TG (Taurog and Dorris 1989). Ultimately the drugs themselves are oxidised and degraded. The effect of thionamides is dependent on their concentration and on the concentration of iodine. At low drug concentration, inhibition of TPO is transient and reversible. In contrast at high drug concentrations their iodination becomes irreversible. The converse is true in the context of iodide concentration: irreversible inhibition of hormone biosynthesis as a result of TPO inactivation by antithyroid drugs is counteracted by high iodine concentrations. This may explain why in countries with a high dietary iodine intake antithyroid drugs are less effective in establishing and maintaining euthyroidism, and relapse following cessation of these drugs is much more common.

Small amounts of antithyroid drugs bind to TG following oxidation thus altering its structure and function. The thionamides may also inhibit TG synthesis and thyroid follicular cell growth. Additionally, PTU but not CBZ or MMI block the peripheral conversion of T_4 to T_3.

II. Immunological Effects

1. Graves' Disease

Hyperthyroid Graves' disease is the commonest form of hyperthyroidism in areas of the world where iodine intake is adequate. The disease is an organ-specific autoimmune disease and as such occurs commonly in association with other members of this group of diseases and in families in which there is commonly a history of Graves' disease or of an organ-specific autoimmune disease. The disease is due to autoantibodies which, by binding to the thyroid follicular cell basement membrane thyrotropin (TSH) receptor, stimulate thyroid cell function by activation of the thyroid follicular cell adenylate cyclase system, which is linked to the TSH receptor (WEETMAN and MCGREGOR 1994). The disease is more common in women, particularly in the childbearing years, and may present for the first time following pregnancy. Characteristically because of the immunological changes that occur during pregnancy, the disease tends to improve at this time though exacerbation is likely in the postpartum period. Untreated disease does, in some individuals, remit spontaneously but observations of the natural history of the disease prior to the availability of appropriate therapies provided clear evidence of significant morbidity and even mortality when untreated. On these grounds the advice to patients is that their disease should be controlled and in Europe the first line of treatment for controlling the disease is still the antithyroid drugs.

2. Drug Action

a) Graves' Disease

In patients with hyperthyroid Graves' disease treated with antithyroid drugs, levels of TSH receptor antibody (but not non-thyroidal autoantibodies, MCGREGOR et al. 1982) can be shown to decline as the disease is treated, whether or not the patient is maintained euthyroid by the addition of thyroxine supplementation (MCGREGOR et al. 1980). Other indirect and fairly nonspecific markers of the aberrant autoimmune response in Graves' disease such as the assessment of circulating levels of T-lymphocyte subsets show clearly that in response to antithyroid drugs there is a return to normal levels of the elevated levels of activated T cells and depressed levels of cytotoxic-suppressor cells demonstrable prior to treatment (LUDGATE et al. 1984; TÖTTERMAN et al. 1987). Additionally, a well-established literature, which long pre-dates these observations, demonstrates that in patients treated with antithyroid drugs there is a significant diminution of the intrathyroidal lymphocyte concentration (YOUNG et al. 1976). A recent study, however (PASCHKE et al. 1995), has failed to confirm this observation.

b) Experimental Studies

No animal models of Graves' disease exist but in animal models of destructive thyroiditis, in which the animals have been maintained euthyroid with T_4, the administration of antithyroid drugs has been shown to reduce the levels of circulating autoantibodies as well as the inflammatory infiltrate in their thyroid glands (RENNIE et al. 1983; HASSMAN et al. 1985). In vitro studies have confirmed the in vivo studies, demonstrating that antithyroid drugs do indeed lead to the inhibition of autoantibody production by lymphocytes at concentrations capable of being achieved within the thyroid gland of patients with hyperthyroid Graves' disease. These effects occur independently of changes in thyroid hormone concentrations within the medium in which the cells are cultured (WEETMAN et al. 1984b). One explanation for this effect, based on considerable data, suggests that antithyroid drugs may be inhibiting the peroxidase enzyme systems of antigen-presenting cells and thus inhibit the presentation of antigens to lymphocytes. The mechanism for this effect may well rely on the ability of MMI to inhibit the generation of oxygen radicals in antigen-presenting cells, since these drugs are potent oxygen radical scavengers (WEETMAN et al. 1984a). There is no evidence to support the view that these drugs interfere with antigen presentation by thyrocytes themselves. An alternative or additional immunological explanation for the immunosuppressive effects of these drugs is the possibility of a direct effect on the thyroid (WEETMAN et al. 1984b; VOLPÉ et al. 1986). In particular, antithryroid drugs inhibit the release of the inflammatory mediators such as reactive oxygen metabolites, prostaglandin E_2 and interleukin-1α and interleukin-6 from thyroid cells themselves (WEETMAN 1992; WEETMAN et al. 1992b). The net effect of the reduction in these inflammatory mediators might be to reduce the lymphocytic infiltrate of the thyroid gland itself and as a result perhaps reduce autoantibody levels.

Extensive, reproducible and consistent data demonstrate without doubt that antithyroid drugs are immunosuppressive. What remains to be established is how important this effect is in contributing to the control of the hyperthyroidism of Graves' disease.

E. Clinical Use

I. Indications

Antithyroid drugs are indicated in situations in which hyperthyroidism results from the overproduction of thyroid hormone in which the aetiology of the disease leading to hyperfunction resides within the thyroid. They have little role to play in the management of the transient hyperthyroidism of destructive thyroiditis, in iodine-induced hyperthyroidism or in factitious hyperthyroidism due to the ingestion of thyroid hormone. In all of these settings the uptake of radioiodine into the thyroid on a thyroid scan will be suppressed. As has been suggested earlier, in the authors' clinical practice antithyroid drugs are the treatment of choice for the first episode of hyperthyroidism due to Graves' disease but radioactive iodine therapy is seen as being preferable in patients with toxic solitary or multinodular goitres. Since over 75% of patients presenting with hyperthyroidism do so because of Graves' disease, the use of antithyroid drug medication is common. Special consideration needs to be given to the use of these drugs in relation to pregnancy, when used in conjunction with radioactive iodine and in the setting of severe hyperthyroidism (thyroid storm), and these issues are considered in subsequent sections.

II. Adverse Effects

Minor adverse events are reported in 5%–10% of the population of patients taking antithyroid medication (Table 2). Most commonly this includes pruritus with or without a rash. Arthralgia and a low-grade fever may also develop. These effects are considered to be due to an allergic reaction to the antithyroid drug and usually occur shortly after the onset of treatment. Two alternative approaches to the management of this situation are possible; either the patient can be advised to persevere with the drug since the symptoms usually abate with time, or if the symptoms are intolerable and not responsive to local treatment then it is worth substituting CBZ for PTU or vice versa. If similar reactions develop with the second preparation there is no option but to consider radioiodine.

The most serious side effect is agranulocytosis, which is rare, being reported in less than 0.25% of patients taking antithyroid medication. It is an idiosyncratic reaction but slightly more common with high-dose therapy. The incidence is no different whether CBZ or PTU are used. It can occur at any time during the treatment course but is much more likely in the first 3 months after the initiation of treatment and seems to be more common in older patients. The exact pathogenesis remains unknown but may be due to lymphocyte sensitisation and subsequent antibody production directed against neutrophils. Agranulocytosis is defined as a neutrophil count of less than 500×10^6/l. The onset is usually very sudden so that routine monitoring of white cell counts is unhelpful. Instead all patients should be warned to seek medical advice if they develop a fever or sore throat which persists for longer than a few days. Treatment consists of immediate withdrawal of the antithyroid drug, determination of the total white cell count and differential count, and supportive measures if indicated. Provided the antithyroid drug is stopped immediately recovery is very likely. Following recovery, recommencement of

Table 2. Side effects of antithyroid drugs

Minor (5%–10%)		
	Common	Pruritis
		Urticarial rash
		Urthralgia
		Fever
	Uncommon	Abnormal taste (methimazole)
		Gastrointestinal upset
		Hypoglycaemia (anti-insulin antibodies)
Major (<0.25%)		
	Rare	Agranulocytosis
	Very rare	Aplastic anaemia
		Thrombocytopenia
		Hepatitis (propylthiouracil)
		Cholestatic jaundice (methimazole)
		Lupus-like syndrome

antithyroid drug therapy is absolutely contra-indicated and treatment with radioiodine becomes the favoured alternative. Other serious side effects such as hepatitis are exceedingly rare but also warrant permanent discontinuation of antithyroid drug treatment.

III. Administration and Use

1. Graves' Disease

a) International Therapeutic Practices

Despite the fact that antithyroid drug treatment has been available since the mid-1940s, we still remain surprisingly ignorant about how best to use these medications (FELDT-RASMUSSEN et al. 1993; ROSS 1993). A number of key questions still cause considerable controversy and as a result practices throughout the world remain variable. A key contributor to resolving the problem is the enormous variability in iodine intake which exists between Japan, North America and Europe. Against this background the questions which require answering are: (1) Are antithyroid drugs or radioiodine the treatment of choice for a first episode of hyperthyroid Graves' disease? If antithyroid drugs are to be the first line of treatment then (2) which is the drug of choice? (3) What is the ideal dose? (4) How frequently should the drug be given and (5) for how long should treatment be maintained?

In a recent survey in which questionnaires were sent to members of the American, European and Japanese Thyroid Associations, 77% of Europeans, 88% of Japanese but only 30% of Americans used drug therapy as first-line treatment for an initial episode of hyperthyroid Graves' disease (GLINOER et al. 1987; SOLOMON et al. 1990; WARTOFSKY et al. 1991 and Table 3). In the United States, therefore, the majority prefer radioiodine. In Europe and Japan either CBZ or MMI is the drug of choice whereas in North America when drugs are used PTU is the drug of choice.

Table 3. Surveys: European vs. American vs. Japanese Thyroid Associations. Treatment of hyperthyroid Graves' disease. (Modified from WARTOFSKY et al. 1991)

Index patient
Female; 43 years; first episode; completed family; diffuse enlarged (40–50 g) thyroid, minimal eye signs

Treatment – first line

	Antithyroid drugs	^{131}I	Surgery
ETA	77%	22%	1%
ATA	30.5%	69%	0.5%
JTA	88%	11%	1%

b) Antithyroid Drugs

α) Dose, Frequency and Duration. Two main regimens are adopted for the administration of antithyroid drugs. In the first, the so-called titration regimen, patients are commenced on a high dose of antithyroid drug treatment until euthyroidism is achieved and then the dose of antithyroid drug is titrated against the clinical and biochemical thyroid status so that patients are maintained on the lowest possible dose of antithyroid drug medication needed to sustain euthyroidism. In contrast, the blocking and replacement regimen relies on the administration of a fixed high dose of antithyroid drug therapy with the subsequent addition of T_4 once euthyroidism is achieved so that the patient is thereafter maintained euthyroid on a combination of antithyroid drug and T_4.

β) Titration Regimen. The adoption of this treatment schedule assumes that by using a smaller dose of medication the risk of likely side effects from the drugs will be minimised. Starting doses of 30–40 mg CBZ per day or 100 mg three times a day of PTU are usual and these are reduced over the subsequent few months as euthyroidism is achieved. Most patients end up being maintained on 5–10 mg CBZ or 50–100 mg PTU a day and may take these doses for up to 2 years. The major disadvantage of such a regimen is the need for relatively frequent re-assessment of thyroid function and, therefore, the need for frequent reattendance at outpatient clinics. Additionally the requirement that patients take medication long term is often associated with problems of poor compliance.

γ) Block and Replacement Regimen. Whether the use of a high dose of antithyroid drug ensures that these agents are therefore able to act not only by inhibiting thyroid hormone synthesis but also by reducing the autoimmune response in Graves' disease remains controversial (Romaldini et al. 1983): There is no doubt, however, that at doses of CBZ of 40 mg daily, the levels of MMI achieved in the thyroid gland during the hyperthyroid phase of the disease (Jansson et al. 1983) are certainly immunosuppressive. An important advantage of this regimen is the fact that once patients are established on a fixed dose of antithyroid drug coupled with T_4, euthyroidism can be maintained without the need for frequent visits to the clinic for clinical and biochemical assessment of their thyroid function. Additionally, at least in environments where iodine intake is normal rather than excessive, it is clear that using such a regimen for longer than 6 months does not increase the likelihood of a more favourable disease outcome (Weetman et al. 1994), though this has not been the experience of all groups (Allannic et al. 1990).

On the grounds, therefore, of reduced need for follow-up and shorter duration of treatment, our preference is for a 6-month block and replacement regimen. Sufficient data exist to suggest that once daily CBZ is as effective as taking the compound more frequently (ROTI et al. 1989) and our own practice is to use CBZ at a dose of 40 mg (2 × 20-mg tablets) once a day for 6 months with the addition of a T_4 supplement (usually of 50–100 μg daily) once euthyroidism has been maintained (usually at 6–8 weeks). The advantage of CBZ over PTU in this setting is that there is not the need with CBZ to take the medication three times daily as is the case with PTU. Patient compliance with once daily medication for only 6 months is excellent. In a large multicentre European study (REINWEIN et al. 1993) in which 10 mg MMI daily was compared with 40 mg MMI daily, with both groups being supplemented with T_4 where needed, remission rates in the two groups of patients were no different and side effects were higher in the group of patients receiving the higher dose of MMI. The study needs to be interpreted with some caution because of the very high drop-out rate of patients from the study and because of the enormous variability in iodine intake across Europe, with some centres involved in the study being in areas of iodine deficiency and others being in areas of relative iodine excess.

c) Resting the Thyroid

The conventional role of adding T_4 to antithyroid medication to maintain euthyroidism was extended in a study by HASHIZUME and collegues, who examined the potential benefits of T_4 itself on reducing the subsequent recurrence of hyperthyroidism (HASHIZUME et al. 1991). Two groups of patients were treated for 6 months with MMI at a dose of 30 mg daily and then divided into two groups which received either a small dose of 10 mg MMI with placebo or a similar dose of MMI in conjunction with 100 μg T_4. The treatment was continued for a year and thereafter the MMI was stopped and the patients continued for a further 3 years with the one group continuing on T_4 alone and the other on placebo (Table 4). Only 1.7% of the T_4-treated group relapsed whereas 34.7% of the placebo-treated group were shown to relapse. Interestingly the TSH receptor antibody levels continued to decline in the group treated with T_4 but not in the group treated with placebo. The authors suggested that T_4 administration resulted in TSH suppression and that this induced a reduction in TSH receptor antibody activity and therefore the

Table 4. Administration of thyroxine in treated Graves' disease. (Modified from HASHIZUME et al. 1991)

MMI + T_4 or placebo – 18 months	
Continue T_4 (0.1 mg) or placebo	
Follow-up 3 years	
Results – in T_4-treated group	
1. ↓ TSH receptor antibodies	
2. Relapse rate	
T_4 group	– 1.7% ($n = 1$)
Placebo group	– 34.7% ($n = 17$)

frequency of relapse of Graves' disease. The term "resting the thyroid" has been coined to describe this phenomenon, whereby giving T_4 exogenously seems to have a dramatically beneficial effect on the subsequent outcome of Graves' disease.

These studies were performed in Japan, an area of high iodine intake, and in a population of patients who differ markedly in their immunogenetic backgrounds as defined by HLA antigens. It has been important therefore to see whether these results could be confirmed elsewhere since the dramatic reduction in relapse rates suggested by HASHIZUME and colleagues would require a major reconsideration of the way in which we use antithyroid drugs in the management of Graves' disease. Initial attempts to repeat these observations have not been encouraging and an increasing number of observations have failed to confirm the results. TAMAI and colleagues (1995) also from Japan, in a not strictly comparable study, examined the influence of the addition of T_4 to MMI on TSH receptor antibody activity. They failed to show any difference in the rate of fall of antibody activity whether patients were treated with MMI alone or MMI with T_4 supplementation. More recently, the first comparable published evidence seems to provide little support for the Hashizume observations, at least in Caucasians in an area of normal iodine intake. In studies from Edinburgh in Scotland (MCIVER et al. 1996), there was no benefit of T_4 administration following withdrawal of antithyroid medication on either the onset or the frequency of recurrence of hyperthyroidism following cessation of treatment. Nor was there any influence of T_4 on TSH receptor antibody activity. The considerable scepticism that has surrounded the concept of "resting the thyroid" is increasingly supported by data which suggest little benefit from such a regimen.

d) Subsequent Follow-up

Having commenced patients on antithyroid drug medication and provided them with the necessary information on the adverse effects and the need to seek urgent medical advice should any such problems arise, patients are then seen again at 6–8 weeks after commencing on antithyroid drug treatment. If a block and replacement regimen is adopted then once euthyroidism is achieved T_4 can be added, and if 4 weeks later patients are clinically and biochemically euthyroid there may be no further need to see them until they have completed their 6-month course of antithyroid medication. In patients being treated with a titration regimen the need to monitor them clinically and biochemically at 4- to 6-week intervals, as their maintenance dose is reduced, requires regular visits throughout the period of treatment, which may be for up to 2 years.

Crucial to the assessment of patients, whatever the regimen, is consideration of their eyes. Whilst clinically apparent Graves' ophthalmopathy may only be present in 50% of patients with hyperthyroid Graves' disease, with this being apparent in the majority of patients around the time of their presentation with hyperthyroidism, nevertheless in a significant proportion ophthalmopathy may develop during the treatment of their hyperthyroidism and patients need to be aware of this possibility and to return to the clinic if problems arise.

In summary, therefore, follow-up of patients is designed to establish clinical and biochemical euthyroidism, to respond to any adverse events, to monitor ophthalmopathy which is present or may develop during treatment, and once treatment is complete to then remain alert to the possibility of subsequent relapse. Whatever the mode of therapy used with antithyroid drugs remission rates of greater than 50% are unlikely to be achieved (Hedley et al. 1989 and Table 5), and are likely to be influenced by iodine intake (Solomon et al. 1987 and Table 6).

e) Prediction of Relapse

A huge literature has evolved on trying to identify clinical, biochemical, immunological or genetic markers which might predict the likelihood of subsequent relapse following treatment with antithyroid drugs for hyperthyroid Graves' disease (Weetman et al. 1986; Schleusener et al. 1989; Benker et al. 1995). The benefits of such information would be enormous in, on the one hand, suggesting that there would be no worth in using antithyroid drugs in some patients because of the certainty of relapse, and on the other one could with confidence reassure patients, having had a course of antithyroid drugs, that long-term follow-up was unnecessary because they were cured. However, no markers have been identified which make such confident statements possible. A few clinical observations have stood the test of time; patients who are older, male, with large goitres, particularly if they fail to reduce in size during the

Table 5. Recurrent hyperthyroidism in Graves' disease – life-table analysis in 434 patients following anti-thyroid drugs. (Modified from Hedley et al. 1989)

Recurrence within (years)	Recurrence rate (%)
1	40
5	58
10	61

Table 6. Remission rates with anti-thyroid drug therapy: continuing influence of iodine intake? (Modified from Solomon et al. 1987)

Year of study	Relapse rate (%)	Slice of bread iodine contents (μg)
1973	86.0	150
1987	49.3	32

course of antithyroid medication, are more likely to relapse and those that do relapse tend to have higher levels of TSH receptor antibody activity at the time of completion of their course of treatment. The considerable effort that has been devoted to looking for markers which predict relapse following antithyroid drugs, particularly those which might provide such an indication before treatment commences, has not born fruit.

f) Subsequent Management

Since at least 50% of patients treated with antithyroid drugs relapse following cessation of their medication, strategies need to be in place for the subsequent management of the recurrence of hyperthyroidism in this group. A significant group of physicians will still resort to further courses of antithyroid medication and even long-term maintenance of such patients on small doses of CBZ with all the inconvenience, cost and compliance problems associated with such an approach. Our own view is to take a very different attitude. We have been impressed in our practice by the significant reduction in the frequency with which we see severe ophthalmopathy in patients with hyperthyroid Graves' disease. This contrasts with our experience with patients referred to us with severe ophthalmopathy from other centres in which very characteristically there is a long history of hyperthyroidism with frequent recurrences following multiple courses of antithyroid drug therapy. We have therefore adopted the approach in which we offer patients only a single course of antithyroid drug medication and if they relapse after 6 months of our blocking and replacement regimen, then depending on their age, thyroid size, and the presence or absence of ophthalmopathy, they are offered either radioiodine ablation or partial thyroidectomy. We are not keen to treat patients who have evidence of active ophthalmopathy with radioactive iodine because of fear of exacerbation of their eye disease (Tallstedt et al. 1992 and Table 7). In this group we prefer to control their disease with antithyroid drugs and then once euthyroid to recommend partial thyroidectomy. Likewise in patients with large goitres in whom radioiodine is unlikely to be effective we recommend partial thyroidectomy. In young women who have yet to complete their families we

Table 7. Occurrence of ophthalmopathy after treatment of Graves' hyperthyroidism. (Modified from Tallstedt et al. 1992)

Patients ($n = 168$)	
Two groups (20–34 years, 35–55 years)	
Random assign – MMI, surgery; ^{131}I	
T_4 – to all in MMI, surgery groups	
– to all ^{131}I who became hypothyroid	
Ophthalmopathy development (within 24 months)	
MMI	10%
Surgery	16%
^{131}I	33%

prefer to recommend partial thyroidectomy but if radioiodine is their preferred choice, then we prescribe this and advise the women not to become pregnant for 6 months after their radioiodine. In using radioiodine we are keen to use an ablative dose so that post-radioiodine hypothyroidism is established early and patients can be treated with T_4 early and thence be discharged from follow-up.

2. Drug Usage with Radioiodine

Because of concern that the use of radioiodine may exacerbate hyperthyroidism (Radioiodine Audit Subcommittee 1995) with marked release of thyroxine due to radiation thyroiditis, there may be an indication for the use of antithyroid drugs in patients with severe hyperthyroidism who are being treated with radioiodine (Cooper 1994). Since patients treated with antithyroid drugs prior to the administration of radioiodine seem to be more resistant to radioactivity, there is a need to consider giving a higher activity of radioiodine in this setting. If antithyroid drugs are to be used they should be discontinued at least 2 days prior to the administration of radioiodine since their effect lasts for 24 h or longer, and if there is the intention to continue the antithyroid medication after the radioiodine this should not be recommenced for at least 3 days after the administration of the dose (Burch et al. 1994). It makes sense in patients who are at risk, that is those with severe disease or who are elderly or known to have heart disease, to cover their radioiodine with antithyroid drugs before and after the administration of the radioiodine as suggested above. If such a regimen is adopted the patients need to be followed carefully in the succeeding 4–8 weeks so that the drugs are stopped before any risk of hypothyroidism results. Preventing hypothyroidism developing may have important implications for the prevention of subsequent ophthalmopathy (Tallstedt et al. 1992, 1994).

3. Drug Usage in Pregnancy

Characteristically patients with hyperthyroid Graves' disease show improvement of their disease during pregnancy with exacerbation in the postpartum period. Against this background the likelihood of problems with hyperthyroidism during pregnancy is small. When women with Graves' disease become pregnant whilst taking antithyroid medication or develop hyperthyroidism during pregnancy, the use of antithyroid drugs in a blocking and replacement regimen is absolutely contraindicated. Whilst the mother may remain euthyroid, the high levels of antithyroid drugs crossing the placenta induce hypothyroidism and goitre formation in the baby. In this setting, therefore, titration of the dose against the mother's thyroid function is essential with the aim of achieving the lowest dose possible to maintain her euthyroid. In many women it may be possible to withdraw antithyroid medication in the third trimester because of the improvement in the disease characteristic of pregnancy. Either CBZ or PTU may be used. Exacerbation in the postpartum period may require larger doses of antithyroid medication and though both CBZ and PTU enter the breast milk there is no contraindication to breast feeding.

4. Thyroid Storm

Thyroid storm is said to exist when the severity of the hyperthyroid state is such that it is life threatening with evidence of major organ failure (TIETGENS and LEINUNG 1995). Whilst exceedingly rare, the situation is fatal if untreated. The pathogenesis remains unknown. The clinical presentation of severe hyperthyroidism often with fever, dysrhythmia, cardiac failure and mental state changes are characteristic. Often a precipitating event can be defined such as infection or severe stresses such as major illness or major surgery. Treatment is designed to correct the hyperthyroidism, treat the precipitating event and, where indicated, treat organ failure. In treating the hyperthyroidism PTU is used to inhibit thyroid hormone synthesis and the peripheral conversion of T_4 to T_3. If PTU cannot be given orally it may need to be given by nasogastric tube. A loading dose of 600–1000 mg is followed by 200–250 mg every 4 h. Once thyroid hormone synthesis has been inhibited by PTU (2 to 3 h after PTU administration), there is a need to block the release of pre-formed thyroid hormone and this is achieved with inorganic iodine. This is administered orally or again by a nasogastric tube as Lugol's solution given as 30 drops/day in three to four divided doses.

F. Conclusions

Antithyroid drugs have been available for clinical use since the 1940s. Used appropriately they are remarkably safe and effective in controlling hyperthyroidism though in the best hands, despite a wide variety of regimens, relapse rates of 50% are the norm. Considerable controversy and ignorance still abound in seeking to define the best way to use these agents. Our view is that we should make their use as simple as possible and use them for as short a time as is possible to achieve the maximum benefit. We aim also to ensure patient cooperation and compliance. In this context using CBZ once a day in a blocking and replacement regimen for a maximum of 6 months is optimal in achieving an acceptable remission rate with minimal patient inconvenience. In those patients that do relapse we believe that disease cure is in their best interest not only because of the subsequent convenience but also because of the reduced likelihood of development or worsening of their ophthalmopathy. Whilst the mechanism of action of these drugs is well understood and likely to be predominantly directed at inhibiting thyroid hormone synthesis, nevertheless a considerable body of evidence has accumulated which suggests that they may also have immunosuppressive effects. That these effects occur is not in doubt but their impact on the control of hyperthyroidism in patients with Graves' disease remains to be established.

References

Allannic H, Fauchet R, Orgiazzi J, Madec AM, Genetet B, Lorcy Y, Le Guerrier AM, Delambre C, Derennes V (1990) Antithyroid drugs and Graves' disease: a prospective randomised evaluation of the efficacy of treatment duration. J Clin Endocrinol Metab 70:675–679

Astwood EB (1943) Treatment of hyperthyroidism with thiourea and thiouracil. JAMA 122:78–89

Benker G, Vitti P, Kahaly G, Raue F, Tegler L, Hirche H, Reinwien D (1995) Response to methimazole in Graves' disease. Clin Endocrinol (Oxf) 43:257–263

Burch H, Solomon BL, Wartofsky L, Burman KD (1994) Discontinuing antithyroid drug therapy before ablation with radioiodine in Graves' disease. Ann Intern Med 121:553–559

Cooper DS (1984) Antithyroid drugs. N Engl J Med 311:1353–1362

Cooper DS (1994) Antithyroid drugs and radioiodine therapy: a grain of (iodized) salt (editorial). Ann Intern Med 121:612–614

Feldt-Rasmussen U, Glinoer D, Orgiazzi J (1993) Reassessment of antithyroid drug therapy of Graves' disease. Annu Rev Med 44:323–334

Franklyn JA (1994) The management of hyperthyroidism. N Engl J Med 330:1731–1738

Glinoer D, Hesch D, Lagasse R, Laurberg P (1987) The management of hyperthyroidism due to Graves' disease in Europe in 1986. Results of an international survey. Acta Endocrinol (Copenh) [Suppl] 285:6–19

Hashizume K, Ichikawa K, Sakurai A, Suzuki S, Takeda T, Kobayashi M, Miyamoto T, Arai M, Nagasawa T (1991) Administration of thyroxine in Graves' disease: effects on the level of antibodies to thyroid stimulating hormone receptors and on the risk of recurrence of hyperthyroidism. N Engl J Med 324:947–953

Hassman R, Weetman AP, Gunn C, Hall R, McGregor AM (1985) The effects of hyperthyroidism on experimental thyroiditis in the rat. Endocrinology 116:1253–1258

Hedley AJ, Young RE, Jones SJ, Alexander WD, Bewsher PD (1989) Antithyroid drugs in the treatment of hyperthyroidism of Graves' disease: long-term follow up of 434 patients. Clin Endocrinol (Oxf) 31:209–218

Jansson R, Dahlberg PA, Johansson H, Lindstrom B (1983) Intrathyroidal concentrations of methimazole in patients with Graves' disease. J Clin Endocrinol Metab 57:129–132

Ludgate ME, McGregor AM, Weetman AP, Ratanachaiyavong S, Lazarus J, Hall R, Middleton G (1984) Analysis of T cell subsets in Graves' disease: alterations associated with carbimazole. Br Med J 288:526–530

McGregor AM, Petersen MM, McLachlan SM, Rooke P, Rees Smith B, Hall R (1980) Carbimazole and the autoimmune response in Graves' disease. N Engl J Med 303:302–307

McGregor AM, Smith BR, Hall R, Collins PN, Bottazzo GF, Petersen MM (1982) Specificity of the immunosuppressive action of carbimazole in Graves' disease. Br Med J 284:1750–1751

McIver B, Rae P, Beckett G, Wilkinson E, Gold A, Toft A (1996) Lack of effect of thyroxine in patients with Graves' hyperthyroidism who are treated with an antithyroid drug. N Engl J Med 334:220–224

Paschke R, Vogg M, Kristoferitsch R, Aktuna D, Wawschinek O, Eber O, Usadel KH (1995) Methimazole has no dose-related effect on the intensity of the intrathyroidal autoimmune process in relapsing Graves' disease. J Clin Endocrinol Metab 80:2470–2474

Radioiodine Audit Subcommittee of the Royal College of Physicians of London (1995) Guidelines on the use of radioiodine in the management of hyperthyroidism. Royal College of Physicians Publication Unit, London

Ratanachaiyavong S, McGregor AM (1985) Immunosuppressive effects of antithyroid drugs. Clin Endocrinol Metab 14:449–466
Rennie DP, McGregor AM, Keast D, Weetman AP, Hall R (1983) The influence of methimazole on thyroglobulin-induced autoimmune thyroiditis in the rat. Endocrinology 112:326–330
Reinwein D, Benker G, Lazarus JH, Alexander WD (1993) A prospective randomised trial of antithyroid drug dose in Graves' disease therapy. J Clin Endocrinol Metab 76:1516–1521
Romaldini JH, Bromberg N, Werner RS (1983) Comparison of effects of high and low dosage regimens of antithyroid drugs in the management of Graves' hyperthyroidism. J Clin Endocrinol Metab 57:563–570
Ross DS (1993) Current therapeutic approaches to hyperthyroidism. Trends Endocrinol Metab 4:281–285
Roti E, Gardini E, Minelli R, Salvi M, Robuschi G, Braverman LE (1989) Methimazole and serum thyroid hormone concentration in hyperthyroid patients: effects of single and multiple daily doses. Ann Intern Med 111:181–182
Schleusener H, Schwander J, Fischer C, Holle R, Holl G, Badenhoop K, Hensen J, Finke R, Bogner U, Mayr WR, Schernthaner G, Schatz H, Pickardt CR, Kotulla P (1989) Prospective multicentre study on the prediction of relapse after antithyroid drug treatment in patients with Graves' disease. Acta Endocrinol (Copenh) 120:689–701
Solomon B, Evaul JE, Burman KD, Wartofsky L (1987) Remission rates with antithyroid drug therapy: continuing influence of iodine intake? Ann Intern Med 107:510–512
Solomon B, Glinoer D, Lagasse R, Wartofsky L (1990) Current trends in the management of Graves' disease. J Clin Endocrinol Metab 70:1518–1524
Tallstedt L, Lundell G, Torring O, Wallin G, Ljunggren J-G (1992) Occurrence of ophthalmopathy after treatment for Graves' hyperthyroidism. N Engl J Med 326:1733–1738
Tallstedt L, Lundell G, Blomgren H, Bring J (1994) Does early administration of thyroxine reduce the development of Graves' ophthalmopathy after radioiodine? Eur J Endocrinol 130:494–497
Tamai H, Hayaki I, Kawai K, Komaki G, Matsubayashi S, Kuma K, Kumagai LF, Nagataki S (1995) Lack of effect of thyroxine administration on elevated thyroid stimulating hormone receptor antibody levels in treated Graves' disease patients. J Clin Endocrinol Metab 80:1481–1484
Taurog A (1991) Hormone synthesis: thyroid iodine metabolism. In: Braverman LE, Utiger RD (eds) Werner and Ingbar's the thyroid, 6th edn. Lippincott, Philadelphia, pp 51–97
Taurog A, Dorris ML (1989) A re-examination of the proposed inactivation of thyroid peroxidase in the rat thyroid by propylthiouracil. Endocrinology 124:3038–3042
Tietgens ST, Leinung MC (1995) Thyroid storm. Med Clin North Am 79:169–184
Totterman TH, Karlsson FA, Bengtsson M, Mendel-Hartvig I (1987) Induction of circulating activated suppressor-like T cells by methimazole therapy for Graves' disease. N Engl J Med 316:15–21
Volpé R, Karlsson A, Jansson R, Dahlberg PA (1986) Evidence that antithyroid drugs induce remissions in Graves' disease by modulating thyroid cellular activity. Clin Endocrinol (Oxf) 25:453–462
Wartofsky L, Glinoer D, Solomon B, Nagataki S, Lagasse R, Nagayama Y, Izumi M (1991) Differences and similarities in the diagnosis and treatment of Graves' disease in Europe, Japan and the United States. Thyroid 1:129–135
Weetman AP (1992) How antithyroid drugs work in Graves' disease. Clin Endocrinol 37:317–318
Weetman AP, McGregor AM (1994) Autoimmune thyroid disease: further developments in our understanding. Endocr Rev 15:788–830

Weetman AP, Holt ME, Campbell AK, Hall R, McGregor AM (1984a) Methimazole inhibits oxygen radical generation by monocytes: a potential role in immunosuppression. Br Med J 288:518–520
Weetman AP, McGregor AM, Hall R (1984b) Evidence for an effect of antithyroid drugs on the natural history of Graves' disease. Clin Endocrinol (Oxf) 20:163–169
Weetman AP, Ratanachaiyavong R, Middleton GW, Hall R, Darke C, McGregor AM (1986) Prediction of outcome in Graves' disease after carbimazole treatment. Q J Med 59:409–419
Weetman AP, Tandon N, Morgan BP (1992b) Antithyroid drugs and release of inflammatory mediators by complement-attacked thyroid cells. Lancet 340:633–636
Weetman AP, Pickerill AP, Watson P, Chatterjee VK, Edwards OM (1994) Treatment of Graves' disease with the block-replace regimen of antithyroid drugs: the effect of treatment duration and immunogenetic susceptibility on relapse. Q J Med 87:337–341
Young RJ, Sherwood MB, Simpson JG, Nicol AG, Michie W, Beck JS (1976) Histometry of lymphoid infiltrate in the thyroid of primary thyrotoxicosis patients. J Clin Pathol 29:398–402

CHAPTER 9

Effect of Lithium on the Thyroid Gland

J.H. LAZARUS

A. Introduction

The history of the introduction of lithium into medicine has been reviewed by JOHNSON (1984). Lithium was discovered in 1817 and accounts for about 0.006% of the earth's crust. It belongs in Group IA in the Periodic Table of Elements but shares some physical properties with magnesium (Group IIA). The main use of lithium in therapeutics is in the treatment and prophylaxis of manic depressive psychosis. In the first half of the twentieth century lithium was used as a salt substitute in patients with cardiac failure but severe toxicity prevented its acceptance. In 1949 J.F.J.CADE, an Australian psychiatrist, noticed that guinea pigs who had been given lithium urate during an investigation into the role of uric acid in manic patients became less startled. This led to the trial administration of lithium to manic depressive patients (CADE 1949) and then to the widely acclaimed studies of SCHOU and colleagues in defining the clinical effectiveness of this ion in psychiatry (SCHOU et al. 1954; SCHOU 1957).

In 1967 the occurrence of goitre in patients receiving lithium was mentioned at a conference in Denmark and these data were reported in 1968 by SCHOU and others (SCHOU et al. 1968). Since then a large number of clinical and experimental studies on the effect of lithium on thyroid physiology have been performed and reviewed (LAZARUS 1986a; BAGCHI and BROWN 1988; DRUMMOND et al. 1988; ST. GERMAIN 1988; HASSMAN and MCGREGOR 1988; KUSHNER and WARTOFSKY 1988; SPAULDING 1989; CHOW and COCKRAM 1990). This chapter will discuss the effects of lithium on thyroid physiology and the clinical effects on thyroid function in psychiatric patients. The clinical usefulness of the drug in the management of thyroid disease is also discussed.

B. Effect on Thyroid Physiology

I. Iodine Concentration

Lithium reduces the radioiodine uptake into rat thyroid in vivo (BURROW et al. 1971) and in vitro (HULLIN and JOHNSON 1970) and a similar depressant effect on the iodide-concentrating mechanism is seen in quail thyroid (DOWNIE et al. 1977) and mouse salivary gland (LAZARUS and MUSTON 1978). Lithium is itself concentrated by the thyroid at levels three to four times that in plasma (BERENS et al. 1970a). The relationship of the thyroidal lithium-concentrating mechanism to the iodide-concentrating process is not clear but lithium has been found to be concentrated in mouse salivary glands, which also actively concentrate iodine, perhaps suggesting a common pathway. In humans, lithium administration has been reported to result in both a reduction and an increase in thyroidal radioiodine uptake (BERENS et al. 1970b). The possible reasons for this are that lithium causes iodide retention and the increase in uptake may also be due to thyroid-stimulating hormone (TSH) secreted as a result of lithium-induced hypothyroidism.

II. Intrathyroidal Effects

There is evidence that lithium inhibits the coupling of iodotyrosines to form iodothyronines in rat thyroid homogenates (see Chap. 4, this volume). However, although thyroid hormone synthesis may be impaired, total iodination is not reduced as total iodoacid concentrations are not changed following lithium administration (MANNISTO 1973). Some workers (COOPER et al. 1970; LJUNGGREN et al. 1971) have not found any intrathyroidal blocking effects and it is probable that they are of less importance than other thyroidal actions of the ion. Indeed, in man there is no effect of lithium on the perchlorate discharge test, although if the sensitivity of this test is increased by iodide administration, positive tests are seen (ANDERSEN 1973). In view of this it is possible that lithium may increase the patient's sensitivity to added iodine, leading to an increase in the thyroid to serum iodide ratio and thereby producing an organification block. Any block produced by lithium alone is very small compared to iodide. Lithium may alter thyroglobulin structure by affecting protein conformation and function (SINGER and ROTENBERG 1973), resulting in the minor iodotyrosine coupling defects, but no inhibitory effect of lithium has been observed on the biosynthesis or degradation of thyroglobulin in the rat (BAGCHI et al. 1978).

III. Effect on Thyroid Hormone Secretion

SEDVALL et al. (1968) were the first to postulate that lithium might act on the thyroid by inhibiting the release of thyroid hormone after noting a reduction in protein-bound iodide in lithium-treated patients when the iodide uptake was increased. A reduction in ^{131}I release rate has been found in rats given lithium (BERENS et al. 1970b) and reduced thyroxine (T_4) release was demonstrated in both euthyroid and hyperthyroid patients receiving the drug (BURROW et al. 1971). T_4 release is controlled by TSH; in sheep and bovine thyroid membranes lithium reduced TSH-stimulated activity by about 50% although basal cyclic AMP (cAMP) levels were not altered (BURKE 1970). The lithium-induced block was inversely related to the magnesium concentration in the medium, suggesting that lithium competes with magnesium at a magnesium-binding site on the adenylate cyclase enzyme. When lithium was given to mice in vivo, it inhibited the action of TSH on dibutyryl cAMP-stimulated ^{131}I release from in vitro mouse thyroid, suggesting that the block is distal to cAMP formation (WILLIAMS et al. 1971). The process of thyroid hormone secretion involves a decrease in colloid droplet formation together with a number of complex steps involving the degradation of thyroglobulin (BJORKMAN and EKHOLM 1990). As mentioned, lithium has little effect on thyroglobulin hydrolysis in the iodine replete state, but does alter tubulin polymerization (BHATTACHARYYA and WOLFF 1976), which may account for its inhibitory effect on hormone secretion.

IV. Effect on Peripheral Thyroid Hormone Metabolism

Under physiological conditions, deiodination accounts for 80% of total T_4 turnover, this process being mediated by three specific deiodinase enzymes (Chap. 4, this volume; HENNEMAN et al. 1994). The significant decrease in T_4 clearance from plasma in patients receiving lithium, first reported over 20 years ago (SPAULDING et al. 1972; CARLSON et al. 1973), may be due to inhibition of thyroid hormone secretion, thereby inducing a decrease in type I 5′ deiodinase activity. Lithium causes a decrease in T_4 deiodination in rat liver (VOSS et al. 1977). Tissue culture experiments examining the effect of lithium on T_4 deiodination have shown significant inhibitory effects of lithium on T_4 to tri-iodothyronine (T_3) conversion in mouse neuroblastoma cells and GH3 cells (ST. GERMAIN 1987). Similar data have been obtained in rats; their clinical relevance is questionable because of the high doses of lithium used in some experiments, although suggestive data have been obtained in man (TERAO et al. 1995).

Recently, administration of lithium to rats for 14 days has been shown to affect intracellular metabolism of thyroid hormones in the frontal cortex of the rat by increasing the type II deiodinase enzyme and decreasing the type III enzyme (BAUMGARTNER et al. 1994a). This raises the question as to whether these effects of lithium on thyroid hormone metabolism in the central nervous system may be involved in the mood-stabilising effects of the drug similar to results obtained for other psychotropic agents (BAUMGARTNER et al. 1994b). However, it is still not clear whether these changes in deiodinase activity result from a direct action of lithium on the brain or from a reduction in serum T_4 levels leading in turn to a rise in type II deiodinase activity.

C. Effect on the Hypothalamic-Pituitary Axis

Lithium is concentrated in the pituitary gland as well as the hypothalamus (PFEIFER et al. 1976) and may interfere with cell metabolism in those tissues as a result of this. In addition there are data to suggest that lithium, which is known to inhibit inositol-1-monophosphatase, thereby altering signal transduction, is capable of exerting significant effects on inositol lipid metabolism in cultured GH3 pituitary cells when these are exposed to lithium concentrations seen in treated patients (DRUMMOND et al. 1988). In cross-sectional studies there are numerous reports (MCLARTY et al. 1975; TANIMOTO et al. 1981; LAZARUS et al. 1981) showing that lithium therapy in psychiatric patients results in an exaggerated TSH response to thyrotrophin-releasing hormone (TRH) in at least 50%–100% of patients (Fig. 1). Approximately 10% of patients so studied have an elevated basal TSH and non-manic patients treated with lithium also have high basal and stimulated TSH levels. Basal prolactin concentrations are not raised in manic and non-manic patients on lithium but they do show exaggerated responses to TRH. While these effects may be due to the feedback effect of reduced thyroid hormone levels, the latter are not always low. The effect of the ion on pituitary thyroid hormone receptors may also be a cause of the observed changes (see below). The enhancing effect of lithium on TRH-induced prolactin release could also be related to a decrease in the sensitivity of dopamine receptors to stimulation by catecholamines, but there are no firm experimental data to support this view at present.

In a recent longitudinal study in which thyroid function was investigated in 12 euthymic bipolar patients who had normal thyroid function and no circulat-

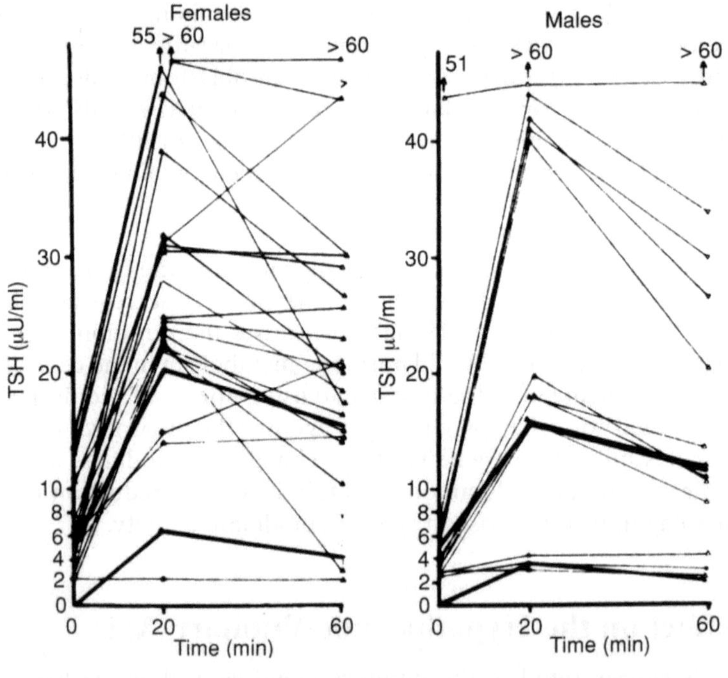

Fig. 1. Serum TSH response to 200 μg i.v. TRH administered at time 0 in 34 male and 39 female patients receiving lithium carbonate. Normal TSH response is shown by *area within the heavy black lines*. Abnormal responses are seen in 49.3% of patients. [From LAZARUS et al. (1981) with permission from Cambridge University Press]

ing thyroid antibodies, a significant rise in basal TSH was found in 83% and a rise in TRH-stimulated TSH was observed in 11 after 12 months of therapy. However, the impairment of the hypothalamic-pituitary axis was temporary in most cases, adjusting to a new level of control during lithium therapy (LOMBARDI et al. 1993). In 28 depressed patients maintained on lithium for a mean of 12 months, it was found that TSH levels were normal and only levels of reverse T_3 were raised (BAUMGARTNER et al. 1995). Interestingly, the efficacy of lithium prophylaxis was significantly correlated with serum T_3 suggesting, in the author's view, an interaction with thyroid hormone metabolism in the brain. TRH tests were not done in this study so it is difficult to compare with others. Nevertheless, the data from this and other groups suggest that TSH and thyroid hormone abnormalities which are seen in lithium therapy do return to normal after years of treatment.

D. Lithium and Cell Function

Lithium has many actions on the cell (LAZARUS 1986b), including effects on ATPase activity, cAMP activity, intracellular enzymes, inositol phospholipid metabolism and cell growth (Table 1). The inhibitory effect of lithium on inositol phospholipid metabolism is mainly mediated by the ability of the cation to inhibit uncompetitively the enzyme inositol (1,4) P2 1-phosphatase (HALLCHER and SHERMAN 1980). This results in alteration of many intracellular inositol metabolites, thus affecting signal transduction. Intense interest in this action of lithium has occurred and it is thought that its action on these pathways particularly located at the site of G proteins may account for the therapeutic effect in manic depression (AVISSAR et al. 1988). Lithium may be capable of modulating the function of G_i proteins coupled to insulin-like growth factor-1 (IGF-1) receptors during the G(1) phase of the FRTL-5 rat thyroid cell cycle (TAKADA et al. 1993). Lithium induces end organ resistance to TSH in intact cells at least partly due to inhibition of adenylate cyclase by lithium. MACNEIL et al. (1993) have suggested that lithium interferes with intracellular cross-talk influences such as inositol metabolism rather than the

Table 1. Effect of lithium on cellular metabolism

Agent	Effect
Na^+K^+ ATPase	Variable Increased in some tissues Decreased in others
Cyclic AMP	Inhibits adenylate cyclase-cAMP system in many tissues, e.g. thyroid, brain, kidney
Intracellular enzymes	Mostly inhibitory
Inositol phospholipid metabolism	Inhibition of inositol-1-monophosphatase
Cell growth	Modulates function of many growth factors

adenylate cyclase enzyme directly. Further work is required to determine the multiple effects of the cation on intracellular signal transduction.

Lithium stimulates DNA synthesis in thyroid cells under basal conditions as well as after stimulation by IGF-1; this growth stimulation may partly explain the goitrogenic action of lithium (TSUCHIYA et al. 1990). Recently, the same group has shown that lithium may require the activation of a particular genistein-sensitive kinase, possibly a tyrosine kinase, to induce cell proliferation in FRTL-5 cells (TAKANO et al. 1994).

E. Immunological Effects on Thyroid Function

Lithium affects many aspects of both cellular and humoral immunity (LAZARUS 1986c; HART 1993). For example, addition of lithium to peripheral human lymphocytes enhanced the response of these cells to mitogens (SHENKMAN et al. 1978). It also stimulates interleukin-2 production, and inhibits suppressor T cells and increases the secretion of immunoglobulins by B cells (WEETMAN et al. 1982). Lithium can either enhance or inhibit mitogen-induced stimulation of lymphocytes in vitro depending upon the concentration of mitogen and lithium used (FERNANDEZ and FOX 1980). The ion is also known to cause involution of the thymus and spleen (JANKOVIC et al. 1979) as well as neutrophilia and lymphopenia (LEVITT and QUEENSBURY 1980).

From the clinical point of view it has been noted that some patients receiving lithium for affective disorders develop newly diagnosed autoimmune disease or suffer exacerbation of existing autoimmune disease although this is not the case for all autoimmune diseases (HART 1993). Numerous studies (EMERSON et al. 1973; LAZARUS et al. 1981; ALBRECHT and HOPF 1982) have noted a high proportion of patients receiving lithium to have detectable antithyroid antibodies and it has been shown that lithium therapy is associated with a rise in antibody levels in patients who have positive antibodies before starting lithium (LAZARUS et al. 1985). In normal control subjects lithium administration does not cause any development of antithyroid antibodies but does induce a rise in soluble interleukin-2 receptor level (RAPAPORT et al. 1994). Although there are many studies of the effect of lithium on thyroid antibodies in humans, it has been less intensively evaluated in animal models of thyroid disease. Lithium, at pharmacologically relevant serum concentrations, augmented the development of autoimmune thyroid disease in female August strain rats immunised with thyroglobulin (Fig. 2). Thyroglobulin antibody production was enhanced during the induction of disease and lithium also caused a more rapid disappearance of these antibodies as the disease resolved. This experiment shows that lithium can exert both positive and negative influences on experimental autoimmune thyroiditis (HASSMAN et al. 1985). It may influence the uptake of thyroglobulin by macrophages and its subsequent presentation to T cells and may stimulate the increased proportion

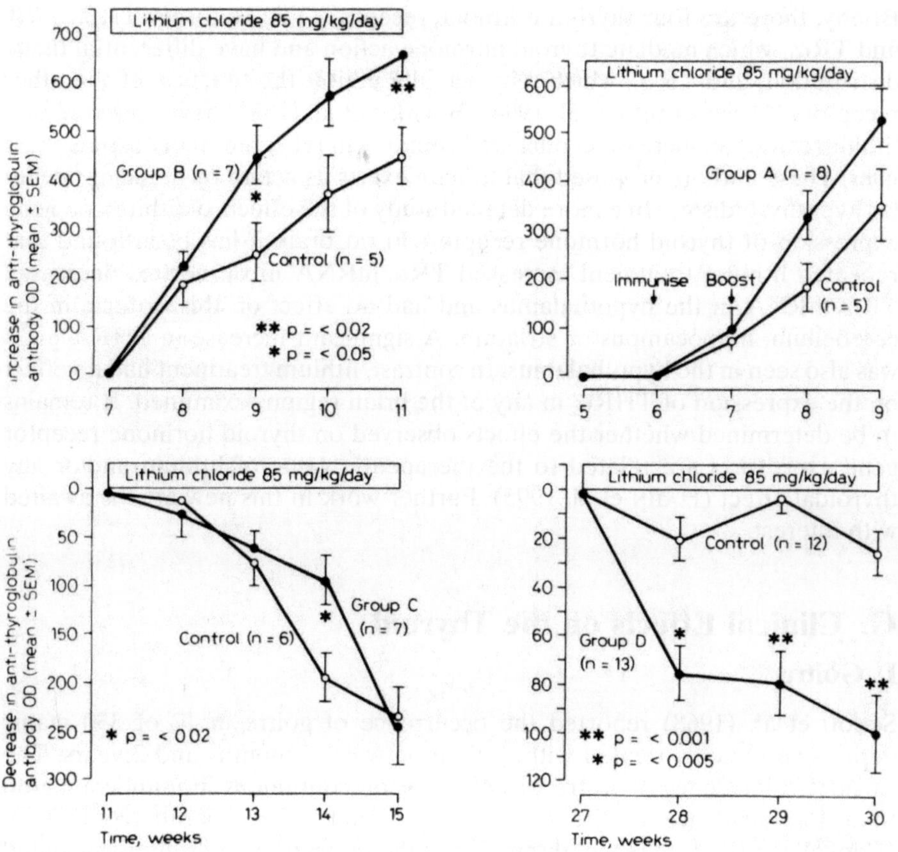

Fig. 2. Influence of lithium on experimental autoimmune thyroid disease in female August rats. Rats were immunised by injection of rat thyroglobulin and Freund's adjuvant (*groups A, B*). Immunological activity was measured by the concentration of circulating antithyroglobulin antibody. [From HASSMAN et al. (1985) with permission from Blackwell Science Publications]

of helper T cells to produce antibody. While there must be caution in the interpretation of animal data in relation to human disease, these experiments suggest that lithium does have significant effects on the course of autoimmune thyroid disease, although the mechanisms are still not clear.

F. Effect on Thyroid Hormone Action

Since the identification and cloning of the thyroid hormone nuclear receptors, much data has emerged on the details of thyroid hormone action (see Chap. 6, this volume). Central to this action is the specific binding of T_3 to these nuclear receptors, thereby initiating transcription and production of messenger RNA.

Briefly, there are four thyroid hormone receptor (TR) isoforms: TRβ_1, *TR*β_2 and TRα_1, which mediate thyroid hormone action and have differential tissue distribution, and TRα_2, which may actually inhibit the function of the other receptors (OPPENHEIMER et al. 1994). BOLARIS et al. (1995) have reported that lithium causes an increase in nuclear T_3 binding in rat cerebral hemisphere and liver. These authors proposed that lithium exerts its action by inducing "cellular hypothyroidism". In a more detailed study of the effects of lithium on gene expression of thyroid hormone receptors in rat brain it has been found that repeated lithium treatment increased TRα_1 mRNA in rat cortex, decreased TRα_1 mRNA in the hypothalamus and had no effect on this isoform in the cerebellum, hippocampus or striatum. A significant increase in THRβ levels was also seen in the hypothalamus. In contrast, lithium treatment had no effect on the expression of THRα_2 in any of the brain regions examined. It remains to be determined whether the effects observed on thyroid hormone receptor gene expression are related to the therapeutic value of lithium and/or any thyroidal effect (HAHN et al. 1995). Further work in this new area is awaited with interest.

G. Clinical Effects on the Thyroid

I. Goitre

SCHOU et al. (1968) reported the occurrence of goitre in 12 of 330 manic depressive patients treated with lithium between 5 months and 2 years. The calculated incidence of goitre was 4%/year on continuous lithium, compared to a 1% incidence in the general population of a separate community (Copenhagen). More recent discussion of the prevalence of lithium-associated goitre is available (WOLFF 1978; MANNISTO 1980; LAZARUS 1986a). There is considerable variation in the estimates due to the population sample, observer experience and method of diagnosing goitre. An overall prevalence in 876 patients was 6.1% (WOLFF 1978) and 5.6% in 1257 patients (MANNISTO 1980). Some groups, however, have found no goitre (SEDVALL et al. 1969; COOPER and SIMPSON 1969; MYERS et al. 1985) while others (FIEVE and PLATMAN 1968; LAZARUS et al. 1981; MARTINO et al. 1982) have found incidence rates of 30%, 37% and 60%, respectively. If imaging techniques such as scintiscanning or ultrasound are used, significant thyroid enlargement was noted when thyroid volume after 3 months of lithium treatment was compared to pretreatment values (LAZARUS and BENNIE 1972). Interestingly, this was observed in normal female volunteers after 28 days of lithium therapy but not in males (PERRILD et al. 1984).

Clinically the goitre is smooth and non-tender. It may develop within weeks of starting lithium therapy (BURROW et al. 1971), but others have stated that it may take months to years of lithium treatment (MANNISTO 1980). The mechanism of thyroid enlargement is due to the initial inhibition of thyroid hormone release (see below), which results in an increase in TSH leading to thyroid enlargement. Although an increase in serum thyroglobulin is seen in subjects with non-toxic goitre, this was not the case in normal women given lithium for 4 weeks (PERRILD et al. 1988). This is consistent with the finding that lithium causes inhibition of endocytosis (MILONI et al. 1983), resulting in accumulation of colloid and thyroglobulin within the thyroid. The chronic effect of lithium on the release of thyroglobulin is not known.

The goitrogenic effect of lithium is also seen in the rat (SANGVI et al. 1975). Here the main histological feature is an increase in follicular diameter and a decrease in follicle cell height (HELTNE and OLLERICH 1973). Limited observations in humans have shown that all follicles had pronounced pleomorphism of the epithelial cells and marked nuclear changes (FAUERHOLDT and VENDSBORG 1981).

II. Hypothyroidism

Hypothyroidism was not a feature of the first patients to be recorded who had goitre associated with lithium therapy, but subsequent case reports then started to appear (ROGERS and WHYBROW 1971). The clinical presentation of hypothyroidism in lithium-treated patients is not different from that seen in other forms of hypothyroidism. Subclinical hypothyroidism may also occur and this should be considered in a patient who is not showing a good response to lithium. Symptoms of the condition may appear within weeks of starting lithium but may not occur for many months or even years and may include the unusual or atypical features such as myxoedema coma (WALDMAN and PARK 1989). The female to male ratio is about 5:1 and it does appear that there is a significantly higher incidence of hypothyroidism in females even when compared to the normally expected higher incidence of this condition in the general population (KUSHNER and WARTOFSKY 1988). Prevalence figures for lithium-induced hypothyroidism vary widely depending on the population studied and on differences in clinical and laboratory evaluation. In a review of 16 reports totalling 4681 patients, the prevalence was 3.4% (range 0%–23.3%; LAZARUS 1986a).

More recently, in following 116 patients for 2 years, BOCCHETTA et al. (1992) concluded that while elevated TSH concentrations were transitory in most patients, the risk of developing hypothyroidism was higher in women with thyroid antibodies. Clearly, the presence of thyroid antibodies is an important determinant of hypothyroidism in lithium-treated patients although the inhibitory action of the drug on thyroid hormone release may account for those cases of hypothyroidism which recover to the euthyroid state. The prevalence of thyroid antibodies in patients on long-term lithium therapy has been reported to vary between 10% and 33% (LAZARUS 1986a) – it now seems unlikely that lithium can significantly induce the de novo production of thyroid antibodies but there is evidence (LAZARUS et al. 1985) that lithium therapy is associated with a rise in antibody titre in patients who already are antibody positive at the start of treatment.

With regard to other factors which may influence the development of hypothyroidism, it has been shown that iodine and lithium can act synergistically to produce hypothyroidism (SHOPSIN et al. 1973). Variations in iodine status, dietary goitrogens, immunogenetic make-up and their interactions in the setting of chronic lithium therapy contribute to the variable pattern of expression of hypothyroidism in different ethnic groups and areas (LEE et al. 1992). Thus the pathogenesis of lithium-induced hypothyroidism is either autoimmune or by direct action of lithium on hormone secretion leading to goitre and hypothyroidism.

III. Hyperthyroidism

Despite the general suppressive effect of lithium on thyroid function, a significant number of cases of hyperthyroidism have been reported. The first case was reported from New Zealand (FRANKLIN 1974). Since then there have been a further 40–50 cases described (LAZARUS 1986a; CHOW and COCKRAM 1990; CHOW et al. 1993; PERSAD et al. 1993; BARCLAY et al. 1994). Review of the clinical characteristics of lithium-associated thyrotoxicosis in 24 patients showed that it occurred after many years of lithium therapy in most but not all patients. The aetiology of the hyperthyroidism included Graves' disease, toxic nodular goitre and silent thyroiditis. Recently a case of granulomatous thyroiditis associated with lithium therapy was described (SINNOTT et al. 1992) and the thyroid histology in another case (MIZUKAMI et al. 1995) showed extensive follicular destruction with no lymphocytic infiltration. Lithium might therefore directly damage thyroid cells with consequent release of throglobulin and thyroid hormones into the circulation.

It is clearly probable that lithium treatment could mask underlying hyperthyroidism by reduction of thyroid hormones such that when lithium is stopped hyperthyroidism will appear. Whether lithium induces autoimmune hyperthyroidism by, for example, producing thyroid-stimulating antibodies is not known and the reported cases have been thought to be chance events. However, BARCLAY et al. (1994), in a careful epidemiological study of 14 cases of lithium-associated thyrotoxicosis from New Zealand, concluded that long-term lithium therapy is associated with an increased risk of thyrotoxicosis. Nine of the 14 patients in this series had autoimmune thyrotoxicosis although TSH receptor antibody measurements were not available. The others had toxic nodular goitre and it is possible that lithium-associated thyrotoxicosis in these patients was due to a maladaptation to disturbed iodine kinetics with a possible escape phenomenon after expansion of the intrathyroidal iodine pool.

An intriguing report of the association of lithium therapy with exophthalmos was made by SEGAL et al. (1973). This eye sign was observed in 10% of his patients and 25% of 73 patients studied by LAZARUS et al. (1981). Both of these reports did not have accurate measurement of the eye changes and the possible mechanisms are unclear. Nevertheless, it is interesting that the eye signs regressed when lithium was discontinued in a case of a bipolar patient who developed thyrotoxicosis with severe exophthalmos while on lithium (BYRNE and DELANEY 1993).

H. Clinical Use in Thyroid Disease

The discovery that the main action of lithium on the thyroid gland is to inhibit thyroid hormone release led to an early successful trial of the drug in hyperthyroidism (TEMPLE et al. 1972a). The secretion rate of iodide and hormonal iodine was reduced by 30%–85% within 12 h of achieving a therapeutic level of lithium. Further studies showed that lithium alone produced a decrease in serum thyroxine concentration of between 21% and 35% after 6–14 days of treatment (TEMPLE et al. 1972b; GERDES et al. 1973; LAZARUS et al. 1974). Unlike iodide, lithium can be given for as long as 6 months to thyrotoxic patients without any danger of the "escape" as seen with iodide (LAZARUS et al. 1974).

When lithium was compared to carbimazole in the treatment of thyrotoxicosis (KRISTENSEN et al. 1976), it was found not to be superior in its ability to achieve rapid control of the disease but combination therapy with lithium and carbimazole was more effective than carbimazole alone in terms of reduction of thyroid hormone concentrations (TURNER et al. 1976; HEDLEY et al. 1978). In view of the earlier reports of synergy between lithium and iodide (SHOPSIN et al. 1973; SPAULDING et al. 1977), the combination of lithium and iodide in the treatment of thyrotoxicosis was studied by BOEHM et al. (1980). They proposed that the effect of lithium in inhibiting colloid droplet formation exerted a maximal effect itself and iodine inhibition of thyroglobulin hydrolysis could not improve on this. Lithium then is an effective agent for rapidly lowering thyroid hormone levels in thyrotoxic patients and may be indicated in patients who cannot receive thiocarbamide antithyroid drugs (EULRY et al. 1977) or for pre-operative preparation (MOCHINAGA et al. 1994; TAKAMI 1994).

When lithium is administered a few days before ^{131}I therapy for hyperthyoidism, thyroid retention of the isotope is increased and hyperthyroidism is ameliorated more rapidly than with ^{131}I alone. However, there is no long-term advantage in the hypothyroid rate. It is possible that this approach may reduce the total body radiation dose to the patient (BROWNLIE et al. 1979). Because of the delayed thyroidal ^{131}I release and the effectiveness of the lithium ^{131}I combination in treating hyperthyroidism, it was suggested that lithium would be a useful adjunct in the management of differentiated thyroid carcinoma. An increase in biological half-life and whole body retention of ^{131}I has indeed been observed (GERSHENGORN et al. 1976), but the clinical outcome of the disease has not been significantly altered and this strategy has not been generally adopted.

Summary

Lithium has many actions on thyroid physiology. The most important is the inhibition of thyroid hormone release. This may result in the development of goitre and hypothyroidism. Independent effects on the hypothalamic pituitary thyroid axis and the receptor-mediated mechanism of thyroid hormone action may contribute to this picture. The effect of lithium on inhibition of cyclic AMP mediated cellular events and its inhibitory effect on the phosphoinositol pathway help to explain the intracellular disturbances but the full mechanisms are still not clear. The immunological influence of lithium on thyroid antibody concentrations leads to a more rapid onset of thyroid autoimmunity characterised usually by goitre and hypothyroidism but possibly also a state of hyperthyroidism in some cases. Lithium is an effective treatment for hyperthyroidism in certain clinical indications and may also be administered in conjunction with ^{131}I in the management of hyperthyroidism or thyroid cancer. However, the long-term results of such therapy do not appear to confer any clinical advantage over conventional treatment. The relationship of the effect of lithium on cerebral thyroid hormone metabolism to the psychotropic effects of the drug is uncertain at present and further research in this area is indicated.

References

Albrecht J, Hopf U (1982) Humoral autoimmune phenomena under long-term treatment with lithium with special regard to thyroidal autoantibodies. Klin Wochenschr 60:1501–1504

Andersen BF (1973) Iodide perchlorate discharge test in lithium-treated patients. Acta Endocrinol (Copenh) 73:35–42

Avissar SS, Schreiber G, Danon A, Belmaker RH (1988) Lithium effects on cyclic AMP and phosphatidylinositol metabolism may promote adrenergic–cholinergic balance. In: Birch NJ (ed) Lithium: inorganic pharmacology and psychiatric use. IRL, Oxford, pp 213–228

Bagchi N, Brown TR (1988) Hypothalamic pituitary regulation of thyroid function. In: Johnson NF (ed) Lithium and the endocrine system. Karger, Lancaster, pp 99–106

Bagchi N, Brown TR, Mack RE (1978) Studies on the mechanism of inhibition of thyroid function by lithium. Biochim Biophys Acta 542:163–169

Barclay ML, Brownlie BEW, Turner JG, Wells EJ (1994) Lithium associated thyrotoxicosis: a report of 14 cases, with statistical analysis of incidence. Clin Endocrinol (Oxf) 40:759–764

Baumgartner A, Campos-Barros A, Gaio U, Hessenius C, Frege I, Meinhold H (1994a) Effects of lithium on thyroid-hormone metabolism in rat frontal-cortex. Biol Psychiatry 36:771–774

Baumgartner A, Dubeyko M, Campos-Barros A, Eravci M, Meinhold H (1994b) Subchronic administration of fluoxetine to rats affects triiodothyronine production and deiodination in regions of the cortex and in the limbic forebrain. Brain Res 635:68–74

Baumgartner A, Vonstuckrad M, Mulleroerlinghausen B, Graf KJ, Kurten I (1995) The hypothalamic-pituitary-thyroid axis in patients maintained on lithium prophylaxis for years – high triiodothyronine serum concentrations are correlated to the prophylactic efficacy. J Affect Dis 34:211–218

Berens SC, Wolff J, Murphy DL (1970a) Lithium concentration by the thyroid. Endocrinology 87:1085–1087
Berens SC, Bernstein RS, Robbins J et al (1970b) Antithyroid effects of lithium. J Clin Invest 47:135–1367
Bhattacharyya B, Wolff J (1976) Stabilization of microtubules by lithium ion. Biochem Biophys Res Commun 73:383–390
Bjorkman U, Ekholm R (1990) Biochemistry of thyroid hormone formation and secretion. In: Greer MA (ed) The thyroid gland. Raven, New York, pp 83–125
Bocchetta A, Bernardi F, Burrai C, Pedditzi M, Loviselli A, Velluzzi F, Martino E, Delzompo M (1992) The course of thyroid abnormalities during lithium treatment – a 2-year follow-up study. Acta Psychiatr Scand 86:38–41
Boehm TM, Burman KD, Barnes S, Wartofsky L (1980) Lithium and iodine combination therapy for thyrotoxicosis. Acta Endocrinol (Copenh) 94:174–183
Bolaris S, Margarity M, Valcana T (1995) Effects of LiCl on triiodothyronine (T-3) binding to nuclei from rat cerebral hemispheres. Biol Psychiatry 37:106–111
Brownlie B, Turner J, Ovenden B, Rogers T (1979) Results of lithium ^{131}I treatment of thyrotoxicosis. J Endocr Invest 2:303–304
Burke G (1970) Effects of cations and ouabain on thyroid adenyl cyclase. Biochem Biophys Acta 220:30–41
Burrow GN, Burke WR, Himmelhoch JM, Spencer RP, Hershman JM (1971) Effect of lithium on thyroid function. J Clin Endocrinol 32:647–652
Byrne AP, Delaney WJ (1993) Regression of thyrotoxic ophthalmopathy following lithium withdrawal. Can J Psychiatry 38:635–637
Cade JFJ (1949) Lithium salts in the treatment of psychotic excitement. Med J Aust 36:349–352
Carlson H, Temple R, Robbins J (1973) Effect of lithium on thyroxine disappearance in man. J Clin Endocr Metab 73:383–390
Chow CC, Cockram CS (1990) Thyroid disorders induced by lithium and amiodarone: an overview. Adv Drug React Acute Poison Rev 9(4):207–222
Chow CC, Lee S, Shek CC, Wing YK, Ahuja A, Cockram CS (1993) Lithium-associated transient thyrotoxicosis in 4 Chinese women with autoimmune-thyroiditis. Aust N Z J Psychiatry 27:246–253
Cooper TB, Simpson GM (1969) Preliminary report of a longitudinal study on the effects of lithium on iodine metabolism. Curr Ther Res 11:603–608
Cooper TB, Wagner BM, Kline NS (1970) Contribution to the mode of action of lithium on iodine metabolism. Biol Psychiatry 2:273–278
Downie SE, Wasnidge C, Floto F, Robinson GA (1977) Lithium-induced inhibition of ^{125}I accumulation by thyroids and growing oocytes of Japanase quail. Poultry Sci 56:1254–1258
Drummond AH, Joels LA, Hughes PJ (1988) Thyrotropin-releasing hormone. In: Johnson NF (ed) Lithium and the endocrine system. Karger, Lancaster, pp 107–122
Emerson CH, Dyson WL, Utiger R (1973) Serum thyrotropin and thyroxine concentrations in patients receiving lithium carbonate. J Clin Endocrinol Metab 36:338–346
Eulry F, Orgiazzi J, Mornex R (1977) Les sels de lithium ont-ils leur place dans le traitement des hyperthyroidies Graves? Nouv Presse Med 6:2955–2958
Fauerholdt L, Vendsborg P (1981) Thyroid gland morphology after lithium treatment. Acta Pathol Microbiol Scand 89:339–341
Fernandez L, Fox R (1980) Pertubation of the human immune system by lithium. Clin Exp Immunol 41:527–532
Fieve R, Platman S (1968) Lithium and thyroid function in manic-depressive psychosis. Am J Psychiat 125:119–122
Franklin LM (1974) Thyrotoxicosis developing during lithium treatment: case report. N Z Med J 79:782
Gerdes H, Littmann K-P, Mahlstedt JK (1973) Die Behandlung der Thyreotoxikose mit Lithium. Dtsch Med Wochenschr 98:1551–1555

Gershengorn MC, Izumi M, Robbins J (1976) Use of lithium as an adjunct to radioiodine therapy of thyroid carcinoma. J Clin Endocrinol Metab 42:105–111
Hahn C-G, Pawlyk AC, Whybrow PC, Tejani-Butt SM (1995) Effects of lithium on gene expression of thyroid hormone receptors (THRS) in rat brain. Proceedings of the annual meeting of Society for Neuroscience, San Diego, California, Nov (abstract)
Hallcher LM, Sherman WR (1980) The effects of lithium ion and other agents on the activity of myoinositol-1-phosphatase from bovine brain. J Biol Chem:10896–10901
Hart DA (1993) Lithium and autoimmune disease: murine models and the human experience. In: Birch NJ, Padgham C, Hughes MS (eds) Lithium in medicine and biology. Marius, Carnforth, UK, pp 165–173
Hassman RA, McGregor AM (1988) Lithium and autoimmune thyroid disease. In: Johnson FN (ed) Lithium and the endocrine system. Karger, Lancaster, pp 135–146
Hassman RA, Lazarus JH, Dieguez C, Weetman AP, Hall R, McGregor AM (1985) The influence of lithium chloride on experimental autoimmune thyroid disease. Clin Exp Immunol 61:49–57
Hedley J, Turner J, Brownlie J, Sadler W (1978) Low dose lithium-carbimazole in treatment of thyrotoxicosis. Aust N Z J Med 8:628–630
Heltne CE, Ollerich DA (1973) Morphometric and electron microscopic studies of goiter induced by lithium in the rat. Am J Anat 136:297
Hennemann G, Docter R, Krenning EP (1994) Thyroid hormone production, transport and metabolism. In: Wheeler MH, Lazarus JH (eds) Diseases of the thyroid. Chapman and Hall London, pp 21–27
Hullin RP, Johnson AW (1970) Effect of lithium salts on uptake of I^{125} by rat thyroid gland. Life Sci 9:9–20
Jankovic B, Popeskovil L, Isakovic K (1979) Cation-induced immunosuppression; the effect of lithium on arthus reactivity, delayed hypersensitivity and antibody production in the rat. In: Muller-Rucholtz W, Muller-Hermelink HK (eds) Function and structure of the immune system. Plenum Press, New York, pp 339–344
Johnson FN (1984) The history of lithium. McMillan, London, pp 1–198
Kristensen O, Harrestrup Andersen H, Pallisgaard G (1976) Lithium carbonate in the treatment of thyrotoxicosis. A controlled trial. Lancet 1:603–605
Kushner JP, Wartofsky L (1988) Lithium-thyroid interactions. An overview. In: Johnnson NF (ed) Lithium and the endocrine system. Karger, Lancaster, pp 74–98
Lazarus JH (1986a) Effect of lithium on the thyroid gland. In: Lazarus JH (ed) Endocrine and metabolic effects of lithium. Plenum, New York, pp 99–124
Lazarus JH (1986b) Lithium and the cell. In: Lazarus JH (ed) Endocrine and metabolic effects of lithium. Plenum, New York, pp 31–54
Lazarus JH (1986c) Other effects of lithium mediated through metabolic pathways. In: Lazarus JH (ed) Endocrine and metabolic effects of lithium. Plenum, New York, pp 187–201
Lazarus JH, Bennie EH (1972) Effect of lithium on thyroid function in man. Acta Endocrinol (Copenh) 70:266–272
Lazarus JH, Muston HL (1978) The effect of lithium on the iodide concentrating mechanism in mouse salivary gland. Acta Pharmacol Toxicol 43:55–58
Lazarus JH, Richards AR, Addison GM, Owen GM (1974) Treatment of thyrotoxicosis with lithium carbonate. Lancet 2:1160–1162
Lazarus JH, John R, Bennie EH, Chalmers RJ, Crockett G (1981) Lithium therapy and thyroid function: a long-term study. Psychol Med 11:85–92
Lazarus JH, Ludgate M, McGregor A, Hassman R, Creagh F, Kingswood C (1985) Lithium therapy induces autoimmune thyroid disease. In: Walfish PG, Wall JR, Volpe R (eds) Autoimmunity and the thyroid. Academic, London, pp 319–320
Lee S, Chow CC, Wing YK, Shek CC (1992) Thyroid abnormalities during chronic lithium treatment in Hong-Kong Chinese – a controlled study. J Affect Dis 26:173–178

Levitt L, Queensberry J (1980) The effect of lithium on murine hematopoiesis in a liquid culture system. N Engl J Med 302:713–719

Ljunggren J-G, Sedvall G, Levin K, Fryo B (1971) Influence of the lithium ion on the biosynthesis of thyroxine and thyroglobulin in the rat. Acta Endocrinol (Copenh) 67:784–792

Lomabardi G, Panza N, Biondi L, Di Lorenzo L, Lupoli G, Muscettola G, Carella C, Bellastella A (1993) Effects of lithium treatment on hypothalamic-pituitary-thyroid axis – a longitudinal study. J Endocrinol Invest 16:259–263

MacNeil S, Wragg MS, Wagner M, Tomlinson S (1993) Investigation of the mechanism of lithium-induced hormone resistance. In: Birch NJ, Padgham C, Hughes MS (eds) Lithium in medicine and biology. Marius, Carnforth, UK, pp 133–141

Mannisto PT (1973) Thyroid iodine metabolism in vitro. II. Effect of lithium ion. Ann Med Exp Biol Fenn 51:42–45

Mannisto PT (1980) Endocrine side-effects of lithium. In: Johnson FN (ed) Handbook of lithium therapy. MTP Press, Lancaster, pp 310–322

Martino E, Placid G, Sardano G, Mariotti S, Fornaro P, Pinchera A, Baschieri L (1982) High incidence of goiter in patients treated with lithium carbonate. Ann Endocr 43:269–276

McLarty D, O'Boyle J, Spencer C, Ratcliffe J (1975) Effect of lithium on hypothalmic-pituitary-thyroid function in patients with affective disorders. Br Med J iii:623–626

Miloni E, Burgi H, Studer H, Siebenhuner L, Lemarchand-Beraud T (1983) Thyroglobulin-rich colloid goitres: a result of the combined action of lithium and methimazole on the rat thyroid. Acta Endocrinol (Copenh) 103:231–234

Mizukami Y, Michigishi T, Nonomura A, Nakamura S, Noguchi M, Takazakura E (1995) Histological features of the thyroid gland in a patient with lithium-induced thyrotoxicosis. J Clin Pathol 48:582–584

Mochinaga N, Eto T, Maekawa Y, Tsunoda T, Kanematsu T, Izumi M (1994) Successful preoperative preparation for thyroidectomy in Graves' disease using lithium alone – report of 2 cases. Surg Today 24:464–467

Myers D, Carter R, Burns B, Armond A, Hussain S, Chengapa V (1985) A prospective study of the effects of lithium on thyroid function and on the prevalence of antithyroid antibodies. Psychol Med 15:55–61

Oppenheimer JH, Schwartz HL, Strait KA (1994) An integrated view of thyroid hormone actions in vitro. In: Weintraub BD (ed) Molecular endocrinology: basic concepts and clinical correlations. Raven, New York, pp 249–268

Perrild H, Hegedus L, Arnung K (1984) Sex related goitrogenic effect of lithium carbonate in healthy young subjects. Acta Endocrinol (Copenh) 106:203–208

Perrild H, Feldt-Rasmussen U, Hegedus L, Baastrup PC (1988) Serum thyroglobulin and thyroid volume during administration of lithium carbonate to healthy young subjects. In: Birch NJ (ed) Lithium: inorganic pharmacology and psychiatric use. IRL, Oxford, pp 183–184

Persad E, Forbath N, Merskey H (1993) Hyperthyroidism after treatment with lithium. Can J Psychiatry 38:599–602

Pfeifer WD, Davis LC, Van der Velde CD (1976) Lithium accumulation in some endocrine tissues. Acta Biol Med Ger 35:1519–1523

Rapaport MH, Schmidt ME, Risinger R, Manji H (1994) The effects of prolonged lithium exposure on the immune-system of normal control subjects – serial serum-soluble interleukin-2 receptor and antithyroid antibody measurements. Biol Psychiatry 35:761–766

Rogers M, Whybrow P (1971) Clinical hypothyroidism occurring during lithium treatment. Two case histories and a review of thyroid function in 19 patients. Am J Psychiatry 128:50–55

Sanghvi I, Shopsin B, Gershon S (1975) The influence of dietary iodine on lithium blood level, serum T_4 and thyroid gland weight. Psycopharmacol Commun 1:437–444

Schou M (1957) Biology and pharmacology of the lithium ion. Pharmacol Rev 9:17–58

Schou M, Juel-Nielsen N, Stromgren E, Voldby H (1954) The treatment of manic psychoses by the administration of lithium salts. J Neurol Neurosurg Psychiatry 17:1257–1264
Schou M, Amdisen A, Jensen S, Olsen T (1968) Occurrence of goitre during lithium treatment. Br Med J iii:710–713
Sedvall G, Jonsson B, Pettersson U, Levin K (1968) Effects of lithium salts on plasma protein bound iodine and uptake of I^{131} in thyroid gland of man and rat. Life Sci 7:1257–1264
Sedvall G, Jonsson B, Petterson U (1969) Evidence of an altered thyroid function in man during treatment with lithium carbonate. Acta Psychiatr Scand 207:59–67
Segal RL, Rosenblatt S, Eliasoph I (1973) Endocrine exophthalmos during lithium therapy of manic depressive disease. N Engl J Med 289:136–138
Shenkman L, Borkowsky W, Holzman RS, Shopsin B (1978) Enhancement of lymphocyte and macrophage function in vitro by lithium chloride. Clin Immunol Immunopathol 10:187–192
Shopsin B, Shenkman L, Blum M, Hollander C (1973) Iodine and lithium-induced hypothyroidism. Documentation of synergism. Am J Med 55:695–699
Singer I, Rotenberg D (1973) Mechanisms of lithium action. N Engl J Med 289:254–260
Sinnott MJ, McIntyre HD, Pond SM (1992) Granulomatous thyroiditis and lithium therapy. Aust N Z J Med 22:84
Spaulding SW (1989) Lithium effects on the thyroid gland. In: Gaitan E (ed) Environmental goitrogenesis. CRC, Boca Raton, pp 149–157
Spaulding SW, Burrow G, Bermudez F, Himmelhoch J (1972) The inhibitory effect of lithium on thyroid hormone release in both euthyroid and thyrotoxic patients. J Clin Endocrinol Metab 35:905–911
Spaulding SW, Burrow GN, Ramey JN, Donabedian RK (1977) Effect of increased iodide uptake on thyroid function in subjects on chronic lithium theapy. Acta Endocrinol (Copenh) 84:290
St. Germain D (1987) Regulatory effect of lithium on thyroxine metabolism in murine neural and anterior pituitary tissue. Endocrinology 120:1430–1436
St. Germain DL (1988) Thyroid hormone metabolism. In: Johnson NF (ed) Lithium and the endocrine system. Karger, Lancaster, pp 123–133
Takada K, Tada H, Takano T, Nishiyama S, Amino N (1993) Functional regulation of GTP-binding protein coupled to insulin-like growth factor-I receptor by lithium during G (1) phase of the rat-thyroid cell-cycle. FEBS Lett 318:245–248
Takami H (1994) Lithium in the preoperative preparation of Graves' disease. Int Surg 79:89–90
Takano T, Takada K, Tada H, Nishiyama S, Amino N (1994) Genistein but not staurosporine can inhibit the mitogenic signal evoked by lithium in rat-thyroid cells (FRTL-5). J Endocrinol 143:221–226
Tanimoto K, Maeda K, Yamaguchi N, Chihara K, Fujita T (1981) Effect of lithium on prolactin responses to thyrotropin-releasing hormone in patients with manic state. Psychopharmacol 72:129–133
Temple R, Berman M, Carlson H, Robbins J, Wolff J (1972a) The use of lithium in Graves' disease. Mayo Clin Proc 47:872–878
Temple R, Berman M, Robbins J, Wolff J (1972b) The use of lithium in the treatment of thyrotoxicosis. J Clin Invest 51:2746–2756
Terao T, Oga T, Nozaki S, Ohta A, Otsubo Y, Yamamoto S, Zamami M, Okada M (1995) Possible inhibitory effect of lithium on peripheral conversion of thyroxine to triiodothyronine – a prospective study. Int Clin Psychopharmacol 10:103–105
Tsuchiya Y, Saji M, Ifsozaki O, Arai M, Tshushima T, Shizume K (1990) Effect of lithium on deoxyribonucleic acid synthesis and iodide uptake in porcine thyroid cells in culture. Endocrinology 126:460–465
Turner JG, Brownlie BEW, Sadler WA, Jensen CH (1976) An evaluation of lithium as an adjunct to carbimazole treatment in acute thyrotoxicosis. Acta Endocrinol (Copenh) 83:86–92

Voss C, Schober H, Hartmann N (1977) Einfluss von lithium auf die in vitro-Dejodierung von L-Thyroxin in der Rattenleber. Acta Biol Med Germ 36:1061–1065
Waldman SA, Park D (1989) Myxedema coma associated with lithium therapy. Am J Med 87:355–356
Weetman AP, McGregor AM, Lazarus JH, Rees Smtih B, Hall R (1982) The enhancement of immunoglobulin synthesis by human lymphocytes with lithium. Clin Immunol 2:400–407
Williams J, Berens, Wolff J (1971) Thyroid secretion in vitro. Inhibition of TSH and dibutyryl cyclic-AMP stimulated ^{131}I release by lithium. Endocrinol 88:1385–1388
Wolff J (1978) Lithium interactions with the thyroid gland. In: Cooper TB, Gershon S, Kline NS et al (eds) Lithium controversies and unresolved issues. Excerpta Medica, Amsterdam, pp 552–564

CHAPTER 10

Amiodarone and the Thyroid

W.M. WIERSINGA

A. Pharmacology of Amiodarone

Amiodarone was synthesized in 1961 by TONDEUR and BINON in the Labaz Laboratories in Belgium. It is a benzofuran derivative related to the obsolete vasodilator khellin. Characteristic structural features of the drug are its high iodine content and its resemblance to thyroxine. It was originally introduced in 1962 in clinical medicine for the treatment of angina pectoris, but later the drug was found to be very efficacious in the treatment of cardiac arrhythmias. It is mainly used as a potent antiarrhythmic drug for the suppression of life-threatening ventricular arrhythmias refractory to other agents. More recently, amiodarone has also been used successfully in the treatment of atrial fibrillation and severe congestive heart failure. The toxicity of the drug, however, precludes widespread prescription in less severe cardiac diseases.

I. Physicochemical Properties

The molecular constitution of amiodarone, a diiodinated benzofuran derivate, is given in Fig. 1. It is an amphophilic drug with hydrophilic (tertiary amine) and lipophilic (benzofuran and diiodinated benzene ring) moieties. It has a normal pK_a for a tertiary amine, indicating that, at physiological pH, amiodarone is essentially ionized. The molecular weight of amiodarone and its main metabolite desethylamiodarone (DEA) are 645.32 and 617.27, respectively. The drug is prescribed as amiodarone hydrochloride (MW 681.82); the salt contains 94.65% of the free base. Amiodarone contains 39.33% iodine by weight, amiodarone chloride 37.25%.

II. Pharmacokinetics

The first pharmacokinetic studies of amiodarone in humans were done by BROEKHUYSEN et al. in 1969 using ^{131}I-labelled amiodarone. Their data indicated a very long elimination half-life, a large volume of distribution and an extensive tissue distribution. Although this study is open to criticism because only total radioactivity was measured, and consequently the fate of iodine rather than of amiodarone was evaluated, subsequent studies in the 1980s using sensitive and specific high-performance liquid chromatography (HPLC)

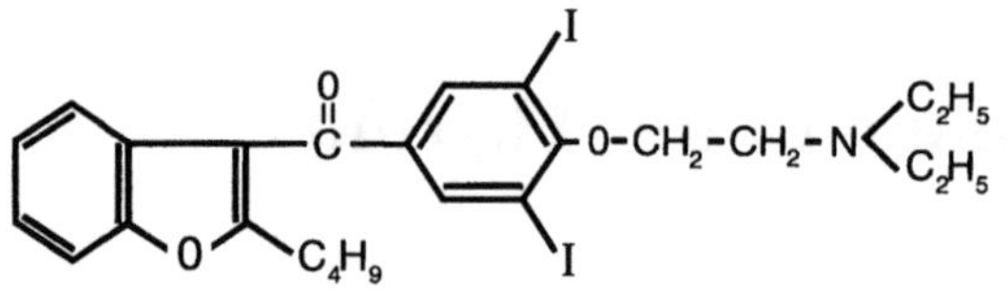

Fig. 1. Molecular constitution of amiodarone (chemical name: 2-butyl-3-[3, 5-diiodo-4-(β-diethylaminoethoxy)-benzoyl] benzofuran)

methods for analysis of amiodarone and DEA have largely confirmed these initial findings (ANDREASEN et al. 1981; PLOMP et al. 1984). The assay of serum amiodarone and DEA by the HPLC method is now widely used (JANDRESKI and VANDERSLICE 1993).

1. Absorption and Bioavailability

Absorption of amiodarone tablets in humans is slow. Following a single 400-mg oral dose peak plasma concentrations of amiodarone (C_{max} 0.37 ± 0.22 μg/ml) are reached after 5 h (t_{max} 4.8 ± 1.5 h); bioavailability was 31 ± 26% (PLOMP et al. 1984). There is a linear relationship between oral dose and plasma concentration with marked variation between subjects. The low oral bioavailability might be due to incomplete absorption across the intestinal mucosa (probably related to poor dissolution characteristics of the drug) (HOLT et al. 1983) or due to first-pass metabolism of amiodarone in the intestinal mucosa (N-dealkylation) and the liver (MASON 1987).

2. Plasma Kinetics

A single intravenous dose of 400 mg amiodarone administered to human volunteers provided the following kinetic data (PLOMP et al. 1984): the decline in plasma amiodarone concentration was best described by a triexponential decay equation with a mean terminal half-life ($t_{1/2}$) of 34 ± 27 h. Mean plasma clearance was 245 ± 120 ml/min, and mean apparent steady-state volume of distribution 376 ± 372 l. Following a single oral dose of 400 mg amiodarone, the $t_{1/2}$ was 32 ± 21 h. In patients on a mean maintenance dose of 440 ± 253 mg for a mean period of 9.1 months, the mean plasma concentrations of amiodarone were 1.85 ± 1.17 μg/ml and of DEA 1.35 ± 0.71 μg/ml, with an overall mean amiodarone/DEA ratio of 1.37. After discontinuation of long-term amiodarone treatment the mean elimination half-lives of amiodarone and DEA were 40 ± 10 days and 57 ± 27 days, respectively (PLOMP et al. 1984). Other studies report essentially similar results (BERGER and HARRIS 1986).

In the circulation amiodarone is bound 96.3 ± 0.6% to plasma proteins, predominantly to albumin (62.1%); the remaining part is carried on a high molecular weight protein, probably β-lipoprotein (BERGER and HARRIS 1986). There is one high-affinity amiodarone binding site per albumin molecule (K_a 5.6×10^6 l/M), and 4.4 additional low-affinity binding sites (K_a 1.9×10^5 l/M), which apparently are not utilized in whole serum (LALLOZ et al. 1984). Amiodarone leaves the plasma to bind extensively with most tissues of the body. The various stages of the distribution phase suggest that the drug is firstly taken up into well-perfused organs, whereas poorly perfused tissues such as fat form the stock or "deep" compartment of amiodarone. The large volume of distribution (106 ± 38 l/kg) is in agreement with the extensive distribution of the drug. The slow turnover of amiodarone from the deep compartment explains the exceptionally long terminal half-life, and results in a low total plasma clearance for amiodarone of the order of 150 ml/min (BERGER and HARRIS 1986).

3. Tissue Distribution

Concentrations of amiodarone and DEA in human tissues obtained at autopsy are reported in various studies; a typical example is given in Table 1. Highest levels are found in adipose tissue, liver and lung; moderate levels occur in heart and kidneys, and lowest levels in muscles, thyroid and brain. The major metabolite DEA follows the same pattern of widespread tissue distribution as the parent drug. Tissue contents of DEA are higher than of amiodarone in all tissues except fat. The steady-state partition coefficient of amiodarone and DEA in fat, liver and pulmonary tissue relative to plasma ranges from 100 to above 1000. The myocardial concentration of amiodarone is 10–50 times that in plasma, but develops slowly indicating the necessity for loading doses (MASON 1987).

As for the subcellular distribution, amiodarone medication induces cytoplasmic multilamellar inclusion bodies in many tissues including human myocardium (SOMANI 1989). Direct and indirect evidence obtained both in vivo and in vitro indicate an intralysosomal localization for amiodarone and DEA (HONEGGER et al. 1993). This comes as no surprise since amiodarone belongs to the group of cationic amphiphilic substances which accumulate in lysosomes.

Table 1. Tissue distribution of amiodarone (A) and desethylamiodarone (DEA) in human autopsies[a]

Tissue	A (μg/g)	DEA (μg/g)	A/DEA
Adipose tissue	316	76	4.2
Liver	391	2354	0.12
Lung	198	952	0.21
Kidneys	57	262	0.22
Heart	40	169	0.24
Muscle	22	51	0.43
Thyroid	14	64	0.22
Brain	8	54	0.15

[a] Figures are mean concentrations of seven to nine observations (HOLT et al. 1983).

4. Metabolism

There appear to be five metabolic pathways which alone or in combination can explain all identified metabolites of amiodarone: N-dealkylation, deiodination, O-dealkylation, hydroxylation and glucuroconjugation (BERGER and HARRIS 1986). Although some quantitative differences exist between species, qualitative differences are minor.

a) N-Dealkylation

The major metabolite is DEA, resulting from N-dealkylation of the parent drug (Fig. 2). Subsequent N-dealkylation leads to the primary amine desdiethylamiodarone, which has been detected in dogs but barely in humans.

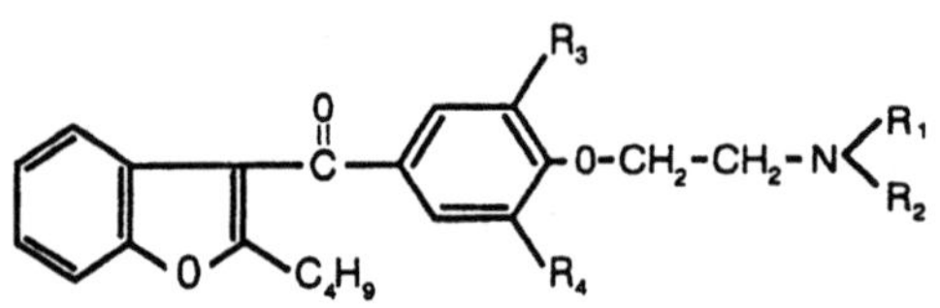

Compound		R_1	R_2	R_3	R_4
1	desethylamiodarone	C_2H_5	H	I	I
2	desdiethylamiodarone	H	H	I	I
3	monoiodoamiodarone	C_2H_5	C_2H_5	I	H
4	desdiiodoamiodarone	C_2H_5	C_2H_5	H	H
5	desethyldesdiiodoamiodarone	C_2H_5	H	H	H

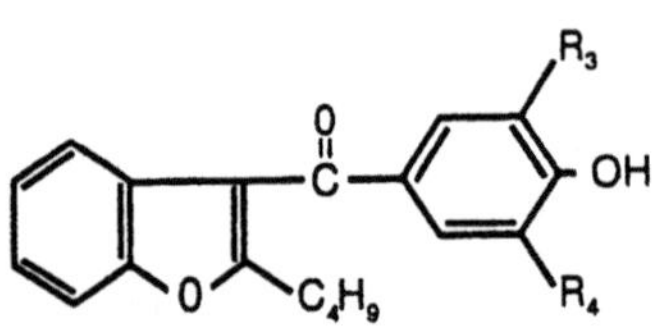

Compound		R_3	R_4
6	L 3373	I	I
7	L 6424	I	H
8	L 3372	H	H

Fig. 2. Molecular constitution of amiodarone metabolites. *Top panel*, deethylated and deiodinated derivates of amiodarone; *bottom panel*, 2-butyl-3(4-hydroxy-benzoyl) benzofuran derivates

In humans, DEA concentration in the portal vein is higher than in the hepatic vein; this suggests that orally administered amiodarone undergoes extensive N-dealkylation during its pass in the gut lumen or across the intestinal mucosa (BERDEAUX et al. 1984). Little DEA is found after acute intravenous or oral dosing. Due to the drug's affinity for adipose tissue and its large volume of distribution, approximately 15 g is necessary to saturate the large body stores (PODRID 1995).

b) Deiodination

The presence of deiodinated amiodarone metabolites might be expected from studies reporting the excretion of free iodide in the urine during amiodarone therapy (ANDREASEN et al. 1981). Monoiodoamiodarone, desdiiodoamiodarone and desethyldesdiiodoamiodarone have indeed been detected in human plasma, lung and liver samples (FLANAGAN et al. 1982; BERGER and HARRIS 1986) (Fig. 2).

The pharmacokinetic profile of organic and inorganic iodine has been determined in healthy subjects after a single oral dose of 600 mg amiodarone (BERGER and HARRIS 1986). Plasma organic iodine reached peak levels of 0.54 mg/l after 5–6 h. The contribution of unchanged amiodarone to plasma organic iodine decreased from 64% at 1 h to 8% at 72 h, and DEA contributed only 14% at 40 h. Unidentified iodinated metabolites of amiodarone therefore composed the main part of plasma organic iodine. Plasma inorganic iodide (usually lower than 0.01 mg/l) reached peak levels of 0.14 mg/l after 4 h, its elimination rate apparently being limited by its rate of formation from organic iodine.

In patients on a maintenance dose of 300 mg amiodarone daily, plasma inorganic iodide was increased 40-fold (from $0.05 \pm 0.01\,\mu$mol/l to over $2\,\mu$mol/l) (RAO et al. 1986). In this study 24-h urinary iodide excretion was increased 40-fold from $270 \pm 50\,\mu$g ($2.14 \pm 0.4\,\mu$mol) to $11\,000 \pm 900\,\mu$g ($87 \pm 7\,\mu$mol). Another study reports similar steady-state data in three patients on a daily amiodarone dose of 3.6, 6.4 and 8.6 mg/kg (STÄUBLI et al. 1983). Only 15%, 11% and 8%, respectively, of the iodine ingested as amiodarone was excreted per 24 h. Thus, for a subject with a body weight of 70 kg, a daily oral dose of 252, 448 or 602 mg amiodarone, respectively, results in a urinary iodide excretion between 14000 and 18000 μg/24 h. This is 47–60 times higher than the upper limit of the optimal daily iodine intake of 150–300 μg recommended by the WHO. The pharmacological quantities of iodine released during the biotransformation of amiodarone consequently must be considered as chronic iodine excess.

c) O-Dealkylation and Hydroxylation

O-dealkylation leads to compound L3373, which is subject to further deiodination (Fig. 2). Hydroxylation may occur in the benzofuran ring. These metabolites so far have not been identified in human tissues.

d) Glucuroconjugation

Using ^{14}C-labelled amiodarone, glucuro- and arylsulphoconjugated metabolites excreted in the bile represented about 55% of the radioactivity in the rat and about 40% in the monkey.

5. Elimination

a) Bile and Other Body Fluids

In all species studied including man, biliary excretion and faecal elimination account for 65%–75% of the ingested drug (BERGER and HARRIS 1986). Amiodarone is extensively metabolized before biliary elimination. Biliary concentrations of amiodarone are 20–50 times higher than the serum amiodarone levels (ANDREASEN et al. 1981). Urinary excretion is a poor elimination route of amiodarone; urinary concentrations of amiodarone and DEA are very low (0.029 mg/l and 0.149 mg/l, respectively) in patients with normal renal function under chronic treatment (HARRIS et al. 1983). Neither amiodarone nor DEA are detected in dialysis fluid in patients on haemodialysis.

Amiodarone and DEA are also excreted in other biological fluids such as sweat, saliva (saliva amiodarone concentrations are about 2% of the corresponding serum levels), tears (amiodarone is excreted into tear fluid above a threshold plasma concentration of 1.2 μg/ml) (NIELSEN et al. 1983), and semen (in which amiodarone and DEA concentrations are in the order of 1 μg/ml).

b) Placental and Milk Transfer

The transplacental transfer of amiodarone and DEA varies from 10% to 15% and from 20% to 22%, respectively (ROBSON et al. 1985). The difference in maternal-fetal transfer between amiodarone and DEA may be explained by differences in protein binding and ionization of both drugs. The placental content of amiodarone is of the order of 30–70 μg/g, and that of DEA is about 300–500 μg/g. Plasma concentrations of amiodarone and DEA in the newborn are about fourfold lower than those in the mother. Amiodarone and DEA are present in breast milk in higher concentrations than in the mother's plasma due to their high lipid solubility and weak basic properties. The milk/plasma ratio of amiodarone would thus increase due to ion-trapping, because the pH of milk (pH 6.8–7.0) is lower than that of plasma (pH 7.4) (PLOMP et al. 1992). Amiodarone concentrations in human breast milk (1.0–13 μg/μl) are higher than of DEA (0.5–5.7 μg/μl), presumably because the metabolite is less lipid soluble and an even weaker base (pK_a 5.6) than the parent drug (pK_a 6.6). The infant's ingestion of amiodarone from breast milk has been estimated as 1.5 mg/kg per day and that of DEA as 0.6 mg/kg per day, which is equivalent to a low maintenance dose of the drug (BERGER and HARRIS 1986).

III. Pharmacology

1. Electrophysiological Effects

The most important direct electrophysiological effect of amiodarone is prolongation of the action potential duration and repolarization time; this prolongation results from inhibition of the potassium ion fluxes that normally occur during phase 2 and 3 of the action potential and from prolongation of the refractory periods (PODRID 1995). These actions, which occur in all cardiac tissue, classify amiodarone as a class III antiarrhythmic agent (SINGH 1983). The prolongation of the repolarization time by amiodarone persists at higher heart rates. Amiodarone is also a weak sodium channel blocker and slows the upstroke velocity of phase 0 of the action potential. This weak class I antiarrhythmic activity reduces the rate of membrane depolarization and impulse conduction (PODRID 1995).

Indirect electrophysiological effects of amiodarone are due to its antiadrenergic action. Amiodarone acts as a non-competitive α- and β-adrenoceptor antagonist. The β-blocking activity results from a reduction in the number of β-adrenergic receptors (VENKATESH et al. 1986a); the α-blocking activity inhibits the slow inward calcium-ion current (PODRID 1995).

DEA was found to be electrophysiologically active in vitro and in vivo largely in a similar way to amiodarone itself (YABEK et al. 1986; VENKATESH et al. 1986a; NATTEL et al. 1988).

2. Haemodynamic Effects

Amiodarone causes smooth muscle relaxation. As a result, it dilates coronary arteries and increases coronary blood flow. Amiodarone also induces peripheral arterial vasodilatation and a decrease in systemic blood pressure and afterload (PODRID 1995). Although amiodarone has a negative inotropic action reducing the force of myocardial contraction, this is offset by the drug's peripheral vascular effects and cardiac output is generally maintained (PODRID 1995). Amiodarone slows the sinus rate directly and indirectly via its antiadrenergic effects. Amiodarone has a favourable effect on the relation between supply and demand for oxygen in patients with ischaemic heart disease (MASON 1987).

IV. Pharmacotherapy

1. Indications for Use

Amiodarone is a highly effective drug against a wide range of cardiac arrhythmias (PODRID 1995). It is primarily used in patients presenting with sustained ventricular tachyarrhythmia, ventricular tachycardia, or ventricular fibrillation refractory to other treatment modalities. It is also effective in suppressing ventricular arrhythmia and in reducing mortality from sudden death and cardiac disease in patients with non-sustained ventricular tachycardia and cardiomyopathy. Amiodarone is a reasonable option if ventricular tachycardia or ventricular fibrillation occurs in a patient who has recently had a myocardial infarction. Amiodarone is effective for atrial fibrillation, although most physicians prefer other drugs in this condition (MIDDLEKAUFF et al. 1992). Lastly, amiodarone is effective in patients with severe congestive heart failure, reducing mortality and hospital admissions (DOVAL et al. 1994; SINGH et al. 1995). Some physicians use amiodarone as an antianginal agent, especially in patients with refractory angina who are not candidates for revascularization (MEYER and AMANN 1993).

2. Dosing Schedules

Dosage forms of amiodarone are tablets (containing 100mg or 200mg amiodarone hydrochloride) or injections (ampoules of 3ml, containing per ml water 50mg amiodarone hydrochloride, 20mg benzylalcohol and 100mg polysorbate 80) (Cordarone). Because of the unique pharmacokinetic properties (large volume of distribution) of amiodarone, the onset of the drug's action is delayed. In order to achieve efficacy of the drug more quickly, a loading dose to saturate the large body stores is frequently required. Recommended dosing schedules of oral amiodarone are as follows (PODRID 1995): for the treatment of ventricular arrhythmias 1200–1800mg/day for 1–2 weeks, then 800mg/day for 2–4 weeks, then 600mg/day for 4 weeks, and 200–400mg/day thereafter; for the treatment of supraventricular arrhythmias the initial dose is 600–800mg/day for 4 weeks, 400mg/day for 2–4 weeks, and 200mg/day thereafter. The duration of loading and the optimal dose vary between patients, dependent on efficacy and toxicity. For the acute management of life-threatening ventricular arrhythmias the intravenous preparation may be helpful, administered as a rapid infusion of 5mg/kg body weight over 15–30min and followed by 1g/24h thereafter.

The onset of drug activity is associated with typical electrocardiographic changes: sinus bradycardia, lengthening of the PR interval, prolongation of the QT interval, and the development of a prominent U wave not due to hypokalaemia. The therapeutic plasma concentration range of amiodarone is not well defined. The lower limit of the therapeutic range appears to be 0.5–1.0μg/ml (LATINI et al. 1984). Low values indicate non-compliance or inadequate dosage. The upper limit of the therapeutic range is difficult to establish in view of the delayed appearance of side effects months or years after a steady state in plasma has been attained (MASON 1987). The minimal dose of amiodarone with sustained antiarrhythmic and haemodynamic activity should be explored (MAHMARIAN et al. 1994).

V. Toxicology

1. Nature of Side Effects

Adverse effects of amiodarone are numerous, involving many organs. Side effects occur in approximately 80% of patients, requiring withdrawal of the drug in 10%–15% (Podrid 1995). The main side effects are as follows (Raeder et al. 1985; Mason 1987; Vrobel et al. 1989; Wilson and Podrid 1991; Podrid 1995):

1. Cardiac: sinus bradycardia, heart block, proarrhythmia. Aggravation of arrhythmia by amiodarone occurs in 2%–3% of patients, an unusually low incidence for an antiarrhythmic drug which is efficacious against ventricular arrhythmia.
2. Pulmonary: dysfunction, pneumonitis. The overall incidence is about 6%–8%. Pulmonary toxicity may occur with the first weeks of treatment, or develops slowly after months or years.
3. Gastrointestinal: anorexia with or without weight loss, nausea with or without vomiting, abdominal discomfort, constipation, foul taste, ageusia. These symptoms are very common (80%).
4. Hepatic: abnormal liver function tests (especially elevated aminotransferase and alkaline phosphatase levels), seen in 25%. Fatal hepatitis has been reported, but is rare.
5. Renal: modest increase in serum creatinine in 8.8% of patients.
6. Neurological: tremor, ataxia, peripheral neuropathy, fatigue and weakness, reported in 48% of patients.
7. Ocular: corneal microdeposits (almost 100%). This universal finding usually does not cause visual disturbances.
8. Dermatological: photosensitivity and unusual blue-gray skin discoloration of exposed areas reported in 55% up to 75%.
9. Thyroidal: thyrotoxicosis or hypothyroidism, occurring in 14%–18% of patients (see Sect. C.II).
10. Genital: epididymitis (11%).
11. Metabolic: increased blood glucose and increased serum lipids.

Potentially fatal adverse effects are pulmonary toxicity (with a mortality rate as high as 23% once the complication occurs), liver failure due to hepatitis (rare), and cardiac reactions (although amiodarone is unique among antiarrhythmic agents because of its minimal proarrhythmic and negative inotropic properties). Unlike other antiarrhythmic agents, amiodarone has not been shown to increase mortality. Neurological, cardiovascular, gastrointestinal and pulmonary side effects are the most common reasons for discontinuation of amiodarone. Although many of the side effects are tolerated by the patients, the accumulation of side effects with longer exposure to amiodarone may become intolerable. Withdrawal of amiodarone for intolerable side effects thus occurs in a large proportion of patients. After discontinuation of amiodarone, its side effects usually disappear slowly; it may take several months until complete resolution is attained, which may be explained by the very long elimination half-life of the drug (which is in the order of 56 days for amiodarone and 129 days for DEA) (HOLT et al. 1983).

2. Pathogenesis of Side Effects

Although adverse reactions are more common in patients with serum amiodarone concentrations greater than 2.5 μg/ml, a great overlap in serum amiodarone concentrations is observed in patients with and without toxic reactions. Early adverse reactions with high loading doses include gastrointestinal and neurological manifestations, which are dose-related and reversible with dosage reduction. The life-threatening pulmonary, cardiac and hepatic toxicity is not related to dosage or serum concentrations of amiodarone (VROBEL et al. 1989). Most side effects, however, develop slowly, and occur after the first half year of therapy. It has been reported that the incidence of some toxic manifestations (especially in the skin and cornea) is related in a log-linear fashion to the total cumulative dose of amiodarone, rather than to the daily dose or total duration of therapy (MASON 1987). This obviously must be related to tissue accumulation of amiodarone or its metabolites, since steady-state serum levels have been attained much earlier. Tissue content of amiodarone and DEA in humans can be judged from the ubiquitous corneal microdeposits (which are related to the total cumulative dose) (NIELSEN et al. 1983; POLLAK et al. 1989), or measured by HPLC in myocardial biopsies (SOMANI 1989). Since amiodarone contains iodine and is taken up in the liver, the increased hepatic attenuation on computed tomography scans provides an indirect measurement of liver amiodarone and DEA content (NICHOLSON et al. 1994).

The mechanism of amiodarone toxicity is multifactorial. Factors involved are the accumulation of amiodarone, DEA or iodine; the development of cellular phospholipidosis secondary to phospholipase inhibition; the formation of free radicals; or immunological injury (PODRID 1995). The early pulmonary toxicity associated with an eosinophilic lung infiltrate is probably due to a hypersensitivity reaction to the drug. Anti-amiodarone antibodies have been detected in the serum of some amiodarone-treated patients, and side effects of amiodarone were prominent in patients with a cumulative dose of amiodarone of >100 g and a concentration of anti-amiodarone antibodies of >0.6 μg/ml (PICHLER et al. 1988). Because the toxic manifestations of amiodarone are observed in many organs, it is tempting to consider one single mechanism responsible for most of the side effects. Amiodarone as an amphiphilic drug has a strong attraction for intralysosomal phospholipids, and the binding of the drug and these phospholipids renders them indigestible by phospholipases. The bound complexes form the intralysosomal multilamellar inclusion bodies, which have been found in lung, liver, heart, skin, corneal epithelium, lymph nodes, peripheral nerve fibres and blood leucocytes of patients treated with amiodarone (VROBEL et al. 1989). It results in a rising tissue to plasma drug ratio with increasing duration of treatment. The findings suggest a drug-induced phospholipidosis with disturbances of lysosomal function as an explanation of the side effects of amiodarone. The theory is in line with the increasing toxicity with time and the relation to the cumulative dosage of amiodarone.

3. Prevention of Side Effects

Prevention of amiodarone toxicity is best performed by limiting treatment to patients with a low risk: benefit ratio and using the lowest dose compatible with clinical control. Most investigators believe that serum amiodarone and DEA concentrations in general do not predict toxic reactions; drug dosage can be adjusted to maintain serum amiodarone concentration above 1.0 μg/ml and below 2.5 μg/ml (VROBEL et al. 1989). Laboratory tests have in general a low predictive value for the development of toxic reactions, although plasma rT_3 levels above 1.62 nmol/l might be strongly predictive of subsequent toxicity according to some but not all studies (see also Sect. D) (NADEMANEE et al. 1982; SINGH and NADEMANEE 1983; STEWART et al. 1984; KERIN et al. 1986).

B. Effects of Amiodarone on Thyroid Hormone Secretion and Metabolism

I. Changes in Plasma Thyroid Hormone Concentrations

1. Human Studies

Amiodarone treatment invariably results in changes in plasma concentrations of thyroid hormones: the effect is observed in every subject to whom the drug is administered (Fig. 3). Typical changes are a decrease in serum T_3 and an increase in serum rT_3, which can be observed 2 weeks after initiation of treatment (BURGER et al. 1976; MELMED et al. 1981). The low T_3 and high rT_3 levels are maintained during chronic administration of amiodarone (PRITCHARD et al. 1975; JONCKHEER et al. 1978; MELMED et al. 1981; AMICO et al. 1984; SANMARTI et al. 1984; WIERSINGA et al. 1986a); there are only two studies which do not find the decrease in serum T_3 in patients on long-term amiodarone therapy (BOROWSKI et al. 1985; FRANKLYN et al. 1985). At steady state, serum T_3 is decreased by 10%–26% and serum rT_3 increased by about 170% (AMICO et al. 1984; NADEMANEE et al. 1986; RAO et al. 1986). Serum free T_3 is approximately 50% lower than in controls (FRANKLYN et al. 1985; WIERSINGA et al. 1986a). The opposite changes in T_3 and rT_3 also occur in subjects on thyroxine substitution, suggesting they are caused by inhibition of type I iodothyronine-5′-deiodinase (BURGER et al. 1976).

Another characteristic feature is the increase in plasma T_4 and of plasma free T_4, again an early phenomenon (BURGER et al. 1976; MELMED et al. 1981). High levels of plasma T_4 and free T_4 are sustained during chronic administra-

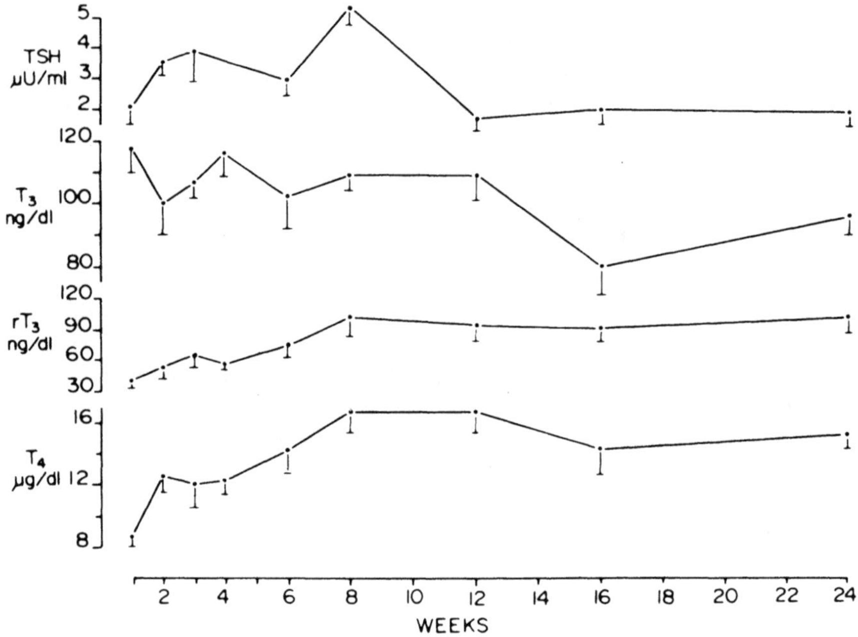

Fig. 3. Changes in thyroid function in ten patients on amiodarone treatment. Each hormone level (shown as means ± SE) was significantly different from the pretreatment value by the end of 3 weeks of treatment. (Reproduced with permission from Melmed et al. 1981)

tion of the drug, being increased on average by 40% (Amico et al. 1984; Franklyn et al. 1985; Nademanee et al. 1986). Serum albumin and serum TBPA (thyroid hormone prealbumin or transthyretin) might be slightly lower in amiodarone-treated patients relative to controls, but the serum concentration of TBG (thyroxine-binding globulin) is not affected by amiodarone therapy (Franklyn et al. 1985). Amiodarone has no influence on the in vitro distribution of the radiolabelled iodothyronines T_4, T_3 and rT_3 amongst their binding proteins in serum, nor are the binding properties of these proteins altered after prolonged treatment with the drug (Lalloz et al. 1984). In accordance, the serum T_3 uptake test (T_3U) is not affected by amiodarone (Jonckheer et al. 1978) (although slightly lower or higher values have been reported (Borowski et al. 1985; Wiersinga et al. 1986a), and the free thyroxine index (calculated as the product of T_4 and T_3U) is increased in line with the increase in total and free plasma T_4 (Amico et al. 1984; Wiersinga et al. 1986a). An apparent dose-response relationship exists between the cumulative dose of amiodarone and plasma T_3, but not with plasma T_4, rT_3, amiodarone or DEA concentrations (Wiersinga et al. 1991).

The course of plasma thyroid-stimulating hormone (TSH) during amiodarone treatment is time dependent. There is an initial rise starting in the first week and lasting for a few months, in which plasma TSH levels may increase above the upper normal limit but in general do not exceed a value of 20 mU/l (BURGER et al. 1976; MELMED et al. 1981). The increased plasma TSH levels return to the normal range after 3 months, although remaining slightly elevated in some cases (MELMED et al. 1981; SANMARTI et al. 1984; NADEMANEE et al. 1986). A trend to lower plasma TSH concentrations has been observed with prolonged continuation of the drug, related to the cumulative dose (JONCKHEER et al. 1978; LAMBERT et al. 1988; WIERSINGA et al. 1991). The TSH response to thyrotrophin-releasing hormone (TRH) is changed according to the change in basal plasma TSH (WIERSINGA et al. 1986a). Plasma TSH increases in hypothyroid patients on stable thyroxine substitution when amiodarone is administered (FIGGE and DLUHY 1990). After withdrawal of amiodarone, it takes a long time before the changes in plasma thyroid hormone concentrations are resolved. Plasma levels of T_4 and rT_3 are still higher and of T_3 lower than pretreatment levels 6 weeks after discontinuation of amiodarone (MELMED et al. 1981).

Benziodarone (with an ethyl group instead of a butyl group but otherwise identical to compound L3373 – see Fig. 2) also decreases serum T_3 and increases serum rT_3 (XANTHOPOULOS et al. 1986).

2. Animal Studies

Amiodarone has been administered to a variety of experimental animals, including male and female Wistar rats, Sprague-Dawley rats, Fisher rats and white New Zealand rabbits. The drug has been given in a dosage ranging from 5 to 200 mg/kg body weight per day for a period of 1–7 weeks. The route of administration was oral (SOGOL et al. 1983; PEKARY et al. 1986; VENKATESH et al. 1986b; KASIM et al. 1987; GØTZSCHE et al. 1989; SCHRÖDER-VAN DER ELST and VAN DER HEIDE 1990; DE JONG et al. 1994), by intraperitoneal injection (KANNAN et al. 1984; PEARCE and HIMSWORTH 1986; CEPPI and ZANINOVICH 1989), or by gastric tube (FRANKLYN et al. 1987; HARTONG et al. 1990; WIERSINGA and BROENINK 1991; YIN et al. 1992; PERRET et al. 1992). In general, these studies are in good agreement with each other and provide similar results as in humans on amiodarone therapy: a decrease in serum T_3 and an increase in serum rT_3 and T_4.

The decrease in serum T_3 is observed in most studies, and ranges from 13% to 70%; it is dose dependent (T_3 decreased by 13%, 36% and 52% in rats treated for 2 weeks with 50, 100 and 150 mg amiodarone/kg per day, respectively) (WIERSINGA and BROENINK 1991). Serum rT_3 increases by 80%–200% (KANNAN et al. 1984; PEARCE and HIMSWORTH 1986; SCHRÖDER-VAN DER ELST and VAN DER HEIDE 1990; PERRET et al. 1992), and serum T_4 by 35%–104% (KANNAN et al. 1984; PEARCE and HIMSWORTH 1986; KASIM et al. 1987; SCHRÖDER-VAN DER ELST and VAN DER HEIDE 1990; WIERSINGA and BROENINK 1991; DE JONG et al. 1994) also largely in a dose-dependent manner (SOGOL et al. 1983; WIERSINGA and BROENINK 1991). When rats are treated with DEA, the decrease in serum T_3 and increase in serum rT_3 are similar to that of an equivalent dose of amiodarone, but DEA does not increase serum T_4 significantly (VENKATESH et al. 1986b; SCHRÖDER-VAN DER ELST and VAN DER HEIDE 1990). Serum amiodarone and DEA are not related to serum T_4, T_3 and rT_3 concentrations.

With some exceptions (SOGOL et al. 1983; CEPPI and ZANINOVICH 1989; PERRET et al. 1992), amiodarone and DEA treatment are associated with an increase in serum TSH (PEKARY et al. 1986; KASIM et al. 1987; FRANKLYN et al. 1987; SCHRÖDER-VAN DER ELST and VAN DER HEIDE 1990); TSH increased by 14%, 93% and 193% when amiodarone was given for 2 weeks in a dose of 50, 100 and 150 mg/kg per day, respectively (WIERSINGA and BROENINK 1991).

II. Changes in Thyroid and Extrathyroidal Tissues

1. Peripheral Tissues

Both amiodarone and DEA treatment in rats cause major changes in tissue contents of thyroid hormones (SCHRÖDER-VAN DER ELST and VAN DER HEIDE 1990). Tissue T_4 concentration increases in liver, kidney, brain and prostate, but not in heart or other organs. Reverse T_3 levels are increased in all tissues except muscle, DEA having a more pronounced effect than amiodarone. Intracellular T_3 is dramatically decreased in all tissues by both amiodarone and DEA. In organs in which no local conversion of T_4 into T_3 occurs (such as muscle), the decrease in tissue T_3 content is in direct proportion to the decrease in plasma T_3. The decrease in T_3 content in other organs can be larger due to a decrease in locally produced T_3 from T_4, as observed in the kidney and particularly in the liver. These findings suggest inhibition of iodothyronine-5′-deiodination. Type I deiodinase catalyses the 5′-deiodination of T_4 into T_3 and of rT_3 into 3,3′-T_2 (see Chap. 4, this volume). Although the mRNA of the gene encoding for type I deiodinase is expressed normally in the liver of amiodarone-treated rats (HUDIG et al. 1994), the activity of the enzyme is inhibited by amiodarone as evident from various studies.

The 5′-deiodinase activity can be assayed by measuring the production of T_3 from T_4 added to a tissue preparation. When rats are pretreated with amiodarone in vivo, the 5′-deiodinase activity in homogenates of liver, heart and kidney is markedly depressed (BALSAM et al. 1978; SOGOL et al. 1983; PEKARY et al. 1986; CEPPI and ZANINOVICH 1989; GØTZSCHE et al. 1989). The decrease is dose dependent (SOGOL et al. 1983). Interestingly, when amiodarone treatment is discontinued, the enzyme activity in liver and kidney is restored within days, but remains depressed in the heart for at least 10 days (GØTZSCHE et al. 1989). In contrast, if amiodarone is added in vitro to liver or heart homogenates of untreated animals, no inhibition of enzyme activity is observed (SOGOL et al. 1983; CEPPI and ZANINOVICH 1989). If amiodarone is added in vitro to isolated hepatocytes of untreated animals, the enzyme activity is dose dependently inhibited (by 36%, 86% and 100% at amiodarone concentrations of 0.6, 6 and 60 μM, respectively – a concentration of 6.6 μM or 4.5 μg/ml falls within the range observed in humans); cellular T_4 uptake was also reduced by amiodarone in this study (AANDERUD et al. 1984).

The discrepancies between the results of in vivo and in vitro experiments and between whole cell preparations and homogenates can be reconciled by assuming that a metabolite of amiodarone (probably DEA) is responsible for direct inhibition of 5′-deiodinase activity and that amiodarone indirectly inhibits 5′-deiodination by decreasing the availability of the substrate T_4. Indeed amiodarone inhibits the active transport of T_4 and T_3 into rat hepatocytes in primary culture (KRENNING et al. 1982).

Finally, amiodarone may affect the number of T_3 receptors (see Chap. 6, this volume). In the heart of amiodarone-treated rats the maximal binding capacity (MBC) of T_3 receptors was decreased by 32% without changes in K_d (GØTZSCHE and ORSKOV 1994); this was not observed in pigs (GØTZSCHE 1993). A recent report describes the mRNAs encoding for the T_3-receptor α_1 and β_1 isoforms in cultured cardiac myocytes: in the presence of isoproterenol, both mRNAs decreased following the addition of 15 μM amiodarone (DRVOTA et al. 1995b).

2. Thyroid

a) In Vitro Studies

DEA is cytotoxic for human thyrocytes in culture; the EC_{50} value is 6.8 ± 1.1 μg/ml and few cells are left after 24-h exposure to 12.5 μg/ml (20 μM). Amiodarone up to 50 μg/ml (77 μM) is less cytotoxic, causing a maximum of a 25% decrease in cell number at 4 days when 5% of amiodarone is converted to DEA (BEDDOWS et al. 1989). Amiodarone at concentrations of ≥75 μM (≥48 μg/ml) has a cytotoxic effect when incubated for 24 h with FRTL-5 cells, a rat thyroid cell line that traps but does not organify iodide; potassium iodide up to 300 μM has no cytotoxic effect (CHIOVATO et al. 1994). The cytotoxic effect of amiodarone in this system is inhibited by dexamethasone and by potassium perchlorate (BRENNAN et al. 1995). In primary cultures of human thyroid follicles that trap and organify iodide, amiodarone is cytotoxic at concentrations of ≥37.5 μM and potassium iodide at >100 μM after 24-h incubation; the cytotoxic effect of amiodarone is partially (and that of potassium iodide completely) abolished by adding methimazole, a drug that inhibits organification (Chap. 8; CHIOVATO et al. 1994). Amiodarone is also cytotoxic for cells such as fibroblast that do not trap iodide. Taken together, these findings suggest a direct cytotoxic effect of amiodarone on thyrocytes in vitro. This is likely to happen also in vivo in view of the substantial tissue accumulation of the drug. Given a plasma amiodarone concentration of 3 μM (1.9 μg/ml) and a thyroid/plasma ratio of the drug ranging from 5 to 25, the thyroid concentration of amiodarone can be calculated as ranging from 15 to 75 μM (9.5–48 μg/ml). These concentrations are cytotoxic in vitro, and are in the same order as those actually observed in amiodarone-treated patients (Table 1).

The cytotoxic effect might be due to cellular vacuolation, suggesting phospholipidosis. The plasma membrane may be involved because both amiodarone and DEA are amphophilic drugs which directly affect the fluidity of membranes, related to ionization (CHATELAINE et al. 1985; FERREIRA et al. 1987).

In rat FRTL-5 cells, amiodarone inhibits TSH-stimulated cell growth at low concentrations (3.75–7.5 μM) that are not cytotoxic (CHIOVATO et al. 1994). In dog thyroid slices, 0.5 mM amiodarone inhibited TSH-stimulated (but not basal) glucose oxidation, phosphate incorporation into phospholipids, and cAMP production. Inhibition by amiodarone, in contrast to that by inorganic iodide, was not prevented by 1 mM methimazole, indicating that the inhibitory effects of amiodarone were not caused by release of iodide (PASQUALI et al. 1990). In isolated dog thyroid cells or membranes, 5–50 μM amiodarone decreased TSH-stimulated (but not basal or forskolin-stimulated) adenylate cyclase activity, and increased TSH binding four- to fivefold. Amiodarone (10–100 μM) further inhibited TSH- and carbachol-stimulated glucose uptake and intracellular [Ca^{2+}] concentration (RANI 1990). These experiments indicate direct effects on the plasma membrane, evident within minutes to hours after exposure to amiodarone. Long-term exposure of human thyroid follicles to amiodarone for 3 days dose dependently decreased the TSH-stimulated production of cAMP, thyroglobulin (Tg) and FT_3 and increased that of FT_4 at doses of >6 μM (MASSART et al. 1989). The fall in Tg and FT_3 can be explained by the inhibition of cAMP, which might be due either to uncoupling between the TSH receptor and cyclase (because amiodarone had no effect on forskolin-stimulated adenylate cyclase) or to the generation of iodide from amiodarone (since high doses of iodide in vitro and in vivo inhibit TSH-stimulated cAMP production). Iodine excess, however, also decreases T_4 production and release. The amiodarone-induced increase in FT_4 production by thyroid follicles is consequently most probably due to inhibition of thyroidal 5′-deiodinase, the same enzyme which catalyses the production of T_3 from T_4 in the liver. The failure to observe this effect in perfused dog thyroid lobes (LAURBERG 1988) is probably related to the short exposure time of 140 min. Amiodarone may need transformation, e.g. into DEA or other metabolites, to exert this effect.

Amiodarone at relatively low doses (10–25 μM) inhibited basal and TSH-stimulated iodide organification by 25%–50% in dog thyroid cells (RANI 1990). In contrast, higher doses of amiodarone (0.1–1 mM) caused only a 20% decrease in iodide metabolism in pig thyroid slices (GLUZMAN et al. 1977). Cultured cells appear to be more sensitive than tissue slices, and the acute effects of amiodarone are unlikely to be due to iodide dissociated from the drug.

b) *In Vivo Studies*

Serial kinetic studies on iodine metabolism were performed in 15 patients taking 300 mg amiodarone daily for 6 months (RAO et al. 1986) (Fig. 4). Plasma inorganic iodide and 24 h urine iodide rose 40-fold at 6 weeks and remained at these high levels thereafter; renal iodide clearance did not change. The urinary excretion is predominantly inorganic iodide, because the urinary excretion of amiodarone and DEA is so small that it contributes only marginally (13 μg/l) to the milligrams of iodide measured. Thyroid iodide clearance fell from 5.93 ± 0.82 to less than 0.5 ml/min. Thyroid absolute iodide uptake rose from 16.3 ± 2.7 to 54.6 ± 5.7 nmol/h after 6 weeks, and then progressively declined to still elevated values of 32.0 ± 4.3 nmol/h at 24 weeks. These findings are identical to the response of the thyroid to chronic excess iodide ingestion. The decrease in thyroid iodide clearance has been called the "escape" phenomenon to limit the acute inhibition of iodine organification produced by large doses of iodide (the Wolff-Chaikoff effect): despite high plasma inorganic iodide, the iodide transport is inhibited, allowing intrathyroidal iodine concentrations to fall below

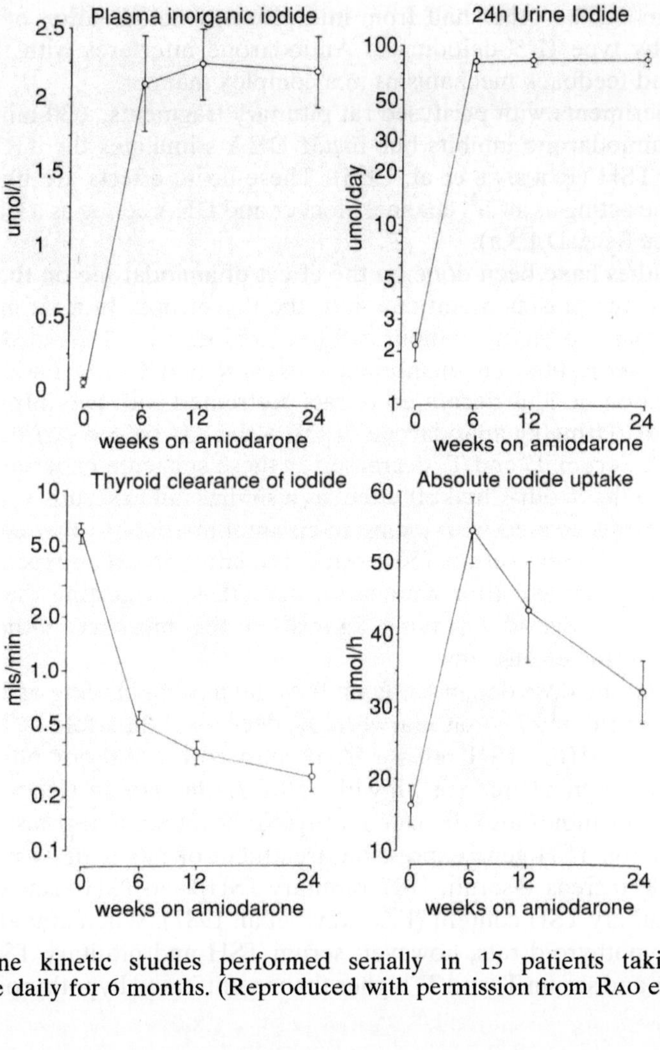

Fig. 4. Iodine kinetic studies performed serially in 15 patients taking 300 mg amiodarone daily for 6 months. (Reproduced with permission from RAO et al. 1986)

the critical level needed to sustain the Wolff-Chaikoff effect (see Chap. 7, this volume). Nevertheless, the absolute iodide uptake remains high, and intrathyroidal iodine is increased three- to fourfold in amiodarone-treated patients when measured by fluorescent excitation analysis (JONCKHEER 1981).

3. Pituitary

Pituitary TSH synthesis and release is predominantly under the control of TRH and thyroid hormones (Chap. 2, this volume). Hypothalamic TRH stimulates TSH-subunit gene expression and TSH release via the phosphatidylinositol pathway. This is counteracted by a direct inhibitory effect of thyroid hormones on TSH gene expression. Nuclear T_3 receptor occupancy in pituitary thyrotrophs is inversely related to serum TSH. Half of the nuclear T_3 is derived from serum T_3, the other half from intrapituitary deiodination of T_4 into T_3 catalysed by type II 5′-deiodinase. Amiodarone interferes with these feed-forward and feedback mechanisms in a complex manner.

In experiments with perifused rat pituitary fragments, a 30-min exposure to 10 μM amiodarone inhibits but 10 μM DEA stimulates the TRH-induced release of TSH (ROUSSEL et al. 1995). These acute effects are likely due to amiodarone acting as a Ca^{2+} channel blocker and DEA acting as a Ca^{2+} channel agonist (see Sect. D.I.3.a).

No studies have been done on the effect of amiodarone on the transport of T_4 across the plasma membrane into the thyrotroph. In a rat growth hormone producing pituitary tumour cell line, amiodarone decreased the transport of T_3 acros the cell membrane (NORMAN and LAVIN 1989). Pituitary 5′-deiodination of T_4 is decreased in rats pretreated with two intraperitoneal injections of 100 mg/kg amiodarone or DEA the day before sacrifice (SAFRAN et al. 1986). Serum T_4 and T_3 decreased in these subacute experiments, obviously due to the Wolff-Chaikoff effect as a similar fall in serum T_4 and T_3 was observed in rats treated with iodine in an amount equal to that contained in amiodarone. Whereas serum TSH rose in the latter group as expected, serum TSH did not increase after amiodarone or DEA, suggesting that the drug functions as a thyroid hormone agonist in the pituitary. Other studies, however, contradict this view.

Amiodarone dose dependently inhibits the in vitro binding of T_3 to nuclei isolated from rat anterior pituitary; the K_a decreased threefold at 1 mM without change in MBC. TSH release from cultured rat anterior pituitary cells increased when incubated for 5 h with >50 μM amiodarone (FRANKLYN et al. 1985). In vivo studies also indicated a thyroid hormone antagonistic effect of amiodarone on TSH gene expression: treatment of rats with 25 mg/kg orally for 3 months increased serum TSH, pituitary TSHβ and TSHα subunit mRNA but not pituitary TSH content (FRANKLYN et al. 1987). When amiodarone was given to hypothyroid rats, however, serum TSH and pituitary TSH mRNA were lower and serum T_4 and T_3 higher than in untreated hypothyroid animals, possibly related to the higher serum T_4 and T_3 levels in the amiodarone-treated group.

The amiodarone-induced changes in TSH release may therefore reflect changes in serum T_3 and T_4, in intrapituitary generation of T_3 from T_4 as well as a direct interaction of amiodarone with nuclear T_3 binding.

III. Changes in Thyroid Hormone Kinetics

1. Human Studies

Short-term treatment with amiodarone (400 mg/day for 3 weeks) decreased T_4 production rate (PR) by 12% and T_4 metabolic clearance rate (MCR) by 25% relative to treatment with 12.5 mg iodide/day; the half-life of serum T_4 increased from 6.6 to 8.1 days, while the distribution volume of T_4 did not change. T_3 PR decreased by 20%, but T_3 MCR and T_3 distribution volume were not affected (LAMBERT et al. 1982). Amiodarone treatment for 5–6 weeks (200–800 mg daily) did not change T_4 kinetics, but decreased T_3 PR by 48% and reduced the percentage of T_4 converted to T_3 from baseline values of 26%–43% to 10%–17% (HERSHMAN et al. 1986). The absence of an effect of amiodarone on T_3 MCR was also found in hypothyroid patients treated for 3 weeks with 400 mg amiodarone and either T_4 or T_3 (ZANINOVICH et al. 1990).

Long-term treatment with amiodarone (200 mg/day for 9 months or longer) in contrast increased T_4 PR by 105%; T_4 MCR was reduced by 18% and the half-life of serum T_4 was 7.3 days (LAMBERT et al. 1982). These patients had a normal or low plasma TSH but were clinically euthyroid; their T_4 PR, although increased with the equivalent of 250 μg T_4 per day, was only 40% of the T_4 PR observed in patients with Graves' hyperthyroidism and equally increased plasma concentrations of T_4 and FT_4. These data were also evaluated by compartmental analysis: short-term amiodarone administration reduced the fractional transfer rate of T_4 between serum and rapidly equilibrating tissues, whereas long-term amiodarone treatment increased fractional rates of T_4 transfer between serum and both rapidly and slowly equilibrating pools sixfold (KAPTEIN et al. 1988). No data are available on rT_3 kinetics in humans.

2. Animal Studies

Amiodarone treatment in rabbits (20 mg/kg per day i.p. for 3 weeks) resulted in an increase in T_4 PR and a decrease in T_4 MCR; T_3 MCR did not change, and although T_3 PR was not significantly reduced the ratio of T_3 PR to T_4 PR was; rT_3 MCR also decreased but rT_3 PR did not alter (KANNAN et al. 1984). Another study in rabbits (10 mg/kg/day i.p. for 6 weeks) confirmed the lower T_4 MCR but found no change in T_4 PR (PEARCE and HIMSWORTH 1986). In rats, treatment with amiodarone or DEA (~30 mg/kg per day orally for 3 weeks) had quantitatively similar results: T_4 PR increased by 32%, T_3 PR by the thyroid decreased by >90%, T_3 PR from peripheral T_4 to T_3 conversion decreased by 49%, but T_4 and T_3 plasma clearance rates did not change

(SCHRÖDER-VAN DER ELST and VAN DER HEIDE 1990). In isolated perfused rat livers obtained from animals pretreated with amiodarone (40 mg/kg per day orally for 3 weeks) and using a two-pool model for describing thyroid hormone kinetics, liver uptake and metabolism of T_3 were unaffected by amiodarone; however, both uptake and metabolism of T_4 were decreased, indicating inhibition of transmembrane T_4 transport and of T_4 5′-deiodination (DE JONG et al. 1994).

Non-deiodinative pathways of T_4 disposal may be enhanced by amiodarone treatment. In one study amiodarone and DEA treatment reduced the urinary excretion of radioactive tracers, and increased the faecal excretion of radioactivity, which is probably a measure of glucuronide and sulphate conjugation of the iodothyronines (SCHRÖDER-VAN DER ELST and VAN DER HEIDE 1990). Decreased deiodination leads to a higher intracellular T_4 content, thereby increasing conjugate production, as has been found with amiodarone and propylthiouracil (DE JONG et al. 1994). T_3 has to be sulphated before 5′-deiodination in rat liver, and therefore T_3 conjugates accumulate when deiodination is inhibited; conjugation is apparently unaffected by amiodarone (DE JONG et al. 1994). Inhibition of deiodination thus does not affect disposal of thyroid hormones in the liver because of a compensating increase in conjugate concentrations. This has been studied in more detail in rabbits treated with amiodarone (200 mg/kg per day i.p. for 3 weeks). It was calculated that the inhibition of the conversion of T_4 into T_3 (from 63% in controls to 29% in amiodarone-treated animals) could be accounted for almost completely by the increased conversion of T_4 to non-deiodinative routes of metabolism (from 29% in controls to 66% under amiodarone) (KANNAN et al. 1990). These non-deiodinative pathways lead to large increases in T_4 conjugates, and possibly also to a modest rise of TETRAC.

IV. Summary

The combined human and animal data allow the following explanation for the observed obligatory effects of amiodarone treatment on thyroid hormone secretion and metabolism (Fig. 5). Amiodarone treatment increases plasma T_4 and rT_3 and decreases plasma T_3; plasma TBG remains unaltered and changes in plasma FT_4 and FT_3 reflect changes in total T_4 and T_3. Plasma TSH is transiently increased, returning to mostly normal values after 3 months. During biotransformation of the drug, pharmacological quantities of iodide are released, increasing plasma inorganic iodide and urinary iodide excretion 40-fold. It results in an increased absolute thyroid iodide uptake, which peaks at 6 weeks and is still twice baseline values at 24 weeks. The chronic iodine excess will transiently inhibit thyroidal synthesis and release of thyroid hormones, explaining the initial decreased T_4 PR and rise of TSH. The thyroid usually escapes from these inhibitory (Wolff-Chaikoff) effects, and T_4 PR and plasma TSH return to normal values.

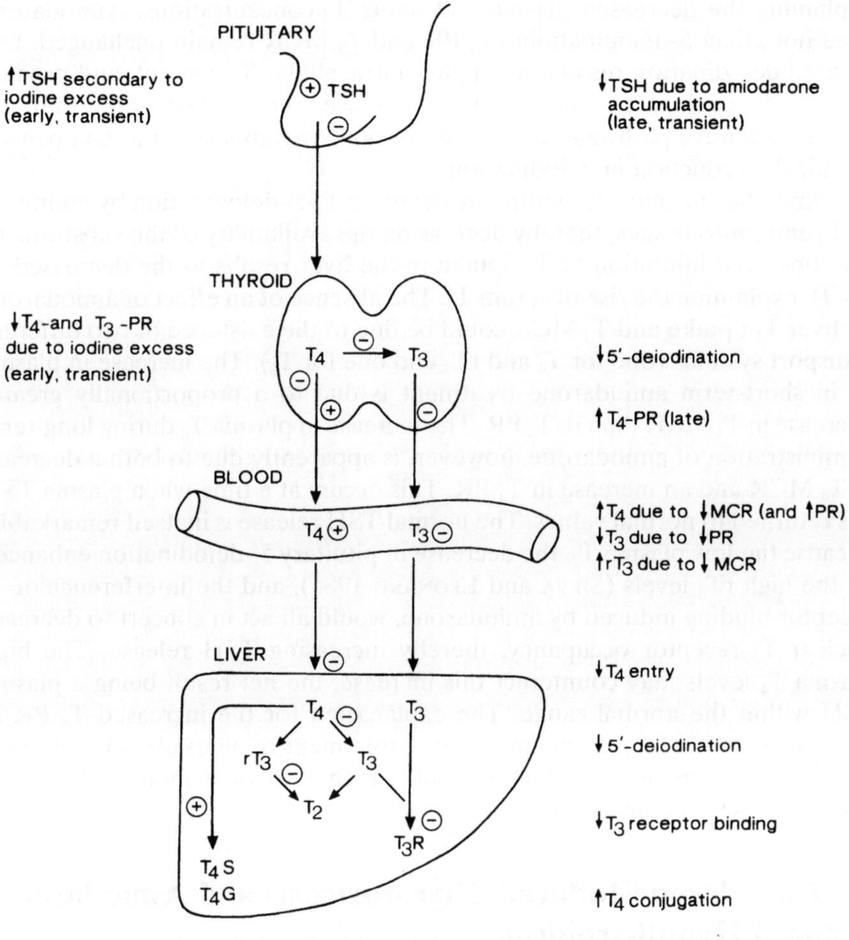

Fig. 5. Early transient (*left column*) and late permanent (*right column*) effects of amiodarone treatment on the secretion and metabolism of thyroid hormones. *PR*, production rate; *MCR*, metabolic clearance rate; T_3R, T_3 receptors; T_4S, T_4 sulfate; T_4G, T_4 glucoronide; ⊕, increase; ⊖, decrease; ↓, inhibition; ↑, stimulation

Apart from its thyroidal effects, however, amiodarone simultaneously affects extrathyroidal thyroid hormone metabolism in a profound manner. Amiodarone, presumably via its metabolite DEA, strongly inhibits type I iodothyronine-5′-deiodinase: like other drugs with diiodo-substituted benzene rings it is a competitive inhibitor of 5′-deiodinase in all tissues. The decreased 5′-deiodination of rT_3 into 3,3′-T_2 results in a decreased rT_3 MCR, explaining the high plasma rT_3 concentrations. The decreased 5′-deiodination of T_4 into T_3, observed in many tissues but most pronounced in the thyroid and in the liver (the main extrathyroidal T_3 production site), results in a decreased T_3 PR, explaining the decreased plasma and tissue T_3 concentrations. Amiodarone does not affect 5-deiodination: rT_3 PR and T_3 MCR remain unchanged. Decreased deiodination results in a higher intracellular T_4 content, and production of T_4 conjugates will therefore increase. Amiodarone may enhance non-deiodinative pathways of thyroid hormone metabolism, thus compensating for the reduction in deiodination.

Amiodarone may also indirectly decrease T_4-5′-deiodination by inhibition of T_4 entry into tissues, thereby decreasing the availability of the substrate T_4. The observed inhibition of T_4 uptake in the liver results in the decreased T_4 MCR, explaining the rise of serum T_4. The absence of an effect of amiodarone on liver T_3 uptake and T_3 MCR could be due to the existence of two different transport systems (one for T_4 and rT_3 and one for T_3). The increase in plasma T_4 in short-term amiodarone treatment is due to a proportionally greater decrease in T_4 MCR than in T_4 PR. The increase in plasma T_4 during long-term administration of amiodarone, however, is apparently due to both a decrease in T_4 MCR and an increase in T_4 PR. This occurs at a time when plasma TSH has returned to normal values. The normal TSH release is in itself remarkable, because the low plasma T_3, the decrease in pituitary 5′-deiodination enhanced by the high rT_3 levels (SILVA and LEONARD 1985), and the interference of T_3 receptor binding induced by amiodarone, would all act in concert to decrease nuclear T_3 receptor occupancy, thereby increasing TSH release. The high plasma T_4 levels may counteract this increase, the net result being a plasma TSH within the normal range. The explanation for the increased T_4 PR in humans receiving long-term amiodarone treatment remains obscure, but may represent a homeostatic adaptation of the thyroid or a modest degree of thyrotoxicosis (see Sect. C.III).

C. Amiodarone-Induced Thyrotoxicosis and Amiodarone-Induced Hypothyroidism

I. Diagnosis

Most patients remain clinically euthyroid during amiodarone treatment, despite the profound changes in thyroid hormone secretion and metabolism provoked by the drug. A subset of amiodarone-treated patients, however, develops amiodarone-induced thyrotoxicosis (AIT) or amiodarone-induced hypothyroidism (AIH).

The clinical diagnosis of AIT or AIH can be very easy if classical symptoms and signs are present. Unfortunately, this is not always the case. The antiadrenergic effects of amiodarone may minimize clinical features. Weight loss, fatigue, tremor and muscle weakness would suggest thyrotoxicosis, but can also be due to gastrointestinal and neurological side effects. An important clue for the diagnosis of AIT is worsening of the cardiac disorder, especially exacerbation of the arrhythmias (BAMBINI et al. 1987; MARTINO et al. 1987; NEWNHAM et al. 1987).

The biochemical diagnosis of AIT or AIH has greatly benefited from the introduction of the sensitive TSH assay: a TSH value within the normal reference range reliably excludes AIT and AIH despite elevated T_4 and FT_4 plasma concentrations (Fig. 6, group 3) (WIERSINGA et al. 1986). An elevated plasma TSH in combination with a low plasma T_4 or FT_4 concentration indicates AIH (group 5); a high TSH but normal T_4 or FT_4 indicates subclinical hypothyroidism (group 4). When plasma TSH is decreased, the values of T_4 or FT_4 in serum do not allow discrimination between subclinical hyperthyroidism (group 2) and overt hyperthyroidism (group 1). If plasma T_3 is elevated, a clear diagnosis of AIT can be made. A normal plasma T_3, however, does not exclude AIT since a normal T_3 is observed in a fair proportion of bona fide cases of

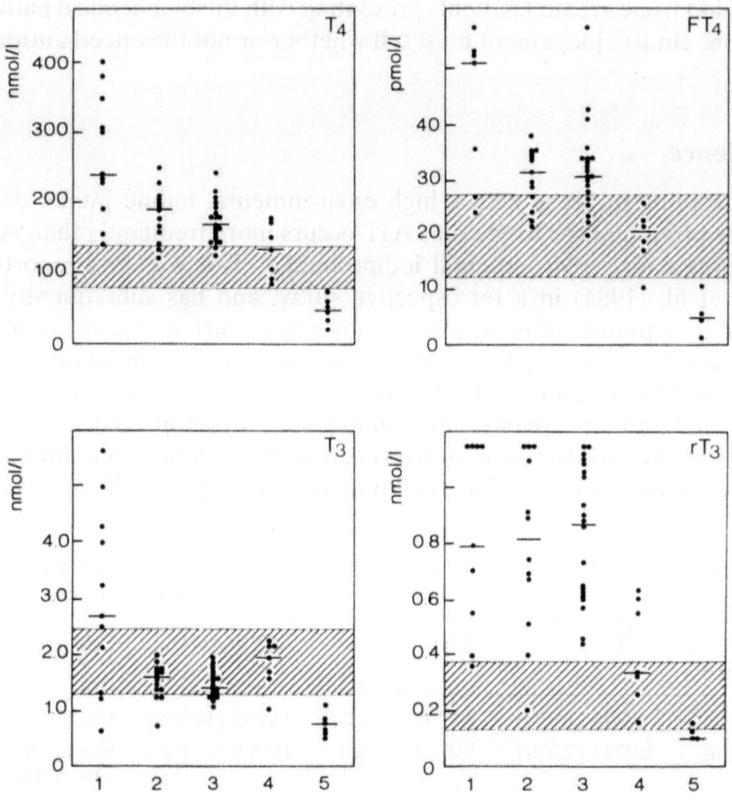

Fig. 6. Plasma thyroid hormone concentrations of 59 patients on long-term amiodarone therapy. Group 1, thyrotoxic (suppressed TSH); group 2, euthyroid but suppressed TSH; group 3, euthyroid and normal TSH; group 4, euthyroid but elevated TSH; group 5, hypothyroid (elevated TSH). Median value in each group is indicated by *a horizontal line*, and *hatched areas* represent the normal reference range. (Reproduced with permission from WIERSINGA and TRIP 1986)

AIT (Wiersinga et al. 1986). AIT thus frequently presents itself as T_4 toxicosis, as is the case in iodide-induced thyrotoxicosis (Jonckheer et al. 1992). The peculiar characteristic of amiodarone of inducing high serum T_4 and FT_4 concentrations consequently prevents a conclusive laboratory diagnosis of AIT in some patients. Measurement of serum markers of tissue thyrotoxicosis has been advocated to solve this problem. Indeed, serum sex hormone-binding globulin (Bambini et al. 1987; Newnham et al. 1987) and Tg (Martino et al. 1987; Newnham et al. 1987; Unger 1988; Weissel 1988; de Rosa et al. 1989) concentrations are higher in AIT than in amiodarone-induced euthyroid hyperthyroxinaemia, but the considerable overlap between groups suggests that these parameters have little to offer in the assessment of individual patients. The same holds true for plasma coenzyme Q10 determination in order to evaluate the metabolic status (Mancini et al. 1989). It follows that in amiodarone-treated patients presenting with the biochemical pattern of T_4 toxicosis, clinical judgement must tell whether or not they need antithyroid treatment.

II. Incidence

Patients residing in areas with a high environmental iodine intake develop AIH more often than AIT, whereas AIT occurs more frequently than AIH in regions with a low environmental iodine intake. This was first reported by Martino et al. (1984) in a retrospective study, and has subsequently been confirmed in a number of prospective studies from various countries in which patients have been followed up to 4.5 years after starting amiodarone (Table 2). The combined incidence of AIT and AIH is rather similar in all regions: 14%–18% of patients treated with amiodarone develop clinical signs and symptoms of thyroid dysfunction, irrespective of ambient iodine intake. Another interesting feature is that AIT may develop up to 3–12 months after

Table 2. Incidence of amiodarone-induced thyrotoxicosis (AIT) and amiodarone-induced hypothyroidism (AIH) in relation to environmental iodine intake

Environmental iodine intake	AIT	AIH	AIT + AIH	Country
High	5/295 (1.7%)	39/295 (13.2%)	44/295 (14.9%)	USA[a], UK[b]
Intermediate	18/229 (7.9%)	13/229 (5.7%)	31/229 (13.6%)	Spain[c], Australia[d], The Netherlands[e]
Low	50/419 (11.9%)	27/419 (6.4%)	77/419 (18.4%)	Italy[f], Belgium[g]

[a] Martino et al. (1984), Amico et al. (1984), Borowski et al. (1985), Nademanee et al. (1986).
[b] Shukla et al. (1994).
[c] Sanmarti et al. (1984).
[d] Newnham et al. (1987).
[e] Trip et al. (1991).
[f] Martino et al. (1984), Foresti et al. (1985).
[g] Chevigné-Brancart et al. (1983).

discontinuation of the drug (JONCKHEER et al. 1973; MARTINO et al. 1985), obviously related to its very long terminal half-life.

In Dutch patients, living in an area with an intermediate iodine intake of 150 μg/day, the calculated probability for AIT was 0.025 after 18 months and 0.355 after 48 months; for AIH, these figures are 0.085 and 0.085, respectively (Fig. 7, upper panel) (TRIP et al. 1991). All cases of AIH had occurred within 18 months after initiation of amiodarone treatment. In contrast, cases of AIT

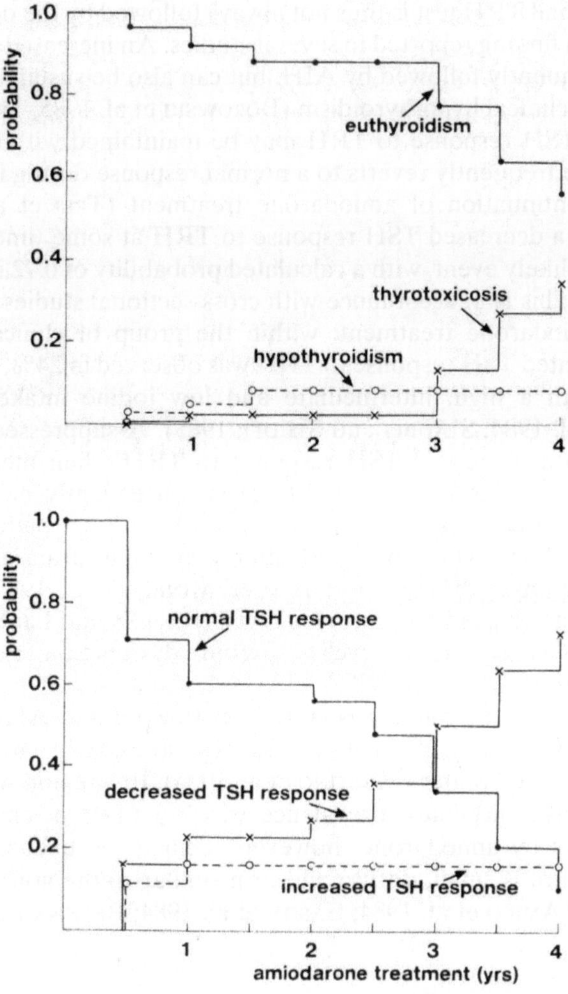

Fig. 7. Probability of developing thyrotoxicosis or hypothyroidism (*upper panel*) and of developing a decreased or an increased TSH response to TRH (*bottom panel*) during amiodarone treatment in patients living in an area of intermediate iodine intake. (Reproduced with permission from TRIP et al. 1991)

continued to occur with longer exposure time to the drug (also reported by CHEVIGNÉ-BRANCART et al. 1983). The probability of remaining clinically euthyroid was 0.56 after 4 years of amiodarone treatment. The probability of maintaining a normal TSH response to TRH during this whole period was substantially lower with a value of 0.10 (Fig. 7, bottom panel). This is due to the occurrence of an increased and especially of a decreased TSH response to TRH in patients without clinical signs and symptoms of thyroid dysfunction, who may be labelled as having subclinical hypothyroidism and hyperthyroidism, respectively.

An abnormal TRH test is thus not always followed by the development of AIH or AIT, a finding reported in several studies. An increased TSH response to TRH is frequently followed by AIH, but can also be sustained without the occurrence of clinical hypothyroidism (BOROWSKI et al. 1985; TRIP et al. 1991). A decreased TSH response to TRH may be maintained without developing AIT, but more frequently reverts to a normal response during further follow-up despite continuation of amiodarone treatment (TRIP et al. 1991). The occurrence of a decreased TSH response to TRH at some time during treatment is a very likely event, with a calculated probability of 0.72 in 4 years (Fig. 7, top panel). This is in accordance with cross-sectional studies in patients on long-term amiodarone treatment: within the group of clinically euthyroid patients, a blunted TSH response to TRH was observed in 24%, 30% and 43% in regions with a high, intermediate and low iodine intake, respectively (MARTINO et al. 1984; STÄUBLI and STUDER 1985). A suppressed plasma TSH (equivalent to a decreased TSH response to TRH when measured with a sensitive assay) (WIERSINGA et al. 1986a) is consequently not a very good indicator of the occurrence of AIT (TRIP et al. 1991). A few patients have been described in whom AIT developed after a previous transient episode of subclinical hypothyroidism (TRIP et al. 1991; MINELLI et al. 1992), or in whom goitre and AIH occurred after previous AIT (KAPLAN and ISH-SHALOM 1991). Sometimes a characteristic cyclic thyroid dysfunction is encountered (SALAMON et al. 1989).

The prevalence of goitre was 60% in both AIH and AIT in an iodine-deficient region of Italy, whereas it was 22% in AIH in an iodine-replete region of the United States (MARTINO et al. 1984). In a region with intermediate iodine intake the goitre prevalence was 7% (TRIP et al. 1991). Newly induced goitres by amiodarone, however, seem to be uncommon; when it occurs, the goitre is small, diffuse and firm similar to the goitres induced by iodine excess (AMICO et al. 1984; EASON et al. 1984; BRENNAN et al. 1987).

III. Pathogenesis

1. Amiodarone-Induced Hypothyroidism

Neither the daily and cumulative doses of amiodarone nor serum protein bound iodine and urinary iodide excretion differ between patients with AIH and those remaining euthyroid (Chevigné-Brancart et al. 1983; Martino et al. 1984; Eason et al. 1984; Nademanee et al. 1986; Wiersinga et al. 1986b; Trip et al. 1991). Although amiodarone is given more frequently to male than to female patients (sex ratio M:F = 2.0:1.0), AIH develops relatively more often in females (M:F = 1.5:1.0) (Chevigné-Brancart et al. 1983; Amico et al. 1984; Martino et al. 1984; Borowski et al. 1985; Trip et al. 1991) and in older patients (Borowski et al. 1985; Chevigné-Brancart et al. 1983). Female sex and the presence of (TPO) antibodies prior to treatment constitute a relative risk of 7.9 and 7.3, respectively, for the subsequent development of AIH; the relative risk of the combination of female sex and TPO or Tg antibodies is 13.5 (95% confidence interval 3.2–57.4) (Trip et al. 1991).

It has been debated whether or not amiodarone is capable of inducing thyroid antibodies. An early report suggested de novo occurrence of TPO antibodies in 6 out of 13 patients after 1 month of treatment; the antibodies had disappeared 6 months after withdrawal of the drug (Monteiro et al. 1986). Other follow-up studies, however, consistently indicate that amiodarone treatment per se is not associated with an increased incidence of TPO and Tg antibodies; this has been reported from regions with a high, intermediate, and low iodine intake (Safran et al. 1988; Weetman et al. 1988; Foresti et al. 1989; Trip et al. 1991; Machado et al. 1992). Circulating thyroid autoantibodies are thus unlikely to appear in amiodarone-treated patients when pretreatment test results are negative. AIH is likely to occur in patients with pre-existing autoimmune thyroid disease, although it may also develop without any evidence of underlying thyroid abnormalities (Hawthorne et al. 1985; Martino et al. 1987, 1994; Trip et al. 1991).

The development of AIH is best explained by a failure of the thyroid gland to escape from the Wolff-Chaikoff effect due to the iodine excess generated by amiodarone. Whereas a normal thyroid is capable of escaping from the inhibitory effects of iodine excess on thyroid hormone synthesis (Chap. 7, this volume), a thyroid gland compromised by an underlying abnormality such as autoimmune thyroiditis may not escape, resulting in a permanently impaired organification. The hallmark in the pathogenesis of AIH appears to be the failure of the thyroid to adapt to chronic iodine excess. The occurrence of AIH relatively early during treatment with amiodarone is in agreement with this view (Chevigné-Brancart et al. 1983; Trip et al. 1991; Martino et al. 1994).

The proposed pathogenesis is further supported by thyroidal radioiodine uptake studies. When iodine intake is increased, thyroid uptake of radioiodine is low (despite a high total iodine uptake by the thyroid gland) due to dilution of the radioisotope by the increased stable iodide pool. A low thyroidal radioiodine uptake is indeed observed in euthyroid and hyperthyroid patients treated with amiodarone, but in AIH patients the uptake is not inhibited and similar to that in subjects without iodine excess (Fig. 8, left panel) (Wiersinga et al. 1986b; Martino et al. 1988). Discharge of radioiodine from the thyroid after administration of perchlorate indicates decreased organification of

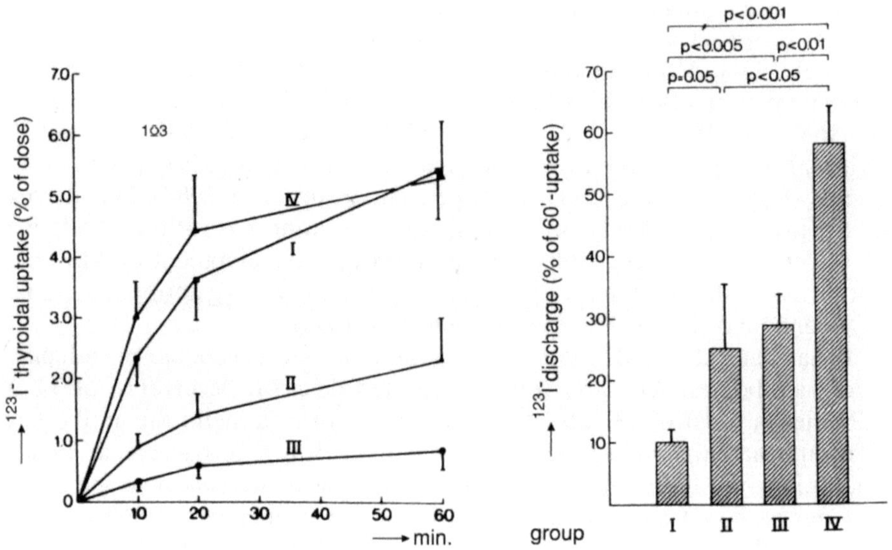

Fig. 8. Thyroidal uptake (*left panel*) and discharge after perchlorate (*right panel*) of $^{123}I^-$ in 30 patients with various cardiac diseases (values as means ± SE). Group I, 11 euthyroid patients (normal TRH test) without iodine excess; group II, 7 euthyroid patients (normal TRH test) with iodine excess due to metrizoate angiography; group III, 7 euthyroid or hyperthyroid patients (TSH response to TRH normal or decreased) with iodine excess due to amiodarone; group IV, 5 hypothyroid patients (TSH response to TRH increased) with iodine excess due to amiodarone. (Reproduced with permission from WIERSINGA et al. 1986b)

thyroidal iodide. The results of the perchlorate discharge tests indicate a severe organification defect in AIH (Fig. 8, right panel) (HAWTHORNE et al. 1985; WIERSINGA et al. 1986b; MARTINO et al. 1988). The preserved radioiodine uptake in AIH might be due to the increased TSH secretion since TSH enhances iodide transport. It is more likely, however, that autoregulatory mechanisms in the thyroid are responsible because thyroid iodide transport varies inversely with iodine intake in hypophysectomized animals. Furthermore, the inhibitory effect of iodine excess on thyroid iodide transport is prevented both in vivo and in vitro if antithyroid drugs are given before or concomitant with the iodide. The implication is that inhibition of transport by iodine excess requires organification of the administered iodide.

From the inverse relationship between the organic iodine content of the thyroid and the activity of the thyroid iodide transport mechanism, it has been speculated that there exists a specific inhibitor of iodide transport in the thyroid (Fig. 9). This hypothetical compound X.I is likely an iodinated lipid; its concentration and action would vary with the total organic iodine content of the thyroid. The severe organification defect observed in AIH is in line with the assumption of a persistent Wolff-Chaikoff effect as the cause of AIH. The organification defect will result in a decrease in thyroidal hormone synthesis,

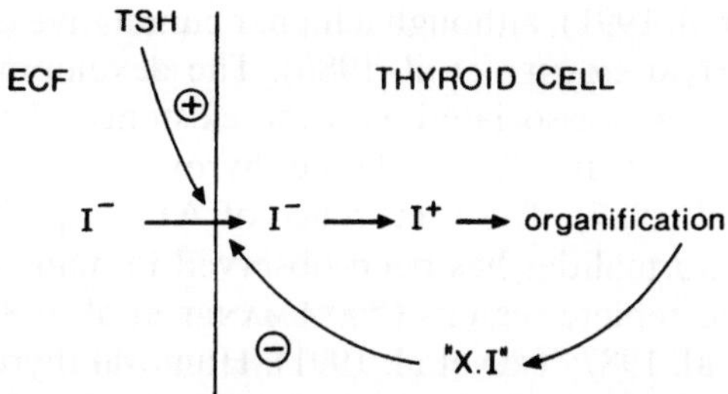

Fig. 9. Inhibition of thyroid iodide transport by iodine excess requires organification of the administered iodide. This inhibition is likely mediated by a specific iodinated compound X.I the concentration and action of which vary with the total organic iodine content of the gland. *ECF*, extracellular fluid. (Reproduced with permission from WIERSINGA et al. 1986b)

but also in a decrease in X.I, explaining the preserved radioiodine uptake in AIH.

Another line of evidence in favour of this interpretation comes from studies of total thyroidal iodine content as measured by X-ray fluorescence. Total thyroidal iodine content is grossly elevated in amiodarone-treated patients who are euthyroid or hyperthyroid; it is, however, within or below the normal range of 14.6 ± 5.0 mg in AIH (FRAGU et al. 1988). Since inorganic iodine comprises only about 0.25% of the total thyroidal iodine, these data are consistent with a decreased organic iodine content in the thyroid in AIH. Patients in whom thyroid iodine content does not increase above the normal range during amiodarone treatment appear at risk for AIH (FRAGU et al. 1988).

Subclinical autoimmune thyroiditis is recognized as an important predisposing factor in making thyroid glands more sensitive to the inhibitory action of excess iodide. The prevalence of autoimmune thyroiditis is relatively high in areas with a high environmental iodine intake, in females, and in old age: these are precisely the factors which predispose to the development of AIH. AIH is consequently to a certain extent predictable from the pretreatment assessment of risk factors like female sex and thyroid antibodies (MARTINO et al. 1987, 1994; TRIP et al. 1991); a personal or family history of thyroid disease may also constitute a risk factor (AMICO et al. 1984).

2. Amiodarone-Induced Thyrotoxicosis

The sex ratio in AIT (M : F = 3.2 : 1.0) is higher than that in euthyroid patients treated with amiodarone (M : F = 2.0 : 1.0), indicating a relative male preponderance in AIT (CHEVIGNÉ-BRANCART et al. 1983; AMICO et al. 1984; MARTINO et al. 1984; BOROWSKI et al. 1985; TRIP et al. 1991). The daily and cumulative doses of amiodarone and the 24-h urinary iodide excretion are also similar in both groups (CHEVIGNÉ-BRANCART et al. 1983; MARTINO et al. 1984; WIERSINGA et al. 1986b; TRIP et al. 1991), although a higher cumulative dose is reported in AIT in one study (NADEMANEE et al. 1986). The development of AIT in an iodine-deficient area was associated with the existence of a diffuse goitre in 29% and a nodular goitre in 38%, while the thyroid was apparently normal in 33% (MARTINO et al. 1987). The occurrence of AIT in patients without preexistent thyroid abnormalities has been observed in many studies, including patients from iodine-replete regions (NADEMANEE et al. 1986; BRENNAN et al. 1987; NEWNHAM et al. 1987; TRIP et al. 1991). Humoral thyroid autoimmunity seems to play no role in the induction of AIT: the incidence of TPO and Tg antibodies as well as of TSH-receptor-stimulating antibodies in amiodarone-treated patients with diffuse or toxic goitre was similar to that observed in spontaneous hyperthyroidism (MARTINO et al. 1986a), and de novo occurrence of TSH receptor antibodies in AIT has not been found (BRENNAN et al. 1987; TRIP et al. 1991). The significance of a reported increase in specific T-cell subsets for the development of AIT is unknown (RABINOWE et al. 1986).

Thyroidal iodine content as measured by X-ray fluorescence is markedly increased in AIT, in both patients with and without goitre (50 ± 19 mg and 55 ± 29 mg, respectively) (FRAGU et al. 1988). Although thyroidal iodine content is higher in AIT than in the patients who remain euthyroid (39 ± 17 mg when treated for 12–60 months), it does not allow accurate prediction of the occurrence of AIT. The thyroidal iodine content in AIT is elevated to the same extent as in iodide-induced thyrotoxicosis (LÉGER et al. 1983). It signifies an excess of organified iodine, and perchlorate discharge tests indeed do not show any major impairment of organification in iodide-induced thyrotoxicosis or in AIT (WIERSINGA et al. 1986b; MARTINO et al. 1988). It is thus reasonable to assume that the iodine excess generated by amiodarone causes AIT.

AIT shares several other characteristics with iodide-induced thyrotoxicosis (FRADKIN and WOLFF 1983): it is more common in males than in females, a goitre is present in ~50%, if the goitre is new it is small, diffuse and firm (LÉGER et al. 1983; EASON et al. 1984; BRENNAN et al. 1987; NEWNHAM et al. 1987), the onset is often acute (NEWNHAM et al. 1987; TRIP et al. 1991), and spontaneous remission frequently occurs (see Sect. C.IV.2). AIT, like iodide-induced thyrotoxicosis, is also more prevalent in iodine-deficient regions than in iodine-replete regions. Previous exposure to iodide may reduce subsequent iodide-induced thyrotoxicosis (FRADKIN and WOLFF 1983), accounting for the rarity of AIT in the United States. This may be related to the sensitivity of the thyroid gland to generate an iodine-induced turn-off signal for hormone biosynthesis (FRADKIN and WOLFF 1983). In subjects accustomed to a high environmental iodine intake, the sensitivity of this autoregulatory mechanism may have increased, rendering the thyroid better able to handle iodine excess: they are relatively resistant to iodide-induced thyrotoxicosis. In iodine-deplete areas, this sensitivity may be diminished: iodine repletion may unmask existing thyroid autonomy in euthyroid patients with Graves' disease or nodular goitre by permitting the autonomous tissue to synthesize and release excessive quantities of thyroid hormone. On the other hand, the extent of iodide excess could, if large enough, override differences in sensitivity.

Subsequent studies have shed more light on this difficult issue. Thyroidal radioiodine uptake is appropriately suppressed in many cases of AIT in view of the dilution of the radioisotope by the increased stable iodide pool, but a normal or even elevated uptake is observed in the majority of patients with an underlying thyroid abnormality like Graves' disease or nodular goitre (LÉGER et al. 1983; MARTINO et al. 1985, 1988; WIERSINGA et al. 1986b). Serum interleukin-6 (IL-6) concentrations in AIT without underlying thyroid abnormalities (574 ± 79 fmol/l) are much higher than in AIT with nodular goitre or Graves' disease (153 ± 46 fmol/l); the latter concentrations are not significantly different from values in spontaneous cases of toxic nodular goitre or Graves' hyperthyroidism (98 ± 10 and 108 ± 18 fmol/l, respectively). IL-6 values in euthyroid patients on amiodarone therapy (51 ± 10 fmol/l) are similar to those of AIH and controls (BARTALENA et al. 1994). These data allow the discrimination of two types of AIT (Table 3). Type I is due to iodine-induced excessive thyroid hormone synthesis, occurring especially in patients with underlying thyroid disease. Type II occurs especially in subjects with apparently normal thyroid glands, and is due to an amiodarone-induced destructive thyroiditis resulting in thyroid cell damage and thyroid hormone release into the circulation.

There are several lines of evidence which support the proposed pathogenesis of AIT type II. Firstly, markedly increased serum IL-6 levels have been found during the thyrotoxic phase of subacute thyroiditis, another thyroid inflammatory process. In some patients with AIT a painful goitre is found, resembling the clinical picture of subacute thyroiditis (GUDBJÖRNSSON et al. 1987; MIASKIEWICZ et al. 1987; LAMBERT et al. 1990). Gallium uptake in the thyroid and the lung of a patient with AIT and pulmonary toxicity is also

Table 3. Proposed pathogenesis of amiodarone-induced thyrotoxicosis. (According to BARTALENA et al. 1994, with some modifications)

	AIT type I	AIT type II
Underlying thyroid abnormality	Yes	No
Goitre	Frequently pre-existent diffuse or nodular goitre	Infrequent, if present small diffuse firm (sometimes tender) goitre
Thyroidal radioiodine uptake	Normal/elevated	Low/suppressed
Serum IL-6	Slightly elevated	Markedly elevated
Pathogenetic mechanism	Excessive thyroid hormone synthesis by iodine excess	Excessive thyroid hormone release by destructive thyroiditis
Subsequent hypothyroidism	No	Possible

compatible with an amiodarone-induced thyroiditis and pneumonitis (Ling et al. 1988). Secondly, like the destructive thyroiditis of subacute and postpartum thyroiditis, AIT can be followed by a mildly hypothyroid stage before euthyroidism is restored (Minelli et al. 1992; Roti et al. 1993). Thirdly, thyroid ultrasonography in patients who had recovered from AIT type II demonstrated an increase in dyshomogeneous echo patterns and hyperechogenecity similar to that in patients after cure of subacute thyroiditis, and obviously the result of the healing of the inflammatory process (Roti et al. 1994). Fourthly, the administration of excess iodine to euthyroid patients with a previous history of AIT did not induce thyrotoxicosis but rather subclinical hypothyroidism, as in patients with a previous episode of subacute thyroiditis (Roti et al. 1992). Finally, and most importantly, the pathology of the thyroid in AIT is characteristic and distinctive from that in thyrotoxicosis due to other causes (Smyrk et al. 1987; Leung et al. 1989; Farwell et al. 1990; Meurisse et al. 1993; Mulligan et al. 1993). Characteristically, small groups of involuted follicles exhibit varying degrees of damage, ranging from degenerative changes in a few lining cells to total follicular destruction. Damaged follicular cells are swollen and feature granular or vacuolated cytoplasm, and also zones of fibrosis. Similar parenchymal and interstitial changes occur in pneumocytes and hepatocytes damaged by amiodarone. Histopathological examination further reveals minimal or no thyroid follicular damage in specimens from amiodarone-treated euthyroid patients, in contrast to severe follicular damage and disruption in AIT type II (Brennan et al. 1995).

AIT type II thus appears to be a drug-induced destructive thyroiditis with subsequent leakage of iodothyronines from damaged and destroyed follicles into the circulation. It is much more likely that amiodarone itself, rather than iodine released during the biotransformation of the drug, is responsible for the destructive lesions (Smyrk et al. 1987; Bartalena et al. 1994). Although high iodide doses have a direct toxic effect on human thyrocytes, inducing necrosis which can be prevented by inhibition of organification (Many et al. 1992), the cytotoxic effect of amiodarone on human thyrocytes occurs independently of effects on iodide organification (Chiovato et al. 1994) (see also Sect. B.II.2.a). Iodine released from amiodarone has a bioavailability different from that of sodium iodide (Briançon et al. 1990). The data suggest that thyroid cytotoxicity produced by amiodarone is mainly due to a direct effect of amiodarone on thyrocytes (especially on lysosomes), but excess iodide released from the drug may contribute to its toxic action.

AIT occurs only in a minority of patients treated with amiodarone. In contrast, most patients remain euthyroid but will develop a suppressed TSH at some time during amiodarone therapy. They have a high probability of a spontaneous return to a normal TSH despite continuation of amiodarone treatment (see Sect. C.II). The implications of this finding are twofold. First, a suppressed plasma TSH is not a good predictor of AIT. Second, the transient presence of a suppressed TSH in euthyroid patients may represent an asymptomatic episode of amiodarone-induced destructive thyroiditis. In view of the gradual accumulation of amiodarone and DEA in tissues, the cytotoxic effect of amiodarone and DEA on thyrocytes will be expressed only when intrathyroidal drug concentrations exceed a certain threshold level (see Sect. B.II.2.a). The time to reach these critical concentrations may depend among other factors on the cumulative dose of amiodarone, explaining the widely different time interval between the start of amiodarone therapy and the onset of AIT. In support of this reasoning is the observation that the TSH response to TRH decreases with increasing cumulative doses of amiodarone in a dose-dependent manner (Fig. 11). The clinically silent destructive thyroiditis may lower the intrathyroidal drug concentration, allowing the repair phase to proceed uninterrupted. This remains, however, speculative at the present time, since the true origin of the transiently suppressed TSH in euthyroid patients on amiodarone therapy is unknown.

IV. Treatment

1. Amiodarone-Induced Hypothyroidism

The logical way to treat AIH is to stop amiodarone therapy. Discontinuation of amiodarone treatment restored euthyroidism after 2–4 months in 12 out of 20 patients. In the remaining eight patients the hypothyroid state was sustained until 5–8 months when thyroxine was instituted; as evident from thyroxine withdrawal 1 year later, these patients all had permanent hypothyroidism (Martino et al. 1987). The transient hypothyroidism was predominantly found in patients without underlying thyroid abnormalities in whom thyroid antibodies were present in 25%, while permanent hypothyroidism occurred exclusively in patients with underlying abnormalities (e.g. Hashimoto's goitre, non-toxic goitre, and ^{131}I therapy for Graves' disease) in whom thyroid antibodies were present in 88%.

In an attempt to shorten the period between discontinuation of amiodarone and restoration of euthyroidism, potassium perchlorate ($KClO_4$) in a single daily dose of 1.0 g has been given for 9–34 days. This led to a prompt restoration of euthyroidism, usually within 2–3 weeks (Martino et al. 1986b; van Dam et al. 1993). Hypothyroidism recurs, however, in about half of the patients 1–10 weeks after withdrawal of $KClO_4$; a second course of $KClO_4$ may then be required, which again is proven to be effective. Because potassium perchlorate acutely blocks the transport of iodide into the thyroid, thereby lowering intrathyroidal iodine content, its favourable therapeutic action in AIH strongly supports the proposed pathogenesis of AIH, i.e. a failure to escape from the inhibitory effect of intrathyroidal iodine excess on thyroid hormone synthesis.

If amiodarone withdrawal is not feasible in view of the patient's cardiac state, euthyroidism can be achieved by treatment with thyroxine, titrating the dose on the level of serum TSH. This usually has the desired outcome, although an occasional fatal case of AIH has been described (MAZONSON et al. 1984).

2. Amiodarone-Induced Thyrotoxicosis

Discontinuation of amiodarone treatment in AIT does not always resolve the thyrotoxic state. While patients with AIT type II become euthyroid within 3–5 months, patients with a diffuse or nodular goitre (AIT type I) usually are still hyperthyroid 6–9 months after discontinuation of the drug (MARTINO et al. 1987). Treatment with antithyroid drugs is not very effective either: after discontinuation of amiodarone, a spontaneous cure of AIT was reached after 7.4 months, not different from that of 7.8 months when propylthiouracil was administered (LÉGER et al. 1983). The poor efficacy of thionamide drugs in AIT has been reported in many studies (WIMPFHEIMER et al. 1982; SIMON et al. 1984; MARTINO et al. 1987; BLOSSEY and PEITSCH 1988; ALTHAUS et al. 1988; BROUSSOLLE et al. 1989), and comes as no surprise in view of the well-known decreased efficacy of antithyroid drugs in patients with hyperthyroidism induced by iodine excess (as in AIT type I) and in thyrotoxicosis induced by destructive thyroiditis (as in AIT type II).

Effective control of AIT thus remains a difficult challenge, especially because these patients often have life-threatening arrhythmias that are resistant to conventional antiarrhythmic drugs, worsen by the development of AIT, and may reappear after discontinuation of amiodarone. Furthermore, ^{131}I therapy is usually not feasible in view of the suppressed thyroidal radioiodine uptake. Propranolol given for symptomatic relief of AIT is sometimes contraindicated by compromising myocardial function, and the combination with amiodarone may give rise to bradycardia and sinus arrest. Under these circumstances surgery might be preferred because it provides immediate and effective control of the thyrotoxic state on the condition that a total or near-total thyroidectomy is performed, and it allows continuation of amiodarone treatment. Although the cardiac state will exclude surgery in some patients, the fear that this group of patients carry a high surgical risk has not materialized. Of the 26 patients who have been reported to undergo surgery because of AIT, none died, euthyroidism was restored in all within 2–15 days, and postoperative morbidity was low (3 cases of hypocalcaemia, 2 cases of dysrhythmia, 1 case of pneumonia) (BRENNAN et al. 1987; BLOSSEY and PEITSCH 1988; FARWELL et al. 1990; MEHRA et al. 1991; MEURISSE et al. 1993; MULLIGAN et al. 1993). One patient was operated on while under local anaesthesia (MEHRA et al. 1991). All patients required postoperative thyroxine treatment.

Non-surgical alternatives, however, are available. One option is treatment with corticosteroids, akin to the favourable effect of steroids on the inflammatory reaction in subacute thyroiditis. Prednisone given in combination with antithyroid drugs improved the clinical state, and serum T_4 and T_3 concentrations had decreased markedly by 10 days; in comparison, treatment with antithyroid drugs alone did not improve the clinical condition nor did it change serum T_4 in 40 days (BROUSOLLE et al. 1989). The results of corticosteroid therapy have been reported in 22 patients, obviously mostly cases of AIT type II (WIMPHEIMER et al. 1982; SIMON et al. 1984; BONNYNS et al. 1989; BROUSOLLE et al. 1989; GEORGES et al. 1992; PECHE et al. 1992; ROTI et al. 1993; BARTALENA et al. 1994). Amiodarone was discontinued in all patients except one, and antithyroid drugs were also given in 16 patients. The daily dose ranged from 15 to 80 mg prednisone or from 3 to 6 mg dexamethasone, administered for 7–12 weeks. This schedule effectively restored euthyroidism in 19 of the 22 patients. However, early discontinuation of steroid therapy after 2–3 weeks was associated with recurrence of the thyrotoxic state, necessitating reintroduction of steroids (WIMPHEIMER et al. 1982; SIMON et al. 1984; ROTI et al. 1993). No recurrences were observed after the final withdrawal of the steroids. Elevated serum IL-6 concentrations return to normal levels within days upon prednisone treatment (BARTALENA et al. 1994), those of serum thyroglobulin after 1 month (BROUSOLLE et al. 1989).

The mechanism by which steroids are effective in AIT is not entirely clear. Dexamethasone inhibits in vitro the cytotoxic effect of amiodarone, and might do so in vivo as well (BRENNAN et al. 1995). Steroids can inhibit the proteolytic action of lysosomes. In destructive thyroiditis the proteolysis of thyroglobulin, mediated by lysosomal enzymes in the follicular cells, is increased probably due to an abnormally high release of lysosomal enzymes. The rapid effect of corticosteroids in AIT type II suggests inhibition of Tg proteolysis due to a lysosomal action (BONNYNS et al. 1989; BROUSOLLE et al. 1989). No good data are available on the efficacy of prednisone in AIT type I.

Another option is potassium perchlorate ($KClO_4$). Besides reducing the cytotoxic effect of amiodarone in vitro (BRENNAN et al. 1995), perchlorate inhibits iodide uptake by the thyroid gland. By doing so, it reduces intrathyroidal iodine content, thereby rendering thionamides more effective. Its use in AIT type I and type II has been pioneered by MARTINO et al. (1986c, 1987). The results, after discontinuation of amiodarone, are as follows. When no treatment was given ($n = 11$) or when methimazole was administered in a daily dose of 40 mg ($n = 17$), all patients were still hyperthyroid at 2 months. When $KClO_4$ in a dose of 1 g daily for 15–45 days was added to methimazole treatment ($n = 27$), 55% of patients with AIT type I ($n = 18$) and 100% of AIT type II ($n = 9$) were euthyroid at 2 months. Euthyroidism was restored within 15–90 days in AIT type I patients with one exception, and within 6–55 days in AIT type II. After the withdrawal of $KClO_4$, methimazole was required only in AIT type I patients.

Others have reported similar results (NEWNHAM et al. 1987), although recurrent thyrotoxicosis was observed after an 8-day course of $KClO_4$, which may be too short a period (DE WEWEIRE et al. 1987). The use of $KClO_4$ has deliberately been limited to a daily dose of 1 g given for a short period in order to minimize the risk of serious side effects (e.g. agranulocytosis), which did not occur. The data suggest that short-term administration of $KClO_4$ shortens the period to reach euthyroidism after discontinuation of amiodarone, both in AIT type II in which spontaneous remission is the rule, and in AIT type I in which it reduces the otherwise prolonged refractoriness to thionamides. Since a prompt control of thyrotoxicosis is essential in cardiac patients, the advantage of the combined therapy of $KClO_4$ and methimazole is self-evident.

Of even greater advantage would be control of AIT despite continuation of amiodarone treatment. This goal can be reached by surgery, but also by medical management. AIT was successfully treated in five patients who continued amiodarone with carbimazole alone (Davies et al. 1992); the reason for the discrepancy with previous descriptions of the ineffectiveness of thionamides in AIT is not clear. Three other patients with AIT were effectively treated with $KClO_4$ and methimazole given simultaneously while treatment with amiodarone was continued; after 40 days, euthyroidism was maintained by methimazole alone (Reichert and de Rooy 1989). Finally, $KClO_4$ and carbimazole restored euthyroidism in two AIT patients within 2 months but the combination therapy was continued until serum TSH values had returned to the normal range, which occurred after 4 and 6 months, respectively; at that time both drugs were stopped and the patients remained euthyroid during follow-up despite continuation of amiodarone (Trip et al. 1994). Nine of these ten patients had AIT type II, which spontaneously remits. The implication of these findings is that it may not be necessary to discontinue amiodarone treatment in AIT type II: a short course of $KClO_4$ and methimazole will rapidly restore euthyroidism, and can be stopped after normalization of serum TSH without great risk of recurrent thyrotoxicosis.

Although effective treatment is available for AIT, the management of individual patients can be extremely difficult. In serious cases plasmapheresis has been tried, which is effective in removing thyroid hormones but cannot be considered as definitive therapy (Uzzan et al. 1991; Aghini-Lombardi et al. 1993). Despite all efforts, some patients do not respond to multidrug treatment with thionamides, potassium perchlorate and steroids; of six patients with life-threatening AIT, four died of thyroid storm (Georges et al. 1992; Peche et al. 1992; Hauptman et al. 1993).

3. Amiodarone Treatment in Pregnancy

Treatment with amiodarone cannot always be avoided in pregnant women. In agreement with the absence of teratotoxicity in experimental animals (Barchewitz et al. 1986; Hill and Reasor 1991), no increased incidence of congenital malformations has been reported so far (Foster and Love 1988; Magee et al. 1995). Exposure of the fetus to amiodarone, however, may result in fetal bradycardia, a prolonged QT interval and hypothyroidism (Widerhorn et al. 1991). The occurrence of fetal hypothyroidism can be expected in view of the transplacental transfer of amiodarone, DEA and iodide. The thyroid state of the infant has been reported in 63 cases, including 17 cases mentioned in discussion sections (summarized by Widerhorn et al.

1991) and 46 cases reported individually (McKenna et al. 1983; Pitcher et al. 1983; Rey et al. 1985, 1987; Robson et al. 1985; Wladimiroff and Steward 1985; Foster and Love 1988; Penn et al. 1985; Arnoux et al. 1987; Laurent et al. 1987; Strunge et al. 1988; de Wolff et al. 1988; Gembruch et al. 1989; Widerhorn et al. 1991; Matsumura et al. 1992; Plomp et al. 1992; Valensise et al. 1992; de Catte et al. 1994; Magee et al. 1995). Amiodarone was administered to the mother mainly because of maternal disease, but in a few cases because of tachycardia and congestive heart failure in the fetus.

The mothers remained euthyroid, and had mostly no evidence of thyroid disease (but thyroid antibodies were not always measured). Abnormal thyroid function was observed in 14% of the children: two neonates (3%) had transient hyperthyroxinaemia, and seven (11%) had AIH associated with goitre in one. AIH in the neonate was not related to the dose and duration of amiodarone treatment in the mother (Magee et al. 1995). Interestingly, in this study the only two infants with an abnormal thyroid function were from mothers who had either compensated hypothyroidism or postpartum thyrotoxicosis. The data suggest a genetically determined susceptibility for the development of AIH in the fetus, in line with the preponderance of AIH in adults with underlying autoimmune thyroid disease. Although the congenital hypothyroidism induced by amiodarone treatment of the mother is likely to be transient (Plomp et al. 1992), it seems too risky to await spontaneous recovery in view of the critical dependence of brain development on thyroid hormones. The majority of infants have been treated with thyroxine, in one instance already started in utero by intra-amniotic administration (de Catte et al. 1994). Euthyroidism was maintained after discontinuation of thyroxine at the age of 5–20 months (de Wolf et al. 1988; Magee et al. 1995). Growth, motor and mental development were normal in some (Strunge et al. 1988; Magee et al. 1995) but impaired in other AIH infants (de Wolf et al. 1988; Plomp et al. 1992).

The case reports demonstrate that amiodarone treatment in pregnancy is feasible and not necessarily associated with an adverse outcome. Even breast feeding has been allowed (Plomp et al. 1992), despite the substantial excretion of amiodarone in milk. However, it seems wise to refrain as much as possible from amiodarone treatment in pregnant and breast feeding women because the fetus and neonate are very sensitive to iodide-induced hypothyroidism. This is further illustrated by the case of a neonate who at 13 h of age was given amiodarone in an oral dose of 10 mg/kg per day and developed AIH on day 13 of life (Hijazi et al. 1992).

4. Amiodarone Treatment of Hyperthyroidism

Whereas on the one hand amiodarone may cause thyrotoxicosis, on the other hand the drug may be used in the treatment of thyrotoxicosis, thus showing its Janus' face. The rationale for amiodarone therapy in Graves' hyperthyroidism and toxic multinodular goitre is the initial albeit transient suppression of thyroidal hormone synthesis and release via the iodine excess generated by the drug, and the inhibition of extrathyroidal T_4 to T_3 conversion. Serum FT_4 and T_3 decreased to a similar extent when amiodarone in a daily dose of 600 mg or iodine in a daily dose of 18 mg (equivalent to that released by amiodarone) was administered for 2 weeks to thyrotoxic patients, associated with symptomatic improvement; the response to carbimazole, started immediately after amiodarone, was, however, delayed in some patients (SHELDON 1983). Other studies have compared a combined regimen of antithyroid drugs (propylthiouracil or methimazole) and amiodarone with that of antithyroid drugs alone (VAN REETH et al. 1987; VAN REETH and UNGER 1991; RAJATANAVIN et al. 1990): in all studies the decrease in serum T_3 and T_4 was faster and greater when amiodarone was added. Patients treated with the combined regimen experienced, in contrast to the conventionally treated group, a return of serum T_3 to normal values within 5 days, and a greater fall in heart rate and gain in body weight; serum rT_3 increased transiently. The combined regimen restored sinus rhythm in one patient with hyperthyroidism and atrial fibrillation within 3 days (CAUCHIE et al. 1988).

It remains questionable, however, whether addition of amiodarone is of much advantage in the management of uncomplicated hyperthyroidism. Administration of amiodarone for longer periods than 3–28 days (the duration of treatment in the above-mentioned studies) carries the risk of aggravation of the thyrotoxic state by escape from the Wolff-Chaikoff effect; this would be particularly unfortunate because the iodine excess renders thionamides less effective and precludes ^{131}I therapy. Amiodarone might be of potential benefit in the treatment of life-threatening thyrotoxicosis such as thyroid storm, especially when cardiac arrhythmias are present, due to both its antiarrhythmic effects and its antithyroid effects exerted simultaneously in the thyroid and extrathyroidal tissues. This application has so far, however, not been reported.

V. Summary

Table 4 summarizes the main characteristics of AIH and AIT. The clinical and biochemical diagnosis of AIH usually poses no problems. The incidence in areas with a high environmental iodine intake is higher than that in iodine-deficient areas (13.2% vs. 6.4%). It occurs more often in females than in males, and relatively early during amiodarone treatment. It is caused by a failure of the thyroid gland to escape from the Wolff-Chaikoff effect (induced by the iodine excess generated from amiodarone), resulting in permanent inhibition of organification. This is more likely to happen in subjects with pre-existent autoimmune thyroiditis. Consequently, AIH is to a certain extent predictable, and females with thyroid antibodies have a high relative risk of developing AIH.

Thyroidal radioiodine uptake is preserved in AIH despite the increased stable iodide pool, which is explained by the drop in an unknown product "X.I" of the organification that normally inhibits iodide uptake. Discon-

Table 4. Characteristics of amiodarone-induced hypothroidism (AIH) and amiodarone-induced thyrotoxicosis (AIT)

	AIH	AIT
Diagnosis	TSH ↑, FT4 ↓	TSH ↓, FT4 ↑, T_3 ↑ or N
Incidence	Iodine-replete areas ♀ > ♂ First years of treatment	Iodine-deplete areas ♂ > ♀ During whole treatment period
Pathogenesis	Failure to escape from Wolff-Chaikoff effect	Type I: iodide-induced thyrotoxicosis Type II: destructive thyroiditis
Predictability	Females with thyroid antibodies	Unpredictable sudden onset
Treatment	T_4, $KClO_4$	Thionamides, $KClO_4$, steroids, thyroidectomy

tinuation of amiodarone will usually restore euthyroidism after 3–4 months, but permanent hypothyroidism may ensue in patients with underlying thyroid disease (as evident from the presence of thyroid antibodies). The time to reach euthyroidism can be shortened by potassium perchlorate, which acts by depleting intrathyroidal iodine stores. Thyroxine is effective in ablating AIH, and allows continuation of amiodarone, which in many patients will be the preferred mode of treatment. Fetal hypothyroidism occurs in 11% of patients treated with amiodarone during pregnancy, and should be treated at once with thyroxine in view of the critical dependency of brain development on thyroid hormones.

The clinical diagnosis of AIT can be difficult; worsening of the underlying cardiac disease and especially the re-occurrence of arrhythmia should arouse the suspicion of AIT. The biochemical diagnosis of AIT is straightforward if TSH is decreased and T_3 increased. If T_3 is not elevated, the biochemical pattern of T_4 toxicosis occurring in some AIT patients may be difficult to distinguish from that in clinically euthyroid patients, who usually have an elevated FT_4 and sometimes a suppressed TSH. The incidence of AIT in areas with a low environmental iodine intake is higher than that in iodine-replete regions (11.9% vs. 1.7%). AIT occurs more often in males than in females, and new cases of AIT continue to occur during the whole duration of treatment.

Two types of AIT have been distinguished. AIT type I occurs in patients with pre-existent diffuse or nodular goitre; thyroidal radioiodine uptake remains inappropriately normal or even elevated, and serum IL-6 levels are moderately increased. AIT type II occurs in the absence of apparent thyroid abnormalities, thyroidal radioiodine uptake is appropriately low or suppressed, and serum IL-6 concentrations are markedly high. Accordingly, a different pathogenesis of both types is proposed. Type I is obviously caused by an increased thyroid hormone synthesis due to overrepletion of intrathyroidal iodine stores by the iodine excess. Type II is most probably the result of a destructive thyroiditis in which thyroid content is released into the circulation, akin to subacute thyroiditis; amiodarone and DEA in view of their cytotoxic effect on thyrocytes (by interference with lysosomes) are more likely to be responsible for the destruction than iodine excess itself. Although a preexistent goitre may predispose to AIT type I, the occurrence of AIT (especially type II) is unpredictable. Thyroid function tests done at regular intervals are of little value for an early diagnosis of AIT in view of its sudden onset and the transient nature of a suppressed TSH in many patients (which may indicate an asymptomatic course of destructive thyroiditis with spontaneous cure).

Treatment of AIT should be tailored to the patient's need, depending on the severity of AIT, which varies from mild to very severe, and on the cardiac condition, which may or may not allow discontinuation of amiodarone treatment. Spontaneous recovery to euthyroidism within 3–5 months after stopping amiodarone is the rule in AIT type II, but the exception in AIT type I. Thionamides are less effective in patients with iodine excess. Combination therapy of thionamides and potassium perchlorate shortens the period until euthyroidism to less than 3 months in type I and less than 2 months in type II. Another option is prednisone, given for 7–12 weeks in combination with thionamides: this schedule is very effective in AIT type II. Since a prompt control of thyrotoxicosis is essential in these cardiac patients, the advantage of the combination of thionamides with potassium perchlorate or corticosteroids is evident. If discontinuation of amiodarone is not permitted, a total or near-total thyroidectomy solves the problem of AIT. Medical control of AIT under continuation of amiodarone can be sometimes achieved by long-term use of thionamides alone, but more often when given initially in combination with potassium perchlorate. The self-limiting nature of AIT type II allows discontinuation of the antithyroid drugs after some months, whereafter the euthyroid state is maintained despite continuation of amiodarone treatment.

D. Amiodarone as a Thyroid Hormone Antagonist

I. Hypothyroid-Like Effects of Amiodarone

1. Heart

Amiodarone is prescribed in clinical medicine for cardiac arrhythmias and angina pectoris. The rationale is given by its pharmacological actions, which include bradycardia, lengthening of the cardiac action potential, and depression of myocardial oxygen consumption. These phenomena are identical to those observed in hypothyroidism (FREEDBERG et al. 1970; ROVETTO et al. 1972; JOHNSON et al. 1973; GAVRILESCU et al. 1976; SHARP et al. 1985). Hypothyroidism produced by thyroidectomy was, in former days, a last resort to treat otherwise irremediable angina pectoris, and can relieve anginal complaints. Hypothyroidism also renders protection against cardiac arrhythmias (CHESS-WILLIAMS and COKER 1989; VENKATESH et al. 1991). The hypothesis has thus been put forward that amiodarone acts through the induction of a local hypothyroid-like state in extrathyroidal tissues, notably the heart (SINGH 1983). In view of the substantial decrease in T_3 in plasma and extrathyroidal tissues induced by amiodarone via inhibition of T_4 5′-deiodination (see Sect. B.II), the hypothesis is quite attractive: it is schematically represented in Fig. 10.

a) Electrophysiological Effects

The electrophysiological changes produced by amiodarone in experimental animals are prevented by the simultaneous administration of T_4 or T_3 (SINGH and VAUGHAN WILLIAMS 1970; PATTERSON et al. 1986). In humans too, the prolongation of the QTc interval induced by amiodarone is abolished by oral administration of T_3, although the therapeutic effect of amiodarone as judged from the frequency of ventricular premature complexes was not lost upon the addition of T_3 (POLIKAR et al. 1986). The proposed hypothesis is not supported, however, by studies with iopanoic acid, a radiographic contrast agent as potent as amiodarone in inhibiting the conversion of T_4 into T_3. Iopanoic acid did not produce bradycardia or QT prolongation in guinea pigs (LINDENMEYER et al. 1984; STÄUBLI and STUDER 1986) nor did it reduce the frequency of ventricular premature complexes in humans (MEESE et al. 1985), despite changes in serum

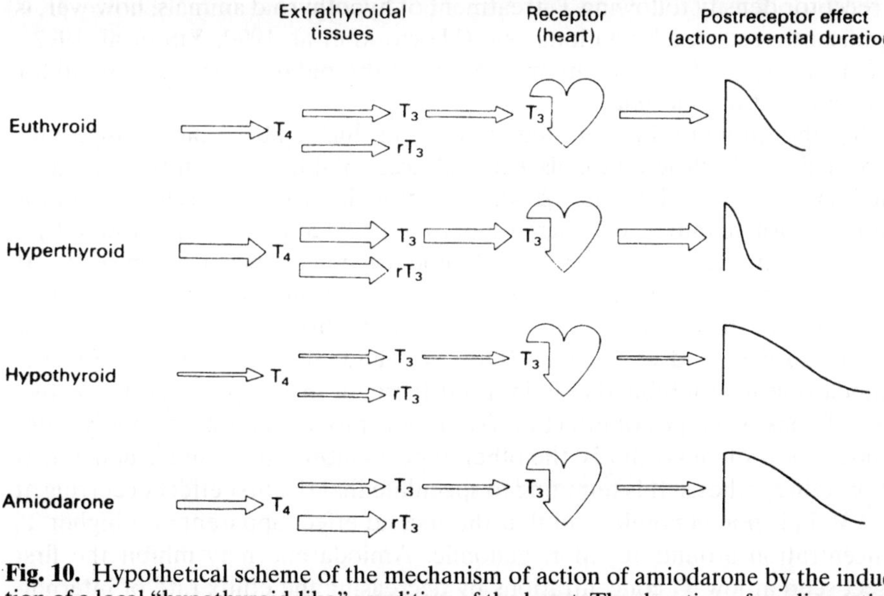

Fig. 10. Hypothetical scheme of the mechanism of action of amiodarone by the induction of a local "hypothyroid-like" condition of the heart. The duration of cardiac action potentials is viewed as a postreceptor effect of nuclear T_3 receptors in the heart. Receptor occupancy is decreased in hypothyroid and in amiodarone-treated patients, resulting in an identical lengthening of the action potential. (Reproduced with permission from WIERSINGA and TRIP 1986)

T_4, T_3 and rT_3 comparable to those during amiodarone treatment. Furthermore, the prolongation by amiodarone of the ventricular refractory period in rats is not related to the thyroid state (LAMBERT et al. 1987), and the antiarrhythmic efficacy of amiodarone in humans is not related to the increase in serum rT_3 (KERIN et al. 1986), although this has been disputed (NADEMANEE et al. 1982).

b) *Effect on* β*-Adrenergic Receptors*

Hypothyroidism reduces the number of β-adrenergic receptors in heart plasma membranes, but does not affect the affinity constant. Amiodarone treatment also reduces the MBC but not the K_d of cardiac β-adrenoreceptors as observed in rats, rabbits, pigs and humans (NOKIN et al. 1983; VENKATESH et al. 1986; BJØRNERHEIM et al. 1991; GØTZSCHE 1993; GØTZSCHE and ORSKOV 1994); the decrease in receptor number is roughly dose dependent, of the order of 14%–45%, which is similar to that in hypothyroidism. Addition of T_3 to the treatment with amiodarone restores the receptor number as well as the heart rate, which is reduced by amiodarone as a function of the cardiac β-adrenoceptor density (PERRET et al. 1992). Iopanoic acid, despite decreasing serum T_3 and T_4 5′-deiodination as potent as amiodarone, did not affect β-adrenoceptor density or heart rate (PERRET et al. 1992). When amiodarone is given to hypothyroid animals, it has no effect on receptor number; the increase in receptor density following T_3 treatment of hypothyroid animals, however, is significantly reduced by amiodarone (HARTONG et al. 1990; YIN et al. 1992). The data suggest that a minimum quantity of thyroid hormone is required for this action of amiodarone.

Further proof of this has been obtained in chick embryo cardiac myocytes (YIN et al. 1994). When the cells were cultured for 48 h in serum-free medium, amiodarone did not influence β-adrenoceptor density. T_3 increased receptor number, with an initial 30% increase between 10^{-14} and 10^{-11} *M*, followed by a second larger increase up to 10^{-7} *M*. Amiodarone in a concentration of 10^{-7} *M* inhibited both effects of T_3. The implications of this finding are twofold. First, it strengthens the notion that amiodarone has no direct effect, independent of T_3, on cardiac β-adrenoceptors (DISATNIK and SHAINBERG 1991). Second, amiodarone may inhibit the T_3-induced increase in receptor density in two ways. T_3 has two types of effect on β-adrenoceptors: one occurs rapidly independent of protein synthesis, the other appears more slowly and is dependent on protein synthesis. It is tempting to speculate that the first effect occurring at 10^{-12} *M* T_3 is non-genomic, and that the second effect apparent at a higher T_3 concentration around 10^{-9} *M* is genomic. Amiodarone may inhibit the first effect seen at low T_3 concentrations by decreasing the efflux rate of internalized β-adrenoceptors to the cell surface, presumably via an extranuclear action of the drug on membranes. The inhibitory effect of amiodarone on the second effect seen at higher T_3 concentrations is likely to be due to a decreased synthesis of β-adrenoceptors via a genomic action of the drug on the T_3-

responsive gene encoding for the β-adrenergic receptor (CHANG and KUNOS 1981; HARTONG et al. 1990; YIN et al. 1994).

Neither amiodarone nor DEA inhibits the in vitro binding of [^{125}I]cyanopindolol to cardiac membranes (GØTZSCHE 1993), although an earlier report did note inhibition (VENKATESH et al. 1986).

c) *Effect on Myosin and Contractility*

Three isoforms of the contractile protein myosin are identified in the heart, differing in their myosin heavy chains (MHC): the V_1 isoenzyme contains two αMHC, has a high Ca^{2+} ATPase activity, and is associated with a high contractile velocity of cardiac fibres; the V_3 isoenzyme contains two βMHC, has a low Ca^{2+} ATPase activity, and is associated with a low contractile velocity; the V_2 isoenzyme is composed of an α/β-heterodimer and is of intermediate activity with regard to Ca^{2+} ATPase and contractile performance. The α- and β-MHC are encoded by separate genes, regulated inversely by T_3 at the transcriptional level. In the heart of euthyroid rats the V_1 isoform predominates: αMHC is expressed at high and βMHC at low levels. In hypothyroidism there is a shift from V_1 to V_3 expression: αMHC decreases and βMHC increases both at the mRNA and protein level. In amiodarone-treated rats a similar shift from V_1 to V_3 is seen, although the decrease in αMHC and the increase in ~30%–40% in βMHC isoforms are less than in hypothyroid animals (WIEGAND et al. 1986; BAGCHI et al. 1987; PARADIS et al. 1991). The changes are found in mRNA and protein levels (with one discrepancy of an amiodarone-induced increase in αMHC mRNA despite a decrease in the V_1 isoenzyme) (FRANKLYN et al. 1987). The effect of amiodarone is abolished by the addition of T_3 (BAGCHI et al. 1987; FRANKLYN et al. 1987; PARADIS et al. 1991). The effect of amiodarone is smaller when given to hypothyroid animals, again suggesting that the effect is thyroid hormone dependent (FRANKLYN et al. 1987; PARADIS et al. 1991).

In line with the changes in myosin isoforms, the Ca^{2+} ATPase activities of myosin decrease in hearts of amiodarone-treated rats, although to a lesser extent than in hearts of hypothyroid rats; the effect of amiodarone is abolished by T_3 (BAGCHI et al. 1987). No effect of amiodarone was observed on Na^+ K^+ ATPase activity. The acute increase in cardiac performance in response to intravenous T_3 is blunted in pigs pretreated with amiodarone (GØTZSCHE 1994). The data indicate that amiodarone impairs myocardial contractility through hypothyroid-like changes in the gene expression of α- and β-MHC. This genomic effect seems to be dependent on thyroid hormones: in chicken cardiac myocytes cultured for 48h, the inotropic response to isoproterenol (not to Ca^{2+}) was inhibited by amiodarone only if T_3 was present in the culture medium (YIN et al. 1994).

Finally, it has been reported that amiodarone treatment increases the number of voltage-operated (dihydropyridine-sensitive) Ca^{2+} channels in rat heart membranes; the effect is smaller but otherwise similar to that observed in hypothyroidism (GØTZSCHE 1994; GØTZSCHE and ORSKOV 1994). It is unknown if this effect is genomic or non-genomic.

2. Liver

a) *Effect on Low-Density Lipoprotein Receptors*

Plasma cholesterol gradually increases from 5.1 ± 0.2 mmol/l before treatment to 6.9 ± 0.8 mmol/l after 30 months of amiodarone treatment in humans. It is associated with an equal increase in apoprotein B, indicating a rise of low-density lipoprotein (LDL) cholesterol. When age- and sex-specific reference values were applied, 30% of the patients had cholesterol values above the 75th percentile before treatment; this number rose to 69% after 2 years of treatment (WIERSINGA et al. 1991). The increase in plasma cholesterol is also described in other studies (ALBERT et al. 1991; POLLAK et al. 1988; KASIM et al. 1990); the negative results of three early studies can be explained by the short treatment period of 6–13 weeks (PRITCHARD et al. 1975; SONNENBLICK et al. 1986; GOTTLIEB and SONNENBLICK 1989), because the rise of plasma cholesterol develops slowly, being significant after 1 year of treatment. Plasma cholesterol was not related to the daily dose of amiodarone or to plasma concentrations of amiodarone, DEA, T_4, T_3, or rT_3; it was directly related to the cumulative dose of amiodarone, and inversely to plasma TSH (Fig. 11) (WIERSINGA et al. 1991). It appears that an increasing cumulative dose of amiodarone has two effects independent of each other: one is a rise of plasma cholesterol not related to plasma thyroid hormone concentrations nor caused by changes in plasma TSH, the other a decrease within the normal range of plasma TSH associated with higher plasma T_4 and lower plasma T_3 values. Both effects apparently are separate manifestations of extensive tissue deposition of the drug and its metabolite, which occurs slowly (Sect. A.II.3).

The hypercholesterolaemic effect of amiodarone, akin to that of hypothyroidism, has been reproduced in a dose-dependent manner in experimental animals (KANNAN et al. 1982; WIERSINGA and BROENINK 1991). Using the rat as a model, it was shown that the amiodarone-induced 60% increase in plasma LDL cholesterol was associated with a decrease in ~50% in hepatic mRNA encoding for the LDL receptor; liver mRNAs encoding for cholesterol 7α-hydroxylase and HMG-CoA reductase (the other key proteins in cholesterol metabolism) did not change (HUDIG et al. 1994). Subsequent studies revealed that the fall in LDL receptor mRNA was not due to increased degradation of the mRNA, and was followed by a decrease of ~45% in liver LDL receptor protein; the decrease in both LDL receptor mRNA and protein was reversed by treatment with T_3 (HUDIG et al. 1997). The data strongly suggest that the hypercholesterolaemic effect of amiodarone is due to a decreased transcription of the T_3-responsive gene encoding for the LDL receptor; precisely the same mechanism is involved in the classical increase in LDL cholesterol in hypothyroidism.

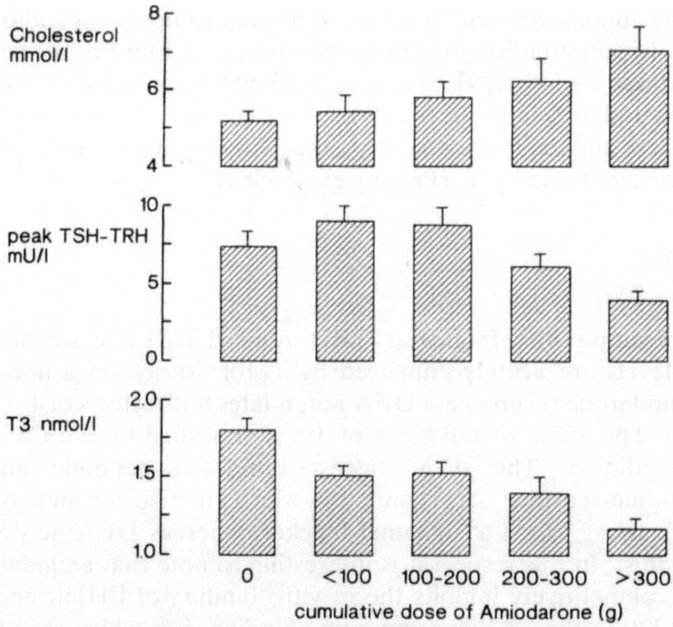

Fig. 11. Increase in plasma cholesterol and decrease in peak TSH response to TRH and in plasma T_3 as a function of the cumulative dosage of amiodarone, observed in euthyroid patients who maintained a normal TRH test during amiodarone therapy. (Reproduced with permission from WIERSINGA et al. 1991)

b) Effect on Lipoprotein Lipase

Treatment with amiodarone in humans results in a slight decrease in plasma triglycerides (WIERSINGA et al. 1991), presumably related to an increase in postheparin lipoprotein lipase activity as hepatic triglyceride lipase does not change (KASIM et al. 1990). This contrasts with the rise of plasma triglycerides during hypothyroidism in humans, which is due to a decreased postheparin lipolytic activity. The situation in the rat is different. In this animal, both amiodarone treatment and hypothyroidism increase serum triglycerides and adipose tissue lipoprotein lipase activity, and decrease hepatic triglyceride lipase activity. Addition of T_3 to the treatment with amiodarone reverses these changes, except hepatic triglyceride lipase activity, which remains low (KASIM et al. 1987).

c) Effect on Other Proteins

Administration of T_3 increases and treatment with amiodarone decreases transcription of the phosphoenolpyruvate carboxykinase gene in rat liver (HARTONG et al. 1987). Another T_3-responsive hepatic gene, "spot 14", encodes for an unknown protein involved in lipid metabolism. Its mRNA is increased by amiodarone with a return to normal values upon addition of T_3; in contrast, hypothyroidism decreases its mRNA, and no further decrease is seen when these hypothyroid rats are treated with amiodarone (FRANKLYN et al. 1989). Amiodarone also decreases the liver content of α-glycerophosphate dehydrogenase and malic enzyme, two other T_3-responsive gene products; the effect can be abolished by T_3 (PEKARY et al. 1986).

3. Pituitary

a) *Effect on TSH*

In perifused rat pituitary fragments, TRH-induced TSH release and intracellular Ca^{2+} levels are acutely enhanced by T_3, obviously via a non-genomic action. Amiodarone reverses but DEA potentiates both effects of T_3 (ROUSSEL et al. 1995). The effect of DEA (as of T_3) is abolished by the Ca^{2+} channel blocker nifedipine. The data suggest rapid non-genomic effects on dihydropyridine-sensitive Ca^{2+} channels in which amiodarone antagonizes the effect of T_3 acting as a Ca^{2+} channel blocker, whereas DEA acts as a Ca^{2+} channel agonist. In this respect it is interesting to note that amiodarone, but not DEA, competitively inhibits the in vitro binding of [^{3}H]nitrendipine or [^{3}H]PN200-110 to the 1,4-dihydropyridine-binding sites which are associated with calcium channels (NOKIN et al. 1986; GØTZSCHE 1993).

Genomic effects of amiodarone on the transcription of the genes encoding for the α- and β-subunits of pituitary TSH have been discussed in Sect. B.II.3. Amiodarone in vitro and in vivo, when given to euthyroid rats, increases the synthesis and release of TSH, as in hypothyroidism, which is reversed by thyroid hormone. Although amiodarone treatment of hypothyroid rats decreased rather than increased TSH synthesis and release (FRANKLYN et al. 1987), this does not necessarily imply a thyroid hormone agonist activity of the drug in view of the higher serum T_4 and T_3 levels in the amiodarone-treated hypothyroid rats than in the untreated hypothyroid rats.

b) *Effect on Prolactin*

In euthyroid rats, amiodarone treatment reduces pituitary prolactin (PRL) mRNA as in hypothyroid animals; neither state, however, affected pituitary PRL content or serum PRL. In hypothyroid rats treated with amiodarone, the reduction in PRL mRNA was less marked. A direct inhibitory effect of $50\,\mu M$ amiodarone on PRL mRNA and PRL release was noted in rat anterior pituitary cells cultured for 24h, which was antagonized by T_3 (FRANKLYN et al. 1987).

c) *Effect on Growth Hormone*

Treatment of euthyroid rats with amiodarone changes neither pituitary growth hormone (GH) mRNA and GH content nor serum GH. In hypothyroid rats, GH mRNA and serum GH are decreased, and restored to normal by amiodarone treatment (FRANKLYN et al. 1987). In cultured rat pituitary GC cells, exposure to amiodarone for 2 days did not influence basal GH mRNA levels; amiodarone, however, dose dependently inhibited the T_3-induced increase in GH mRNA, evident already at $1 \mu M$ (NORMAN and LAVIN 1989). The effect on GH mRNA paralleled the inhibitory effect of amiodarone on nuclear T_3 binding in these cells, indicating competitive antagonism of amiodarone to thyroid hormone action. It could be overcome by an excess of T_3. Finally, the stimulatory effects of T_3 on [^{3}H]thymidine incorporation in rat pituitary GH3 cells are inhibited by amiodarone at concentrations of $\geq 0.5 \mu M$ (GOLDFINE et al. 1982).

The various hypothyroid-like effects of amiodarone and their reversibility by thyroid hormone are summarized in Table 5.

II. Amiodarone as a T_3 Receptor Antagonist

1. Inhibition of T_3 Binding to Nuclear T_3 Receptors

Amiodarone and DEA are strongly lipophilic substances. They are therefore easily dissolved in ethanol, but come out of solution in a hydrophylic environment. This may explain conflicting reports on the in vitro effect of amiodarone on the binding of T_3 to its nuclear receptor proteins. Amiodarone does not appreciably affect the binding of T_3 to nuclei isolated from rat liver (SOGOL et al. 1983; WILSON 1989), but DEA exerts an inhibitory effect with a K_d value of $8.6 \mu M$ (LATHAM et al. 1987). Similarly, amiodarone does not (but DEA does) inhibit the T_3 binding to nuclear T_3 receptors isolated from rat and pig hearts (K_d atrium $35 \mu M$, ventricle $27 \mu M$ – LATHAM et al. 1987; GØTZSCHE and

Table 5. Hypothyroid-like effects of amiodarone in various tissues

Tissue effect	Hypothyroidism	Amiodarone	Amiodarone + T_3
Heart			
QTc interval	↑	↑	N
Heart rate	↓	↓	N
β-Adrenoceptor density	↓	↓	N
Ca^{2+} ATPase activity of myosin	↓	↓	N
DHP-sensitive Ca^{2+} channels	↑	↑	
Liver			
LDL receptor density	↓	↓	N
Triglyceride lipase activity	↓	↓	↓
Spot 14 mRNA	↓	↑	N
Adipose tissue			
Lipoprotein lipase activity	(↑)	↑	N
Pituitary			
TSH synthesis and release	↑	↑	N
PRL mRNA	↓	↓	N
GH mRNA	↓	↓*	N

↑, increase; ↓, decrease; N, return to normal; (↑), increase not significant; ↓*, decrease not of basal but only of T_3-induced increase; for full explanation, see text.

ORSKOV 1994). In isolated rat anterior pituitary cells amiodarone inhibited the in vitro T_3 binding dose dependently, and in a competitive manner as tested at 1 mM (FRANKLYN et al. 1985). In rat pituitary tumour cells amiodarone also acted as a competitive antagonist to nuclear T_3 binding with a K_d of 1.6 μM (NORMAN and LAVIN 1989). This study was done in the presence of a vehicle consisting of (vol/vol) 88.8% H_2O, 9.3% Tween-80 and 1.9% benzylalcohol (cf. Sect. A.IV.2) in order to keep amiodarone in solution. Tween-80 itself, however, is a competitor of T_3 binding (BAKKER et al. 1994), and the reported effect may be due to Tween-80 and not to amiodarone. The effect of DEA in pituitary cells has not been studied.

Further studies employing the chicken α_1-T_3 receptor (TRα_1) and the rat β_1-T_3 receptor (TRβ_1) expressed in *E. coli* have shed more light on this issue (BAKKER et al. 1994; VAN BEEREN et al. 1995). Amiodarone and DEA stayed in solution up to $10^{-4} M$ when 0.05% Triton X-100 was added to the incubation buffer. DEA, but not amiodarone, had a clear inhibitory effect on the binding of T_3 to its receptors, being slightly greater with respect to TRβ_1 than to TRα_1 (Table 6). The type of inhibition differs for the two T_3 receptors. DEA is a non-competitive inhibitor of T_3 binding to TRβ_1 (it decreases dose dependently K_a as well as MBC), whereas it is a competitive inhibitor of T_3 binding to TRα_1 (decreasing dose dependently K_a but not MBC). The K_i for the binding of DEA to the occupied TRβ_1 is 30 μM, but DEA has almost no effect on the occupied TRα_1. The effect of DEA on the unoccupied TRβ_1 and TRα_1 is progressively stronger as DEA concentrations rise. The intracellular concentrations of DEA reached in vivo are high enough (50–500 μM/cell) (BERGER and HARRIS 1986) for the drug to be able to interfere with T_3 action. A recent study employing human TRβ_1 expressed in insect cells reports non-competitive inhibition of amiodarone at 0.25–2 μM and competitive inhibition at 2–8 μM (DRVOTA et al. 1995a).

Table 6. Characteristics of the inhibition of the binding of $[^{125}I]T_3$ to the α_1-T_3 receptor and β_1-T_3 receptor by amiodarone and its analogues[a] in vitro. (Reproduced with permission from VAN BEEREN et al. 1996)

	α_1-T_3 receptor		β_1-T_3 receptor	
	IC_{50} ($10^{-5} M$)	Inhibition	IC_{50} ($10^{-5} M$)	Inhibition
Amiodarone	>20		>20	
Desethylamiodarone	4.7 ± 0.9	Competitive	2.7 ± 1.4[b]	Non-competitive
Desdiethylamiodarone	3.7 ± 0.9	Competitive	1.9 ± 0.3[b]	Non-competitive
Monoiodoamiodarone	>20		>20	
Desdiiodoamiodarone	16.2 ± 5.6	Competitive	9.1 ± 2.1[b]	Non-competitive
L3373 (two iodine atoms)	3.8 ± 1.0	Competitive	3.6 ± 0.5	Competitive
L6424 (one iodine atom)	11.3 ± 5.7		10 ± 2.0	
L3372 (no iodine atom)	No inhibition		No inhibition	

[a] For the molecular constitution, see Fig. 2.
[b] Values lower than those of TRα_1.

2. Structure-Function Relationship

The molecular conformations of amiodarone, DEA and benziodarone are similar (Fig. 12): the carbonyl oxygen is *s-trans* to the benzofuran C(2)-C(3) double bond, the phenyl ring is in a twist conformation about the carbonyl bridge to the benzofuran ring system, the ethoxy side chain is perpendicular to the phenolic ring, the *n*-butyl side chain is folded back over the iodophenyl ring and the amine is protonated in amiodarone and DEA. There is a change from *+gauche* (amiodarone) to *–gauche* (DEA) in the 2-side chain and *N*-ethylamino group, which causes these two structures to have different overall conformations (CODY and LUFT 1989).

In order to understand how these drugs might act as inhibitors of thyroid hormone responsive enzymes and of T_3-receptor binding, computer graphics modelling studies have been carried out to compare their molecular structures with those of iodothyronines. T_4 and T_3 are observed only in the skewed conformation because the bulky *ortho*-tyrosyl iodines restrict flexibility. Reverse T_3, being more flexible with only a single tyrosyl substituent, has been observed in an antiskewed conformation. Amiodarone and its analogues are in twist conformation. The iodophenolic ring of amiodarone can be matched with either the tyrosyl or the phenolic ring of skewed T_4 or antiskewed rT_3. The best fit with T_4 was obtained by superposition of the phenolic (outer) ring of T_4 (CODY and LUFT 1989). Another computational analysis also reports that superimposing the benzoylbenzofuran moiety of amiodarone on the inner ring

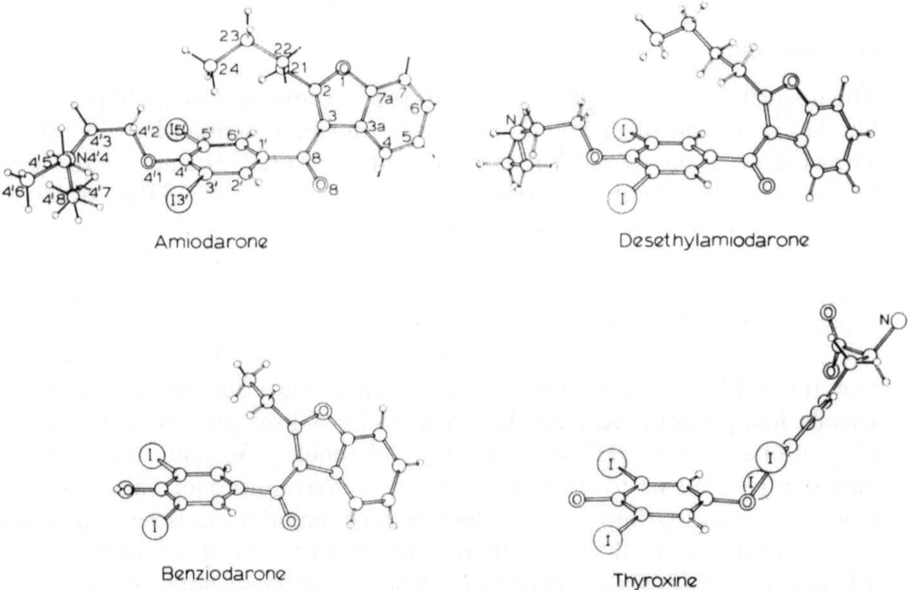

Fig. 12. Molecular conformation of amiodarone, DEA, benziodarone and T_3. (Reproduced with permission from CODY and LUFT 1989)

of T_3 and the diiodophenyl group on the outer ring provides the largest overlap of molecular volumes and gives the closest match of functional groups between amiodarone and T_3 (Chalmers et al. 1992). Other models, however, cannot be excluded.

To obtain more insight into the structure-function relationship of the interaction between amiodarone metabolites and T_3 receptors, several amiodarone analogues have been tested: compounds obtained by dethylation of amiodarone, compounds obtained by deiodination of amiodarone, and benzofuran derivatives with various iodination grades (Table 6). The results are as follows (van Beeren et al. 1996): removal of one or two ethyl groups of amiodarone results in compounds with strong but almost equal potency of inhibiting T_3 receptor binding, whereas removal of one or two iodine atoms of amiodarone has a lower potency in this respect. The strong inhibition of the benzofuran derivative L3373 is lost upon deiodination. The analogues act as competitive inhibitors to the $TR\alpha_1$, and as non-competitive inhibitors to the $TR\beta_1$ (except L3373 which was competitive). All tested analogues preferentially interfere with T_3 binding to unoccupied receptors. The implications of these findings for the structure-activity relationship are: (1) the size of the diethyl substituted nitrogen-group and of the two bulky iodine atoms in the amiodarone molecule hamper the binding of amiodarone at the T_3-binding site of T_3 receptors; and (2) differences in the hormone-binding domain of $TR\alpha_1$ and $TR\beta_1$ are likely to account for the competitive or non-competitive nature of inhibition of T_3 binding by amiodarone analogues.

III. Summary

The majority of the effects of amiodarone in various tissues are hypothyroid-like in nature and reversible by thyroid hormone, as summarized in Table 5. The evidence is most solid for the prolongation of the QTc interval, the lower heart rate, reduced β-adrenoceptor density, decreased Ca^{2+}ATPase of myosin in the heart, and reduced LDL receptor density in the liver. The evidence is less complete for dihydropyridine-sensitive Ca^{2+} channels and the triglyceride and lipoprotein lipase activities. The findings are sometimes contradictory, especially in the case of pituitary effects.

The observations allow a number of generalizations about the hypothyroid-like effects of amiodarone. First, the effect of amiodarone is usually less pronounced than that of hypothyroidism (observed for myosin, Ca^{2+} ATPase and DHP-sensitive Ca^{2+} channels). Second, the effect of amiodarone appears to be dependent on thyroid hormone. This is inferred from the following findings: (1) the effect of amiodarone is less marked in hypothyroid animals than in euthyroid animals (observed for myosin and β-adrenoceptors); (2) the effect of amiodarone in vitro may not be present in the absence of T_3 (observed for β-adrenoceptors, myocyte contractility and GH mRNA). Third, the effect of amiodarone cannot be explained solely by the inhibition of T_4 conversion into T_3, because other drugs such as iopanoic acid equally potent in inhibiting type I 5′-deiodination do not induce hypothyroid-like effects (observed for heart rate, QTc interval and β-adrenoceptors). Fourth, although the inhibitory actions of amiodarone concern T_3-dependent tissue effects, some T_3-responsive genes may not be affected by amiodarone (e.g. HMGCoA reductase and cholesterol 7α-hydroxylase). Fifth, the effects of amiodarone can be genomic or non-genomic. Good evidence exists for the genomic effect on α- and β-myosin heavy chains in the heart and on the LDL receptor in the liver: transcription of the involved genes is modulated by amiodarone qualitatively similar to the changes in hypothyroidism. The effect on β-adrenoceptor density is probably a mixed one: the early decrease in receptor number may be mediated by non-genomic effects on membranes, resulting in a low efflux rate of internalized β-adrenoceptors to the cell surface, while the late decrease in receptor number may be genomic by interference with the gene encoding for β-adrenoceptors, resulting in a decreased synthesis of receptors. The effect on dihydropyridine-sensitive Ca^{2+} channels in view of its rapidity and the electrophysiological effects are likely to be non-genomic.

Amiodarone thus appears to have multiple site of actions, resulting in tissue effects that are usually T_3 dependent. Non-genomic effects of amiodarone may be related to membrane changes (see Sects. A.III.1, A.V.2 and B.II.2a), resulting in alterations in ion channels and cellular fluxes. Inhibition of type I 5′-deiodinase, the most familiar effect of amiodarone, may be a non-genomic effect, resulting in markedly decreased tissue T_3 concentrations. This is dramatic in the heart: T_3 content is 1.55 ± 0.46 nmol/kg in euthyroid rat hearts and 0.06 ± 0.08 nmol/kg in amiodarone-treated rat hearts (Gøztsche and Orskov 1994). The low tissue concentrations of T_3 may enhance the inhibitory effect of DEA on the binding of T_3 to nuclear T_3 receptors, because DEA and the other amiodarone metabolites preferentially interfere with unoccupied T_3 receptors. In view of the slow accumulation of DEA in tissues it is conceivable that the genomic effects of amiodarone develop slowly. This is in good agreement with the clinical experience that the hypercholesterolaemic effect of amiodarone, mediated via a reduced transcription of the LDL receptor gene in the liver, becomes evident gradually dependent on the cumulative dose of amiodarone.

DEA is a non-competitive inhibitor of the binding of T_3 to the β_1-T_3 receptor (IC_{50} 27 μM), and a competitive inhibitor for the α_1-T_3 receptor (IC_{50} 47 μM). The intracellular concentrations of DEA reached in vivo are high enough (50–500 μM) for the drug to be able to interfere with T_3 binding. Decreased nuclear T_3 receptor occupancy will explain modulation of transcription by amiodarone, but other mechanisms (such as interference with dimerization of receptors) are not excluded. The precise mechanism in which DEA interferes with the transcription of T_3-responsive genes thus remains to be elucidated. Structural similarities between amiodarone, DEA and T_3 certainly favour the idea that DEA competes with T_3 at or close to the T_3-binding site of α_1- and β_1-T_3 receptors. In view of the structural similarities the drug may theoretically act as a thyroid hormone agonist (explaining some of the conflicting data in the literature), but the overriding conclusion from both in vitro and in vivo studies is that the drug behaves mainly as a thyroid hormone antagonist. The available studies provide good evidence for the hypothesis that one of the mechanisms of action of amiodarone is the induction of a local "hypothyroid-like" condition in many tissues, notably in the heart. DEA rather than amiodarone itself seems to be responsible for the hypothyroid-like actions. The drug appears to meet the criteria of a thyroid hormone antagonist.

References

Aanderud S, Sundsfjord J, Aarbakke J (1984) Amiodarone inhibits the conversion of thyroxine to triiodothyronine in isolated rat hepatocytes. Endocrinology 115: 1605–1608
Aghini-Lombardi F, Mariotti S, Fosella PV, Grasso L, Pinchera A, Braverman LE, Martino E (1993) Treatment of amiodarone iodine-induced thyrotoxicosis with plasmapheresis and methimazole. J Endocrinol Invest 16:823–826
Albert SG, Alves LE, Rose EP (1991) Effect of amiodarone on serum lipoprotein levels. Am J Cardiol 68:259–261
Althaus B, Bucker H, Schön H, Vogt T (1988) Therapieresistenz einer Amiodaron-induzierten Hyperthyreose. Schweiz Med Wochenschr 118:1176–1181
Amico JA, Richardson V, Alpert B, Klein I (1984) Clinical and chemical assessment of thyroid function during therapy with amiodarone. Arch Intern Med 144:487–490
Andreasen F, Aegerback H, Bjerregaard P, Gotzche H (1981) Pharmacokinetics of amiodarone after intravenous and oral administration. Eur J Clin Pharmacol 19:293–299
Arnoux P, Seyral P, Llurens M et al (1987) Amiodarone and digoxin for refractory fetal tachycardia. Am J Cardiol 59:166–167
Bagchi N, Brown TR, Schneider DS, Banerjee SK (1987) Effect of amiodarone on rat heart myosin isoenzymes. Circ Res 60:621–625
Bakker O, van Beeren HC, Wiersinga WM (1994) Desethylamiodarone is a noncompetitive inhibitor of the binding of thyroid hormone to the thyroid hormone β_1-receptor protein. Endocrinology 134:1665–1670
Balsam A, Ingbar SH, Sexton F (1978) The influence of fasting, diabetes, and several pharmacological agents on the pathways of thyroxine metabolism in rat liver. J Clin Invest 62:415–424
Bambini G, Aghini-Lombardi F, Rosner W, Khan S, Martino E, Pinchera A, Braverman LE, Safran M (1987) Serum sex hormone-binding globulin in amiodarone treated patients. A marker for tissue thyrotoxicosis. Arch Intern Med 147:1781–1785
Barchewitz G, Harris L, Mazue G (1986) Toxicology. In: Harris L, Roncucci R (eds) Amiodarone. Médicine et Sciences Internationales, Paris, pp 181–202
Bartalena L, Grasso L, Brogioni S, Aghini-Lombardi F, Braverman LE, Martino E (1994) Serum interleukin-6 in amiodarone-induced thyrotoxicosis. J Clin Endocrinol Metab 78:423–427
Beddows SA, Page SR, Taylor AH, McNerney R, Whitley GStJ, Johnstone AP, Nussey SS (1989) Cytotoxic effects of amiodarone and desethylamiodarone on human thyrocytes. Biochem Pharmacol 38:4397–4403
Berdeaux A, Roche A, Labaille T, Giroux B, Edouard A, Giudicelli J (1984) Tissue extraction of amiodarone and its metabolite in man after a single oral dose. Br J Clin Pharmacol 18:759–763
Berger Y, Harris L (1986) Pharmacokinetics. In: Harris L, Roncucci R (eds) Amiodarone. Médicine et Sciences Internationales, Paris, pp 45–98

Bjørnerheim R, Frøysaker T, Hanson V (1991) Effects of chronic amiodarone treatment on human myocardial β-adrenoceptor density and adenylate cyclase response. Cardiovasc Res 25:503–509
Blossey HC, Peitsch W (1988) Indication for subtotal thyroidectomy in patients with amiodarone-(iodine-) related hyperthyroidism. Wiener Med Wochenschr 18:444–447
Bonnyns M, Sterling I, Renard M, Bernard R, Demaret B, Bourdoux P (1989) Dexamethasone treatment of amiodarone-induced thryotoxicosis with or without persistent administration of the drug. Acta Cardiol 44:235–243
Borowski GD, Garofano CD, Rose LI, Spielman SR, Rotmensch HR, Greenspan AM, Horowitz LN (1985) Effect of long-term amiodarone therapy on thyroid hormone levels and thyroid function. Am J Med 78:443–450
Brennan MD, Heerden JA van, Carney JA (1987) Amiodarone-associated thyrotoxicosis: experience with surgical management. Surgery 102:1062–1067
Brennan MD, Erickson DZ, Carney JA, Bahn RS (1995) Nongoitrous (type I) amiodarone-associated thyrotoxicosis: evidence of follicular disruption in vitro and in vivo. Thyroid 5:177–183
Briançon C, Halpern S, Telenczak T, Fragu P (1990) Changes in ^{127}I mice thyroid follicle studied by analytical ion microscopy: a key for the comprehension of amiodarone-induced thyroid diseases. Endocrinology 127:1502–1509
Broekhuysen J, Laruel R, Sion R (1969) Recherches dans la série des benzofurannes. XXXVII. Étude comparée du transit et du métabolisme de l'amiodarone chez diverses espèces animales et chez l'homme. Arch Int Pharmacodyn 177:340–359
Brousolle C, Ducottet X, Martin C, Barbier Y, Bornet H, Noel G, Orgiazzi J (1989) Rapid effectiveness of prednisone and thionamides combined therapy in severe amiodarone iodine-induced thyrotoxicosis. Comparison of two groups of patients with apparently normal thyroid glands. J Endocrinol Invest 12:37–42
Burger A, Dinichert D, Nicod P, Jenny M, Lemarchand-Béraud T, Vallotton MB (1976) Effect of amiodarone on serum triiodothyronine, reverse triiodothyronine, thyroxin, and thyrotropin. J Clin Invest 58:255–259
Cauchie P, Decaux G, Unger J (1988) Treatment of atrial fibrillation associated with hyperthyroidism by amiodarone and methimazole. Int J Cardiol 19:123–124
Ceppi JA, Zaninovich AA (1989) Effects of amiodarone on 5′-deiodination of thyroxine and triiodothyronine in rat myocardium. J Endocrinol 121:431–434
Chalmers DK, Munro SLA, Iskander MN, Craik DJ (1992) Models for the binding of amiodarone to the thyroid hormone receptor. J Comput Aided Mol Design 6:19–31
Chang HY, Kunos G (1981) Short term effects of triiodothyronine on rat heart adrenoceptors. Biochem Biophys Res Commun 100:313–320
Chatelaine P, Laruel R, Gillard M (1985) Effect of amiodarone on membrane fluidity and Na^+/K^+ ATPase activity in rat brain synaptic membranes. Biochem Biophys Res Commun 129:148–154
Chess-Williams R, Coker SJ (1989) Ventricular fibrillation is reduced in hypothyroid rats with enhanced myocardial alpha-adrenoceptors responsiveness. Br J Pharmacol 98:95–100
Chevigné-Brancart M, Vandalem JL, Hennen F (1983) Étude prospective de l'incidence des dysthyroidies survenant chez des patients traites par amiodarone. Rev Med Liege 38:269–275
Chiovato L, Martino E, Tonacchera M, Santini F, Lapi P, Mammoli C, Braverman LE, Pinchera A (1994) Studies on the in vitro cytotoxic effect of amiodarone. Endocrinology 134:2277–2282
Cody V, Luft J (1989) Structure-activity relationships of antiarrhythmic agents: crystal structure of amiodarone hydrochloride and two derivatives, and their conformational comparison with thyroxine. Acta Cryst 45B:172–178
Davies PH, Franklyn JA, Sheppard MC (1992) Treatment of amiodarone induced thyrotoxicosis with carbimazole alone and continuation of amiodarone. Br Med J 305:224–225

de Catte L, de Wolf D, Smitz J, Bougatef A, de Schepper J, Foulon W (1994) Fetal hypothyroidism as a complication of amiodarone treatment for persistent fetal supraventricular tachycardia. Prenat Diagn 14:762–765

de Jong M, Docter R, van der Hoek H, Krenning E, van der Heide D, Quero C, Plaisier P, Vos R, Hennemann G (1994) Different effects of amiodarone on transport of T_4 and T_3 into the perfused rat liver. Am J Physiol 266 (Endcrinol Metab 29):E44–E49

de Rosa G, Testa A, Valenza O, Maussier ML, Cecchini L, Calla C, Troucone L (1989) Thyroid toxicity during amiodarone therapy. Eur J Int Med 1:29–35

de Weweire A, Unger Ph, Delwicke F, Unger J (1987) Failure to control hyperthyroidism with a thionamide after $KClO_4$ withdrawal in a patient with amiodarone associated thyrotoxicosis. J Endocrinol Invest 10:529

de Wolf D, de Schepper J, Verhaaren H, Deneyer M, Smitz J, Sacre-Smits L (1988) Congenital hypothyroid goiter and amiodarone. Acta Paediatr Scand 77:616–618

Disatnik MH, Shainberg A (1991) Regulation of beta-adrenoceptors by thyroid hormone and amiodarone in rat myocardiac cells in culture. Biochem Pharmacol 40:1043–1048

Doval HC, Nuh DR, Grancelli HO, Perrone SV, Bortman GR, Curiel R (1994) Randomised trial of low-dose amiodarone in severe congestive heart failure. Lancet 344:493–498

Drvota V, Carlsson B, Häggblad J, Sylven C (1995a) Amiodarone is a dose-dependent noncompetitive and competitive inhibitor of T_3 binding to thyroid hormone receptor subtype β_1, whereas disopyramide, lignocaine, propafenone, metoprolol, dl-sotalol and verapamil have no inhibitory effect. J Cardiovasc Pharmacol 26: 222–226

Drvota V, Brönnegard M, Hägblad J, Barkhem T, Sylven C (1995b) Downregulation of thyroid hormone receptor subtype mRNA levels by amiodarone during catecholamine stress in vitro. Biochem Biophys Res Commun 211:991–996

Eason RJ, Croxson MS, Lim TMT, Evans MC (1984) Goitre and thyroid dysfunction during chronic amiodarone treatment. N Z Med J 97:216–219

Farwell AP, Abend SL, Huang SKS, Patwardhan NA, Braverman LE (1990) Thyroidectomy for amiodarone induced thyrotoxicosis. JAMA 263:1526–1528

Ferreira J, Chatelaine P, Caspers J, Ruysschaert JM (1987) Ionization state of amiodarone mediates its mode of interaction with lipid bilayers. Biochem Pharmacol 36:4245–4250

Figge J, Dluhy RG (1990) Amiodarone-induced elevation of thyroid stimulating hormone in patients receiving levothyroxine for primary hypothyroidism. Ann Intern Med 113:553–555

Flanagan RJ, Storey GCA, Holt DW, Farmer PB (1982) Identification and measurement of desethylamiodarone in blood plasma specimens from amiodarone-treated patients. J Pharm Pharmacol 34:638–643

Foresti V, Parisio E, Scolari N, Carini L, Lovagnini-Scher CA (1985) Amiodarone and antithyroid antibodies. Ann Intern Med 103:157–158

Foresti V, Pepe R, Parisio E, Scolari N, Zubani R, Bianco M (1989) Antithyroid antibodies during amiodarone treatment. Acta Endocrinol (Copenh) 121:203–206

Foster CJ, Love HG (1988) Amiodarone in pregnancy. Case report and review of the literature. Int J Cardiol 20:307–316

Fradkin JE, Wolff J (1983) Iodide-induced thyrotoxicosis. Medicine (Baltimore) 62:1–20

Fragu P, Schlumberger M, Davy JM, Slama M, Berdeaux A (1988) Effects of amiodarone therapy on thyroid iodine content as measured by X-ray fluorescence. J Clin Endocrinol Metab 66:762–769

Franklyn JA, Davis JR, Gammage MD, Littler WA, Ramsden DB, Sheppard MC (1985) Amiodarone and thyroid hormone function. Clin Endocrinol (Oxf) 22:257–264

Franklyn JA, Gammage MD, Sheppard MC (1987) Amiodarone and thyroid hormone effects on anterior pituitary gene expression. Clin Endocrinol (Oxf) 27:373–382

Franklyn JA, Green NK, Gammage MD, Ahlquist JAO, Sheppard MC (1989) Regulation of α- and β-myosin heavy chain messenger RNAs in the rat myocardium by amiodarone and by thyroid status. Clin Sci 76:463–467

Freedberg AS, Papp JG, Vaughan Williams EM (1970) The effect of altered thyroid state on atrial intracellular potentials. J Physiol 207:357–370

Gavrilescu S, Luca C, Lungu G, Deutsch G (1976) Monophasic action potentials of right atrium and the electrophysiologic properties of AV conducting system with hypothyroidism. Br Heart J 38:1350–1354

Gembruch U, Manz M, Bald R, Rüddel H, Redel DA, Schlebusch H, Nitsch J, Hansman M (1989) Repeated intravascular treatment with amiodarone in a fetus with refractory supraventricular tachycardia and hydrops fetalis. Am Heart J 118:1335–1338

Georges JL, Normand JP, Lenormand ME, Schwob J (1992) Life-threatening thyrotoxicosis induced by amiodarone in patients with benign heart disease. Eur Heart J 13:129–132

Gluzman BE, Coleoni AH, Targovnik HM, Niepomniszcze H (1977) Effects of amiodarone on thyroid iodine metabolism in vitro. Acta Endocrinol (Copenh) 85:781–790

Goldfine ID, Maddux B, Woeber KA (1982) Effects of amiodarone on L-triiodothyronine stimulation of [^{3}H]thymidine incorporation into GH_3 cells. J Endocrinol Invest 5:165–168

Gottlieb S, Sonnenblick M (1989) Effect of amiodarone on blood lipids. Am J Cardiol 63:1540

Gøtzsche LBH (1993) β-Adrenergic receptors, voltage-operated Ca^{2+} channels, nuclear triiodothyronine receptors and triiodothyronine concentration in pig myocardium after long-term low-dose amiodarone treatment. Acta Endocrinol (Copenh) 129:337–347

Gøtzsche LBH (1994) Acute increase in cardiac performance after triiodothyronine: blunted response in amiodarone-treated pigs. J Cardiovasc Pharmacol 23:141–148

Gøtzsche LBH, Orskov H (1994) Cardiac triiodothyronine nuclear receptor binding capacities in amiodarone treated, hypo- and hyperthyroid rats. Eur J Endocrinol 130:281–290

Gøtzsche LSBH, Boye N, Laurberg P, Andreasen F (1989) Rat heart thyroxine 5′-deiodinase is sensitively depressed by amiodarone. J Cardiovasc Pharmacol 14:836–841

Gudbjörnsson B, Kristinsson A, Geirsson G, Hreidarsson AB (1987) Painful autoimmune thyroiditis occurring on amiodarone therapy. Acta Med Scand 221:219–220

Harris L, Hind C, McKenna W, Savage C, Krikler S, Storey G, Holt D (1983) Renal elimination of amiodarone and its desethyl metabolite. Postgrad Med J 59:440–442

Hartong R, Wiersinga WM, Lamers WH, Plomp TA, Broenink M, van Beeren MH (1987) Effects of amiodarone on thyroid hormone responsive gene expression in rat liver. Horm Metab Res [Suppl] 17:34–43

Hartong R, Wiersinga WM, Plomp TA (1990) Amiodarone reduces the effect of T_3 on beta-adrenergic receptor density in rat heart. Horm Metab Res 22:85–89

Hauptman PJ, Mechanick J, Lansman S, Gass A (1993) Fatal hyperthyroidism after amiodarone treatment and total lymphoid irradiation in a heart transplant recipient. J Heart Lung Transplant 12:513–516

Hawthorne GC, Campbell NPS, Geddes JS, Ferguson WR, Postlethwaite W, Sheridan B, Atkinson AB (1985) Amiodarone-induced hypothyroidism. A common complication of prolonged therapy: a report of eight cases. Arch Intern Med 145:1016–1019

Hershman JM, Nademanee K, Sugawara M, Pekary AE, Ross R, Singh BN, DiStefano JG III (1986) Thyroxine and triiodothyronine kinetics in cardiac patients taking amiodarone. Acta Endocrinol (Copenh) 111:193–199

Hijazi ZM, Rosenfeld LE, Copel JA, Kleinman CS (1992) Amiodarone therapy of intractable atrial flutter in a premature hydropic neonate. Pediatr Cardiol 13:227–229

Hill DA, Reasor MJ (1991) Effects of amiodarone administration during pregnancy in Fisher 344 rats. Toxicology 65:259–269

Holt DW, Tucker GT, Jackson PR, Storey GCA (1983) Amiodarone pharmacokinetics. Am Heart J 106:843–847

Honegger UE, Zuehlke RD, Scuntaro S, Schaefer MHA, Toplak H, Wiesman UN (1993) Cellular accumulation of amiodarone and desethylamiodarone in cultured human cells. Biochem Pharmacol 45:349–356

Hudig F, Bakker O, Wiersinga WM (1994) Amiodarone-induced hypercholesterolemia is associated with a decrease in liver LDL receptor mRNA. FEBS Lett 341:86–90

Hudig F, Bakker O, Wiersinga WM (1997) Triiodothyronine prevents the amiodarone-induced decrease in the expression of liver low density lipoprotein receptor gene. Endocrinol 152:413–421

Jandreski MA, Vanderslice WE (1993) Clinical measurement of serum amiodarone and desethylamiodarone by using solid-phase extraction followed by HPLC with a high-carbon reversed-phase column. Clin Chem 39:496–500

Johnson PN, Freedberg AS, Marshall JM (1973) Action of thyroid hormone on the transmembrane potentials from sinoatrial node cells and atrial muscle cells in isolated atra of rabbits. Cardiology 58:273–289

Jonckheer MH (1981) Amiodarone and the thyroid gland. A review. Acta Cardiol 36:199–205

Jonckheer MH, Blockx P, Kaivers R, Wijffels G (1973) Hyperthyroidism as a possible complication of the treatment of ischemic heart disease with amiodarone. Acta Cardiol Belg 28:192–200

Jonckheer MH, Blockx P, Broeckaert I, Cornette C, Beckers C (1978) "Low T_3 syndrome" in patients chronically treated with an iodine-containing drug, amiodarone. Clin Endocrinol (Oxf) 9:27–35

Jonckheer MH, Velkeniers B, Vanhaelst L, van Bleck M (1992) Further characterization of iodide-induced hyperthyroidism based on the direct measurement of intrathyroidal iodine stores. Nucl Med Commun 13:114–118

Kannan R, Pollak A, Singh BN (1982) Elevation of serum lipids after chronic administration of amiodarone in rabbits. Atherosclerosis 44:19–26

Kannan R, Ookhtens M, Chopra IJ, Singh BN (1984) Effects of chronic administration of amiodarone on kinetics of metabolism of iodothyronines. Endocrinology 115:1710–1716

Kannan R, Chopra IJ, Ookhtens M, Singh BN (1990) Effect of amiodarone on non-deiodinative pathway of thyroid hormone metabolism. Acta Endocrinol 122:249–245

Kaplan J, Ish-Shalom S (1991) Goiter and hypothyroidism during re-treatment with amiodarone in a patient who previously experienced amiodarone-induced thyrotoxicosis. Am J Med 90:750–752

Kaptein EM, Egodage PM, Hoopes MT, Burger AG (1988) Amiodarone alters thyroxine transfer and distribution in humans. Metabolism 37:1107–1113

Kasim SE, Bagchi N, Brown TR, Khilnani S (1987) Effect of amiodarone on serum lipids, lipoprotein lipase, and hepatic triglyceride lipase. Endocrinology 120:1991–1995

Kasim SE, Bagchi N, Brown TR, Khilnani S, Jackson K, Steinman RT, Lehmann MH (1990) Amiodarone-induced changes in lipid metabolism. Horm Metab Res 22:385–388

Kerin NZ, Blevins RD, Benaderet D, Faitel K, Jarandilla R, Garfinkel C, Klein S, Rubenfire M (1986) Relation of serum reverse T_3 to amiodarone antiarrhythmic efficacy and toxicity. Am J Cardiol 57:128–130

Krenning EP, Docter R, Bernard B, Visser T, Hennemann G (1982) Decreased transport of thyroxine (T_4), 3,3′,5-triiodothyronine (T_3) and 3,3′,5′-triiodothyronine

(rT_3) into rat hepatocytes in primary culture due to a decrease of cellular ATP content and various drugs. FEBS Lett 140:229–233

Lalloz MRA, Byfield PGH, Greenwood RM, Himsworth RL (1984) Binding of amiodarone by serum proteins and the effects of drugs, hormones and other interacting ligands. J Pharm Pharmacol 36:366–372

Lambert MJ, Burger AG, Galeazzi RL, Engler D (1982) Are selective increases in serum thyroxine (T_4) due to iodinated inhibitors of T_4 monodeiodination indicative of hyperthyroidism? J Clin Endocrinol Metab 55:1058–1065

Lambert C, Vermeulen M, Cardinal R, Lamontagne D, Nadeau R (1987) Lack of relation between the ventricular refractory period prolongation by amiodarone and the thyroid state in rats. J Pharmacol Exp Ther 242:320–325

Lambert M, Burger AG, DeNayer P, Beckers C (1988) Decreased TSH response to TRH induced by amiodarone. Acta Endocrinol (Copenh) 118:449–452

Lambert M, Unger J, DeNayer P, Broket C, Gangji D (1990) Amiodarone-induced thyrotoxicosis suggestive of thyroid damage. J Endocrinol Invest 13:527–530

Latham KR, Sellitti DF, Goldstein RE (1987) Interaction of amiodarone and desethylamiodarone with solubilized nuclear thyroid hormone receptors. J Am Coll Cardiol 9:872–876

Latini R, Tognoni G, Kates RE (1984) Clinical pharmacokinetics of amiodarone. Clin Pharmacokinet 9:136–156

Laurent M, Betremieux P, Biron Y, Lellelloco A (1987) Neonatal hypothyroidism after treatment by amiodarone during pregnancy. Am J Cardiol 60:142

Laurberg P (1988) Amiodarone inhibits T_4 and T_3 secretion but does not affect T_4 deiodination to T_3 in perfused dog thyroid lobes. Thyroidology 1:1–4

Léger AF, Fragu P, Rougier P, Laurent MF, Tubiana M, Savoie JC (1983) Thyroid iodine content measured by X-ray fluorescence in amiodarone-induced thyrotoxicosis: concise communication. J Nucl Med 24:582–585

Leung WH, Pun KK, Lau CP, Wong CK, Wang C (1989) Amiodarone-induced thyroiditis. Am Heart J 118:848–849

Lindenmeyer M, Spörri S, Stäubli M, Studer A, Studer H (1984) Does amiodarone affect heart rate by inhibiting the intracellular generation of triiodothyronine from thyroxine? Br J Pharmacol 82:275–280

Ling MCC, Dake MD, Okerlund MD (1988) Gallium uptake in the thyroid gland in amiodarone-induced hyperthyroidism. Clin Nucl Med 13:258–259

Machado HB, da Silca MEP, Pincho B (1992) Long-term amiodarone therapy and antithyroid antibodies. Am J Cardiol 69:971–972

Magee LA, Downar E, Sermer M, Boulton BC, Allen LC, Koren G (1995) Pregnancy outcome after gestational exposure to amiodarone in Canada. Am J Obstet Gynecol 172:1307–1311

Mahmarian JJ, Smart FW, Moyé LA, Young JB, Francis MJ, Kingry CL, Verani MS, Pratt CM (1994) Exploring the minimal dose of amiodarone with antiarrhythmic and hemodynamic activity. Am J Cardiol 74:681–686

Mancini A, Marinis L de, Calabro F, Sciuto R, Oradei A, Lippa S, Sandric S, Littarru GP, Barbarino A (1989) Evaluation of metabolic status in amiodarone-induced thyroid disorders: plasma coenzyme Q10 determination. J Endocrinol Invest 12: 511–516

Many MC, Mesthdagh C, van den Hove MF, Denef JF (1992) In vitro study of acute toxic effects of high iodide doses in human thyroid follicles. Endocrinology 131: 621–630

Martino E, Safran M, Aghini-Lombardi F et al (1984) Environmental iodine intake and thyroid dysfunction during chronic amiodarone therapy. Ann Intern Med 101:28–34

Martino E, Aghini-Lombardi F, Lippi F, Baschieri L, Safran M, Braverman LE, Pinchera A (1985) Twenty-four hour radioactive iodine uptake in 35 patients with amiodarone associated thyrotoxicosis. J Nucl Med 26:1402–1407

Martino E, Marchia E, Aghini-Lombardi F, Antonelli A, Lenziardi M, Concetti R, Fenzi GF, Baschieri L, Pinchera A (1986a) Is humoral thyroid autoimmunity relevant in amiodarone-induced thyrotoxicosis? Clin Endocrinol (Oxf) 24:627–633
Martino E, Mariotti S, Aghini-Lombardi F, Lenziardi M, Morabito S, Baschieri L, Pinchera A, Braverman L, Safran M (1986b) Short term administration of potassium perchlorate restores euthyroidism in amiodarone iodine-induced hypothyroidism. J Clin Endocrinol Metab 63:1233–1236
Martino E, Aghini-Lombardi F, Mariotti S, Lenziardi M, Baschieri L, Braverman LE, Pinchera A (1986c) Treatment of amiodarone associated thyrotoxicosis by simultaneous administration of potassium perchlorate and methimazole. J Endocrinol Invest 9:201–207
Martino E, Aghini-Lombardi F, Mariotti S, Bartalena L, Lenziardi M, Ceccarelli C, Bambini G, Sofran M, Braverman LE, Pinchera A (1987) Amiodarone iodine-induced hypothyroidism: risk factors and follow-up in 28 cases. Clin Endocrinol (Oxf) 26:227–237
Martino E, Bartalena L, Mariotti S, Aghini-Lombardi F, Ceccarelli C, Lippi F, Piga M, Loviselli A, Braverman LE, Safran M, Pinchera A (1988) Radioactive iodine thyroid uptake in patients with amiodarone-iodine-induced thyroid dysfunction. Acta Endocrinol (Copenh) 119:167–173
Martino E, Aghini-Lombardi F, Bartalena L, Grasso L, Loviselli A, Velluzzi F, Pinchera A, Braverman LE (1994) Enhanced susceptibility to amiodarone-induced hypothyroidism in patients with thyroid autoimmune disease. Arch Intern Med 154:2722–2726
Mason JW (1987) Amiodarone. N Engl J Med 316:455–466
Massart C, Hody B, Condé D, Leclech G, Nicol M (1989) Effect of amiodarone and propranolol on the functional properties of human thyroid follicles cultured in collagen gel. Mol Cell Endocrinol 62:113–117
Matsumura LK, Born D, Kunii IS, Franco DB, Maciel RMB (1992) Outcome of thyroid function in newborns from mothers treated with amiodarone. Thyroid 2:279–281
Mazonson PD, Williams ML, Cantley LK, Daldorf FG, Utiger RD, Foster JR (1984) Myxedema coma during long-term amiodarone therapy. Am J Med 77:751–754
McKenna WJ, Harris L, Rowland E, Whitelaw A, Storey G, Holt D (1983) Amiodarone therapy during pregnancy. Am J Cardiol 51:1231–1233
Meese R, Smitherman TC, Croft CH, Burger AH, Nicod P (1985) Effect of peripheral thyroid hormone metabolism on cardiac arrhythmias. Am Heart J 55:849–851
Mehra A, Widerhorn J, Lopresti J, Rahimtoola S (1991) Amiodarone-induced hyperthyroidism: thyroidectomy under local anesthesia. Am Heart J 122:1160–1161
Melmed S, Nademanee K, Reed AW, Hendrickson JA, Singh BN, Hershman JM (1981) Hyperthyroxinemia with bradycardia and normal thyrotropin secretion after chronic amiodarone administration. J Clin Endocrinol Metab 53:997–1001
Meurisse M, Hamoir E, D'Silva M, Joris J, Hennen G (1993) Amiodarone-induced thyrotoxicosis: is there a place for surgery? World J Surg 17:622–627
Meyer BJ, Amann FW (1993) Additional antianginal efficacy of amiodarone in patients with limiting angina pectoris. Am Heart J 125:996–1001
Miaskiewicz SL, Amico JA, Follansbee WP, Levey GS (1987) Amiodarone-associated thyrotoxicosis masquerading as painful thyroiditis. Ann Intern Med 107:118–119
Middlekauff HR, Wiener I, Saxon LA, Stevenson WG (1992) Low-dose amiodarone for atrial fibrillation: time for a prospective study? Ann Intern Med 116:1017–1020
Minelli R, Gardini E, Bianconi L, Salvi M, Roti M (1992) Subclinical hypothyroidism, overt thyrotoxicosis and subclinical hypothyroidism: the subsequent phases of thyroid function in a patient chronically treated with amiodarone. J Endocrinol Invest 15:853–855

Monteiro E, Galvao-Teles A, Santos ML, Mourao L, Correia MJ, Lopo Tuna J, Ribeiro C (1986) Antithyroid antibodies as an early marker for thyroid disease induced by amiodarone. Br Med J 292:227–228

Mulligan DC, McHenry CR, Kinney W, Esselstyn CB (1993) Amiodarone-induced thyrotoxicosis: clinical presentation and expanded indications for thyroidectomy. Surgery 114:1114–1119

Nademanee K, Singh BN, Hendrickson J, Reed AW, Melmed S, Hershaw TM (1982) Pharmacokinetic significance of serum rT_3 levels during amiodarone treatment: a potential method for monitoring chronic drug therapy. Circulation 66:202–211

Nademanee K, Singh BN, Hendrickson JA, Hershman JM (1986) Amiodarone, thyroid hormone indexes, and altered thyroid function: long-term serial effects in patients with cardiac arrhythmias. Am J Cardiol 58:981–986

Nattel S, Davies M, Quantz M (1988) The antiarrhythmic efficacy of amiodarone and desethylamiodarone, alone and in combination, in dogs with acute myocardial infarction. Circulation 77:200–208

Newnham HH, Chosick N, Topliss DJ, Harper RW, Le Grand BA, Stockigt JR (1987) Amiodarone-induced hyperthyroidism: assessment of the predictive value of biochemical testing and response to combined therapy using propylthiouracil and potassium perchlorate. Aust N Z J Med 18:37–44

Nicholsen AA, Caplin JL, Steventon DM (1994) Measurement of tissue-bound amiodarone and its metabolites by computed tomography. Clin Radiol 49:14–18

Nielsen CE, Andreasen F, Bjerregaard P (1983) Amiodarone induced cornea verticillata. Acta Ophthalmol (Copenh) 61:474–480

Nokin P, Clinet M, Schoenfeld P (1983) Cardiac β-adrenoceptor modulation by amiodarone. Biochem Pharmacol 32:2473–2477

Nokin P, Clinet M, Swillens S, Deliseé C, Meysmans L, Chatelain P (1986) Allosteric modulation of [^{3}H]nitrendipine binding to cardiac and cerebral cortex membranes by amiodarone. J Cardiovasc Pharmacol 8:1051–1057

Norman MF, Lavin TN (1989) Antagonism of thyroid hormone action by amiodarone in rat pituitary tumor cells. J Clin Invest 83:306–313

Paradis P, Lambert C, Rouleau J (1991) Amiodarone antagonizes the effects of T_3 at the receptor level: an additional mechanism for its in vivo hypothyroid-like effects. Can J Physiol Pharmacol 69:865–870

Pasquali D, Tseng FY, Rani CSS, Field JB (1990) Inhibition of intermediary metabolism by amiodarone in dog thyroid slices. Am J Physiol 259 (Endocrinol Metab 22):E529–E533

Patterson E, Walden KM, Khazaeli MB, Montgomery DG, Lucchesi BR (1986) Cardiac electrophysiologic effects of acute and chronic amiodarone administration in the isolated perfused rabbit heart: altered thyroid hormone metabolism. J Pharmacol Exp Ther 239:179–184

Pearce CJ, Himsworth RL (1986) The effect of amiodarone on thyroxine kinetics. Clin Endocrinol (Oxf) 24:107–112

Peche R, Abramowicz M, Unger J (1992) Failure to respond to dexamethasone with fatal consequences, after initial response to multidrug treatment in a case of amiodarone-associated thyrotoxicosis. Am J Med 93:702–703

Pekary AE, Hershman JM, Reed AW, Kannan R, Wang YS (1986) Amiodarone inhibits T_4 to T_3 conversion and α-glycerophosphate dehydrogenase and malic enzyme levels in rat liver. Horm Metab Res 18:114–118

Penn IM, Barrett PA, Pannikote V, Barnaby PF, Campbell IB, Lyons NR (1985) Amiodarone in pregnancy. Am J Cardiol 56:196–197

Perret G, Yin YL, Nicolas P, Pussard E, Vassy R, Uzzan B, Berdeaux A (1992) Amiodarone decreases cardiac β-adrenoceptors through an antagonistic effect on 3,5,3′-triiodothyronine. J Cardiovasc Pharmacol 19:473–478

Pichler WJ, Schindler L, Stäubli M, Stadler BM, de Weck AL (1988) Anti-amiodarone antibodies: detection and relationship to the development of side effects. Am J Med 85:197–202

Pitcher D, Leather HM, Storey GCA, Holt DW (1983) Amiodarone in pregnancy. Lancet i:597–598

Plomp TA, van Rossum JM, Robles de Medina EO, van Lier T, Maes RAA (1984) Pharmacokinetics and body distribution of amiodarone in man. Arzneimittelforschung/Drug Res 34:513–520

Plomp TA, Vulsma T, Vijlder JJM de (1992) Use of amiodarone during pregnancy. Eur J Obstet Gynecol Reprod Biol 43:201–207

Podrid PJ (1995) Amiodarone: reevaluation of an old drug. Ann Intern Med 122:689–700

Polikar R, Goy JJ, Schlapfer J, Lemarchand-Béraud T, Biollaz J, Magnenat P, Nicod P (1986) Effect of oral triiodothyronine during amiodarone treatment for ventricular premature complexes. Am J Cardiol 59:987–991

Pollak PT, Sharma AD, Carruthers SG (1988) Elevation of serum cholesterol and triglyceride levels during amiodarone therapy. Am J Cardiol 62:562–565

Pollak PT, Sharma AD, Carruthers SG (1989) Correlation of amiodarone dosage, heart rate, QT interval and corneal microdeposits with serum amiodarone and desethylamiodarone concentrations. Am J Cardiol 64:1138–1143

Pritchard DA, Singh BN, Hurley PJ (1975) Effects of amiodarone on thyroid function in patients with ischemic heart disease. Br Heart J 37:856–860

Rabinowe SL, Larsen PR, Antman EM, George KL, Friedman PL, Jackson RA, Eisenbarth GS (1986) Amiodarone therapy and autoimmune thyroid disease. Increase in a new monoclonal antibody-defined T cell subset. Am J Med 81:53–57

Raeder EA, Podrid PJ, Lown B (1985) Side effects and complications of amiodarone therapy. Am Heart J 109:975–983

Rajatanavin R, Chaiburkit LO, Kongsuksai A, Teeravaniathorn U, Himathongkam T (1990) The effect of amiodarone on the control of hyperthyroidism by propylthiouracil. Clin Endocrinol (Oxf) 33:193–203

Rani CSS (1990) Amiodarone effects on thyrotropin receptors and responses stimulated by thyrotropin and carbachol in cultured dog thyroid cells. Endocrinology 127:2930–2937

Rao RH, McReady VR, Spathis GS (1986) Iodine kinetic studies during amiodarone treatment. J Clin Endocrinol Metab 62:563–567

Reichert LJM, de Rooy HAM (1989) Treatment of amiodarone induced hyperthyroidism with potassium perchlorate and methimazole during amiodarone treatment. Br Med J 298:1547–1548

Rey E, Duperron L, Gautheir R, Lemsy M, Grignon A, Le Lorier J (1985) Transplacental treatment of tachycardia-induced fetal heart failure with verapamil and amiodarone. Am J Obstet Gynecol 153:311–312

Rey E, Bachrach LK, Buttow GN (1987) Effects of amiodarone during pregnancy. Can Med Assoc J 136:959–960

Robson DJ, Jeeva Raj MV, Storey GCA, Holt DW (1985) Use of amiodarone during pregnancy. Postgrad Med J 61:75–77

Roti E, Minelli R, Gardini E, Bianconi L, Gavaruzzi A, Ugolotti G, Neri TM, Braverman LE (1992) Iodine-induced subclinical hypothyroidism in euthyroid subjects with a previous episode of amiodarone-induced thyrotoxicosis. J Clin Endocrinol Metab 75:1273–1277

Roti E, Minelli R, Gardini E, Bianconi L, Braverman LE (1993) Thyrotoxicosis followed by hypothyroidism in patients treated with amiodarone. A possible consequence of a destructive process in the thyroid. Arch Intern Med 153:886–892

Roti E, Bianconi L, De Chiara F, Minelli R, Tosi C, Gardini E, Salvi M, Braverman LE (1994) Thyroid ultrasonography in patients with a previous episode of amiodarone induced thyrotoxicosis. J Endocrinol Invest 17:259–262

Roussel JP, Grazzini E, Guipponi M, Astier H (1995) Dihydropyridine-like effects of amiodarone and desethylamiodarone on thyrotropin secretion and intracellular calcium concentration in rat pituitary. Eur J Endocrinol 133:489–498

Rovetto MJ, Jalmarson AC, Morgan HE (1972) Hormonal control of cardiac myosin adenosine triphosphatase in the rat. Circ Res 31:397–409
Safran M, Fang SL, Bambini G, Pinchera A, Martino E, Braverman LE (1986) Effects of amiodarone and desethylamiodarone on pituitary deiodinase activity and thyrotropin secretion in the rat. Am J Med Sci 292:136–141
Safran M, Martino E, Aghini-Lombardi F, Bartalena L, Balzano S, Pinchera A, Braverman LE (1988) Effect of amiodarone on circulating antithyroid antibodies. Br Med J 297:456–457
Salamon E, Rowe RC, Faiman C (1989) Amiodarone-related cyclic thyroid dysfunction. Can Med Assoc J 141:1247–1249
Sanmarti A, Permanyer-Miralda G, Castellanos JM, Foz-Sala M, Galard RM, Soler-Soler I (1984) Chronic administration of amiodarone and thyroid function: a follow-up study. Am Heart J 108:1262–1268
Schröder-van der Elst JP, van der Heide D (1990) Thyroxine, 3,5,3′-triiodothyronine, and 3,3′,5′-triiodothyronine concentrations in several tissues of the rat: effects of amiodarone and desethylamiodarone on thyroid hormone metabolism. Endocrinology 127:1656–1664
Sharp NA, Neel DS, Parson PL (1985) Influence of thyroid hormone levels on the electrical and mechanical properties of rabbit papillary muscles. J Mol Cell Cardiol 17:119–132
Sheldon J (1983) Effects of amiodarone in thyrotoxicosis. Br Med J 286:267–277
Shukla R, Jowett NI, Thompson DR, Pohl JEF (1994) Side effects with amiodarone therapy. Postgrad Med J 70:492–498
Silva JE, Leonard JL (1985) Regulation of rat cerebrocortical and adenohypophyseal type II 5′-deiodinase by thyroxine, triiodothyronine, and reverse triiodothyronine. Endocrinology 116:1627–1635
Simon C, Schlienger JL, Cherfan J, Roul G, Vignon F, Chabrier G, Imler M (1984) Efficacité de la dexaméthasone dans le traitement de l'hyperthyroïdie à l'amiodarone. Presse Med 13:2767
Singh BN (1983) Amiodarone: historical development and pharmacologic profile. Am Heart J 106:788–797
Singh BN, Nademanee (1983) Amiodarone and thyroid function: clinical implications during antiarrhythmic therapy. Am Heart J 106:857–869
Singh BN, Vaughan Williams EM (1970) The effect of amiodarone, a new anti-anginal drug, on cardiac muscle. Br J Pharmacol 39:657–667
Singh SN, Fletcher RD, Fisher SG, Singh BN, Lewis HD, Deedwania PC, Massie BM, Colling C, Lazzeri D (1995) Amiodarone in patients with congestive heart failure and asymptomatic ventricular arrhythmia. N Engl J Med 333:77–82
Smyrk TC, Goellner JR, Brennan MD, Carney JA (1987) Pathology of the thyroid in amiodarone-associated thyrotoxicosis. Am J Surg Pathol 11:197–204
Sogol PB, Hershman JM, Reed AW, Dillmann WH (1983) The effects of amiodarone on serum thyroid hormones and hepatic thyroxine 5′-monodeiodination in rats. Endocrinology 113:1464–1469
Somani P (1989) Basic and clinical pharmacology of amiodarone: relationship of antiarrhythmic effects, dose and drug concentrations to intracellular inclusion bodies. J Clin Pharmacol 29:405–412
Sonnenblick M, Gottlieb S, Goldstein R, Abraham AS (1986) Effect of amiodarone on blood lipids. Cardiology 73:147–150
Stäubli M, Studer H (1985) Amiodarone-treated patients with suppressed TSH test are at risk of thyrotoxicosis. Klin Wochenschr 63:168–175
Stäubli M, Studer H (1986) The effects of amiodarone on the electrocardiogram of the guinea-pig are not explained by interaction with thyroid hormone metabolism alone. Br J Pharmacol 88:405–410
Stäubli M, Bircher J, Galeazzi RL, Remund H, Studer H (1983) Serum concentrations of amiodarone during long-term therapy. Relation to dose, efficacy and toxicity. Eur J Clin Pharmacol 24:485–494

Stewart JR, Westveer DC, van Dam D, Gordon S, Timmis GC (1984) The relationship of serum amiodarone and reverse T_3 levels to drug efficacy and side effects. J Am Coll Cardiol 3:606

Strunge P, Frandsen J, Andreasen F (1988) Amiodarone during pregnancy. Eur Heart J 9:106–109

Trip MD, Wiersinga WM, Plomp TA (1991) Incidence, predictability, and pathogenesis of amiodarone-induced thyrotoxicosis and hypothyroidism. Am J Med 91: 507–511

Trip MD, Düren DR, Wiersinga WM (1994) Two cases of amiodarone-induced thyrotoxicosis successfully treated with a short course of antithyroid drugs while amiodarone was continued. Br Heart J 72:266–268

Unger J (1988) Serum thyroglobulin concentration may be a clue to the mechanism of amiodarone-induced thyrotoxicosis. J Endocrinol Invest 11:684

Uzzan B, Pussard E, Leon A et al (1991) The effects of plasmapheresis on thyroid hormone and plasma drug concentrations in amiodarone-induced thyrotoxicosis. Br J Clin Pharmacol 31:371–372

Valensise H, Civitella C, Garzetti GG, Romanini C (1992) Amiodarone treatment in pregnancy for dilatative cardiomyopathy with ventricular malignant extrasystole and normal maternal and neonatal outcome. Prenat Diagn 12:705–708

van Beeren HC, Bakker O, Wiersinga WM (1995) Desethylamiodarone is a competitive inhibitor of the binding of thyroid hormone to the thyroid hormone α_1-receptor protein. Mol Cell Endocrinol 112:15–19

van Beeren HC, Bakker O, Wiersinga WM (1996) Structure-function relationship of the inhibition of the T_3 binding to α_1- and β_1-thyroid hormone receptor by amiodarone analogues. Endocrinology 137:2007–2814

van Dam EWCM, Prummel MF, Wiersinga WM, Nikkels RE (1993) Treatment of amiodarone-induced hypothyroidism with potassium perchlorate. Neth J Med 42:21–24

van Reeth O, Unger J (1991) Effects of amiodarone on serum T_3 and T_4 concentrations in hyperthyroid patients treated with propylthiouracil. Thyroid 1:301–306

van Reeth O, Decoster C, Unger J (1987) Effect of amiodarone on serum T_4 and T_3 levels in hyperthyroid patients treated with methimazole. Eur J Clin Pharmacol 32:223–227

Venkatesh N, Padburg JF, Singh BN (1986a) Effects of amiodarone and desethylamiodarone on rabbit myocardial beta-adrenoreceptors and serum thyroid hormones – absence of relationship to serum and myocardial drug concentrations. J Cardiovasc Pharmacol 8:989–997

Venkatesh N, Al-Sarraf L, Hershman JM, Singh BN (1986b) Effects of desethylamiodarone on thyroid hormone metabolism in rats. Comparison with the effects of amiodarone. Proc Soc Exp Biol Med 181:233–236

Venkatesh N, Lynch JJ, Uprichard ACG, Kitzen JM, Singh BN, Lucchesi BR (1991) Hypothyroidism renders protection against lethal ventricular arrhythmias in a conscious canine model of sudden death. J Cardiovasc Pharmacol 18:703–710

Vrobel TR, Miller PE, Mostow ND, Rakita L (1989) A general overview of amiodarone toxicity: its prevention, detection and management. Prog Cardiovasc Dis 31:393–426

Weetman AP, Bhandal SK, Burrin JM, Robinson K, McKenna W (1988) Amiodarone and thyroid autoimmunity in the United Kingdom. Br Med J 297:33

Weissel M (1988) Suppression of thyroglobulin secretion in amiodarone-induced thyrotoxicosis. J Endocrinol Invest 11:53–55

Widerhorn J, Bhandari AK, Bughi S, Rahimtoola SH, Elkayam U (1991) Fetal and neonatal adverse effects profile of amiodarone treatment during pregnancy. Am Heart J 122:1162–1166

Wiegand V, Wagner G, Kreuzer H (1986) Hypothyroid-like effect of amiodarone in the ventricular myocardium of the rat. Basic Res Cardiol 81:482–488

Wiersinga WM, Trip MD (1986) Amiodarone and thyroid hormone metabolism. Postgrad Med J 62:909–914

Wiersinga WM, Broenink M (1991) Amiodarone induces a dose-dependent increase of plasma cholesterol in the rat. Horm Metab Res 23:95–96

Wiersinga WM, Endert E, Trip MD, Verhaest-de Jong N (1986a) Immunoradiometric assay of thyrotropin in plasma: its value in predicting response to thyroliberin stimulation and assessing thyroid function in amiodarone-treated patients. Clin Chem 32:433–436

Wiersinga WM, Touber JL, Trip MD, van Royen EA (1986b) Uninhibited thyroidal uptake of radioiodine despite iodine excess in amiodarone-induced hypothyroidism. J Clin Endocrinol Metab 63:485–491

Wiersinga WM, Trip MD, van Beeren MH, Plomp TA, Oosting H (1991) An increase in plasma cholesterol independent of thyroid function during long-term amiodarone therapy. A dose-dependent relationship. Ann Intern Med 114:128–132

Wilson BD (1989) Does amiodarone inhibit T_3 binding to solubilized nuclear receptors in vitro? Horm Metab Res 21:483–488

Wilson JS, Podrid PJ (1991) Side effects from amiodarone. Am Heart J 121:158–171

Wimpfheimer C, Stäubli M, Schädelin J, Studer H (1982) Prednisone in amiodarone-induced thyrotoxicosis. Br Med J 284:1835–1836

Wladimiroff JW, Steward PA (1985) Treatment of fetal cardiac arrhythmias. Br J Hosp Med 34:134–140

Xanthopoulos B, Koutras DA, Boukis MA, Piperingos GD, Kitsoponides J, Souvatzoglou A, Moulopoulos SD (1986) The effect of benziodarone on the thyroid hormone levels and the pituitary-thyroid axis. J Endocrinol Invest 9:337–339

Yabek SM, Kato R, Singh BN (1986) Effects of amiodarone and its metabolite, desethylamiodarone, on the electrophysiologic properties of isolated cardiac muscle. J Cardiovasc Pharmacol 8:197–207

Yin YL, Perret GY, Nicolas P, Vassy R, Uzzan B, Tod M (1992) In vivo effects of amiodarone on cardiac β-adrenoceptor density and heart require thyroid hormones. J Cardiovasc Pharmacol 19:541–545

Yin Y, Vassy R, Nicolas P, Perret GY, Laurent S (1994) Antagonism between T_3 and amiodarone on the contractility and the density of β-adrenoceptors of chicken cardiac myocytes. Eur J Pharmacol 261:97–104

Zaninovich AA, Bosco SC, Fernandez-Pol AJ (1990) Amiodarone does not affect the distribution and fractional turnover of triiodothyronine from the plasma pool, but only its generation from thyroxine in extrathyroidal tissues. J Clin Endocrinol Metab 70:1721–1724

CHAPTER 11

Effects of Other Pharmacological Agents on Thyroid Function

C.A. MEIER and A.G. BURGER

A. Introduction

Pharmacological agents can modulate thyroid function at all levels, as illustrated in Fig. 1. Glucocorticoids, somatostatin, dopaminergic (dopamine, bromocriptine) and antidopaminergic agents (e.g. metoclopramide, droperidol) can all alter pituitary thyroid-stimulating hormone (TSH) secretion when present in pharmacological doses, as discussed in Chap. 2, this volume. Iodine, antithyroid drugs, lithium and amiodarone all have effects on thyroidal hormone production and these agents are discussed in detail in Chaps. 7–10, this volume. Steroids, diuretics, heparin and non-steroidal anti-inflammatory drugs have effects on thyroid hormone transport, thereby altering the total, but not free, hormone levels, as detailed in Chap. 5, this volume. However, additional substances are rare but important modulators of thyroid function and thyroid hormone metabolism, and they are the subject of the present chapter. At the level of the thyroid, sulphonamides, op'DDD, aminogluthethimide, cyanate, selenium, noradrenaline, cytokines and growth hormone influence hormonogenesis at various steps (Fig. 2). The early steps involved in thyroid hormone metabolism through a system of three different organ-specific deiodinases are subject to interference by iodinated drugs, propylthiouracil (PTU), β-adrenoceptor blockers and glucocorticoids. In addition, the final degradation of thyroid hormones can be altered by a variety of microsomal enzyme inducers, such as antiepileptics and rifampicin. These interactions are of particular interest when dealing with patients on exogenous thyroid hormone therapy. Finally, knowledge about the drugs known to interfere with intestinal thyroxine absorption (sucralfate, ferrous sulphate, cholestyramine, colestipol, aluminum hydroxide) is of equal importance in the management of the latter group of patients.

B. Effects of Various Drugs on Thyroidal Hormonogenesis

Early reports of sulphonamides interfering with thyroid hormone synthesis have been documented, but none of the currently used sulphonamides is

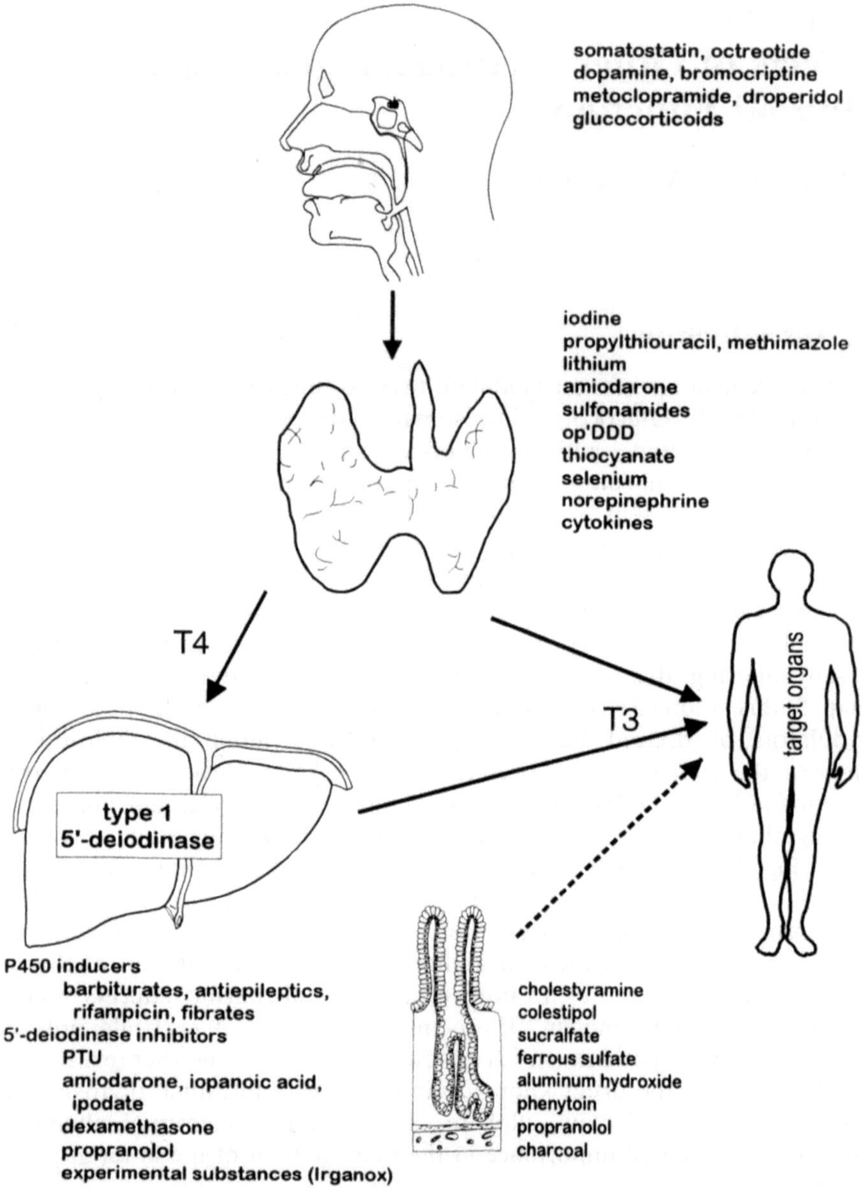

Fig. 1. Possible sites of drug interference with thyroid function

known to maintain this effect. Inhibitors of steroidogenesis have been reported also to affect thyroid function, including aminogluthetimide and op'DDD. However, these effects are not well documented and are unlikely to have a direct influence on thyroid synthesis or release (BROWN et al. 1986).

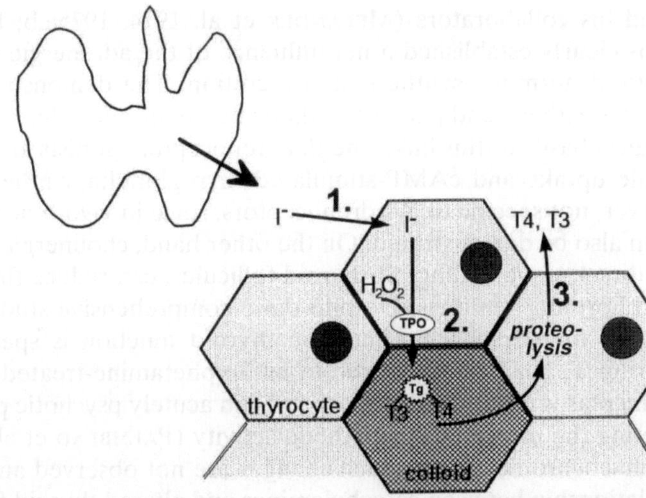

Fig. 2. Schematic illustration of a thyroid follicle: *1*, trapping of iodide by the iodide pump at the basolateral membrane of the follicular cell; *2*, thyroid hormone synthesis at the apical cell membrane; *TPO*, thyroid peroxidase; *TG*, thyroglobulin; *3*, secretion of thyroid hormones after proteolysis of thyroglobulin

Regarding dietary effects, the thiocyanates are of particular interest. Their effects as an inhibitor of iodide trapping are well known and have even been used therapeutically. Also, in severe iodine deficiency areas, thiocyanate-rich food (cassawa roots, brassica vegetables) inhibits the already low iodine uptake of the thyroid and greatly increases the severity of the clinical picture of cretinism (Bourdoux et al. 1978). Even in countries of moderate iodine intake such as Denmark, smoking – which can result in considerably increased thiocyanate levels – is positively correlated with increased thyroid size and slightly higher serum TSH levels (Hegedus et al. 1985).

Another ingredient of nutrients, the selenium ion, may have a protective effect on the thyroid. Thyroid hormone synthesis is obligatorily linked to an oxidative stress which is related to the peroxidative iodination of thyroglobulin. Thyroid glutathione peroxidase is responsible for the reduction of excess H_2O_2 and superoxide. It is a selenoprotein and is markedly decreased in severe selenium deficiency. In rats, it has been clearly documented that selenium deficiency, together with iodine deficiency, can lead to cell death, and it has been postulated that in these highly stimulated thyroids the protection from the oxidative stress is insufficient. In the human this might be a relevant factor explaining iodine-deficient myxoedematous cretinism presenting with an atrophic thyroid, a clinical finding known to occur in areas of combined iodine and selenium deficiency (Thilly et al. 1992; Dumont et al. 1994; Contempré et al. 1995).

The relation between the sympathetic nervous system and thyroid function has been a constant area of clinical and research interest. The work of

MELANDER and his collaborators (MELANDER et al. 1974, 1975a,b; EKHOLM et al. 1975) has clearly established a net influence of the adrenergic nervous system on thyroid hormone synthesis and secretion. The demonstration of interfollicular sympathetic and parasympathetic nerve terminals has provided the morphological basis for this link. The β_2-adrenoceptor agonists are able to stimulate iodide uptake and cAMP-stimulated thyroglobulin synthesis. The effect is, however, not specific to β_2-adrenoceptors, since in vivo α-adrenergic stimulation can also be demonstrated. On the other hand, cholinergic stimuli, through their direct nerve endings at thyroid follicules, can reduce the secretion of thyroid hormones in dogs. Despite these comprehensive studies, evidence in humans for adrenergic effects on thyroid function is sparse. An increase in serum T_4 has been observed in an amphetamine-treated patient and transient increases in serum T_4 are observed in acutely psychotic patients, possibly reflecting the increased sympathetic activity (PALMBLAD et al. 1979). However, in phaeochromocytomas such changes are not observed and proof for a causal relationship between catecholamines and altered thyroid function in man is still lacking.

Several cytokines have been shown to alter thyroid hormone secretion and metabolism. Administration of interferons, interleukins (IL) and granulocyte-macrophage colony-stimulating factor has been associated with a high frequency of transient hypo- and hyperthyroidism during treatment (BURMAN et al. 1986; HOEKMAN et al. 1991; REICHLIN 1993). Although these cytokines may elicit either the appearance of or an increase in thyroid autoantibody titres, these changes are not always associated with thyroid dysfunction, which may conversely also occur in the absence of antibodies, possibly through direct effects on the thyroid gland as discussed below. It is nevertheless advisable that patients scheduled to receive cytokine treatments should be screened for thyroid antibodies since positive patients may be at higher risk of developing thyroid dysfunction.

Interferons, IL-1 and tumour necrosis factor-α are known to inhibit iodine organification and hormone release, as well as to modulate thyroglobulin production and thyrocyte growth (SATO et al. 1990; MOORADIAN et al. 1990; CHOPRA et al. 1991; YAMAZAKI et al. 1993). In contrast to interferon-α and interleukin-2, interferon-γ has been shown to increase the expression of the major histocompatibility complex class II molecules on the cell surface, which is thought to be a crucial event in the perpetuation of autoimmune diseases (KRAIEM et al. 1990; KASUGA et al. 1991). IL-2 is used experimentally in the immunotherapy of cancer, which results in transient thyroid dysfunction in 15%–40% of the patients. Hypo- and hyperthyroidism have been observed, but the occurrence of transient hyperthyroidism followed by a hypothyroid phase, compatible with silent thyroiditis, has also frequently been reported (SCHWARTZENTRUBER et al. 1991; VASSILOPOULOU-SELLIN et al. 1992; VIALETTES et al. 1993). Thyroid function sometimes normalises during, but always after, stopping the cytokine treatment.

C. Effects of Drugs on Thyroid Hormone Metabolism

I. Deiodination

Over 80% of thyroidal hormone secretion consists of thyroxine (T_4), an inactive prohormone that requires activation by peripheral deiodination as illustrated in Fig. 1 and detailed in Chap. 4, this volume. The type, distribution and sensitivity to pharmacological agents of the three deiodinase systems are illustrated in Fig. 3. The type 1 5′-deiodinase is mainly present in liver and kidney and is primarily responsible for the conversion of L-T_4 into the active hormone L-triiodothyronine (L-T_3); 5′-deiodinase type 2 is more restricted in its expression (pituitary, brain) and is also capable of converting T_4 into T_3. However, this enzyme is quantitatively much less important than the type 1 enzyme and is thought to be particularly important in raising the local concentrations of T_3. Finally, the type 3 deiodinase removes the inner-ring iodine

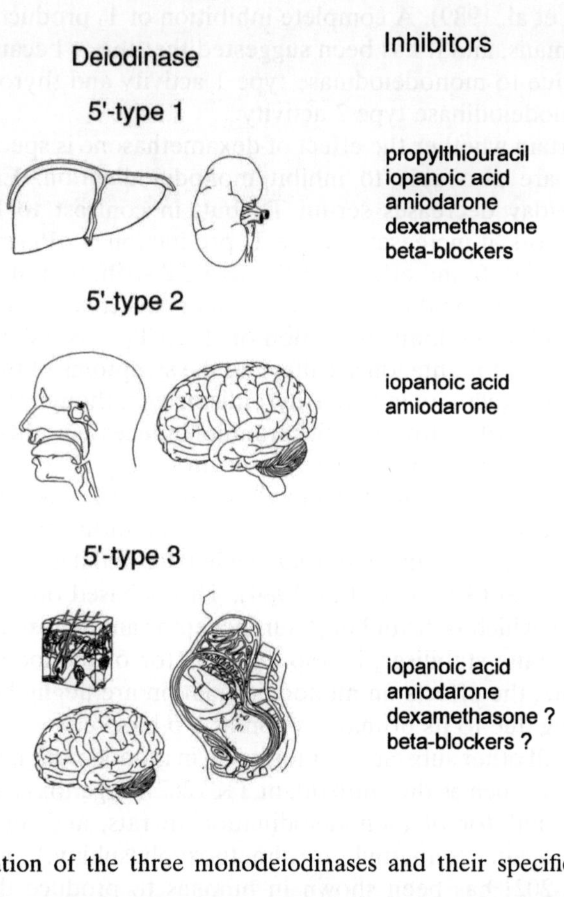

Fig. 3. Localisation of the three monodeiodinases and their specific and unspecific inhibitors

atoms and is hence not involved in the production of T_3. However, similar to the type 1 and 2 deiodinases, the type 3 enzyme is important for thyroid hormone inactivation and the recycling of iodine. All three enzymes were recently cloned and form the family of selenocysteine-containing deiodinases (BERRY et al. 1991; MANDEL et al. 1992; SALVATORE et al. 1995; DAVEY et al. 1995).

So far, there are few drugs increasing outer- or inner-ring monodeiodination although growth hormone (GH) is a possible candidate. Inhibitors of monodeiodination can be separated into iodinated and non-iodinated ones and, also, into specific inhibitors and non-specific inhibitors affecting all three enzymes. The specific inhibitors for deiodinase type I activity are PTU and reverse T_3; for deiodinase type II activity inhibitors are T_4, reverse T_3 and 3′,5′-diiodothyronine (VISSER et al. 1983).

The inhibition of T_4 to T_3 conversion by PTU is well established. With relatively high doses of PTU (600 mg/day) one observes a fall by one-third of the serum T_3 levels, an effect which can be clinically beneficial (NOGIMORI et al. 1986; LOPRESTI et al. 1989). A complete inhibition of T_3 production cannot be obtained in humans, and it has been suggested that this is because circulating T_3 is not only due to monodeiodinase type 1 activity and thyroidal secretion but also to monodeiodinase type 2 activity.

It is not certain whether the effect of dexamethasone is specific or if other glucocortcoids are also able to inhibit monodeiodination. Eight to 12 mg dexamethasone/day decreases serum T_3, but, in contrast to PTU and the iodinated inhibitors, it increases reverse T_3 production (LOPRESTI et al. 1989). In rats it also has profound effects on the tissue distribution of T_3 (CAVALIERI et al. 1984). The hormonal changes seen under this treatment are therefore multifactorial with a predominant action on T_4 to T_3 conversion.

All β-adrenoceptor antagonists alleviate the symptoms of the sympathetic nervous system overactivity in hyperthyroidism, even though there are differences in drug sensitivity. However, propranolol induces a gradual fall of serum T_3 levels with a concomitant increase in serum reverse T_3 levels, and kinetic studies have proven that it interferes in vivo with T_4 to T_3 conversion, and that the increase in reverse T_3 is due its decreased metabolism (FABER et al. 1979). The effect of propranolol can be reproduced in vitro and it is likely to act at the cell membrane level (SHULKIN et al. 1984). This is based on the observation that the D-form, which is devoid of β-adrenoceptor antagonistic activity but is a plasma membrane stabiliser, is also an inhibitor of monodeiodination. In clinical medicine, the effects on monodeiodination are negligible, the beneficial effects being due to its primary action as a β-blocker.

There are still other substances interfering in monodeiodination. A chemical used in plastics such as the antioxidant TK 12627 (Irganox) has been shown to be a weak inhibitor of monodeiodination in rats, and an experimental lipid-lowering agent [dimethyl α-(dimethoxyphosphinyl) p-chlorobenzyl phosphate, SR-202] has been shown in humans to produce the changes in serum hormone levels seen with inhibitors of monodeiodination, e.g. a decrease in serum total and free T_3, an increase in serum total and free T_4 and an increase in serum reverse T_3 without major changes in serum TSH levels (SHULKIN et al. 1984; LIANG et al. 1993).

Among iodinated drugs, the most important clinical inhibitor of monodeiodination is amiodarone, which is discussed in depth in Chap. 11. The other two iodinated compounds are iopanoate and ipodate (ROTI et al. 1988; BURGI et al. 1976). Both are excellent inhibitors of T_4 to T_3 conversion and are the only ones to be markedly effective in humans; however, they inhibit all three deiodinases to different extents, but there is no biochemical proof that they are specific inhibitors of monodeiodination. For iopanoic acid, affinity labelling of monodeiodinase type 1 and type 2 with *N*-bromoacetyl-L-thyroxine has shown that the drug is unable to block the active site of the enzyme and thus it cannot be considered a specific inhibitor of these two enzymes. Nevertheless, both are potent inhibitors of T_4 to T_3 conversion and are used for such purposes in clinical medicine (ROTI et al. 1988).

II. Microsomal Oxidation

The potent cytochromes 450 are a group of enzymes responsible for most hepatic drug oxidation (BROSEN 1990; ZIEGLER 1993). They are also called mixed function oxygenases. The system is tightly linked to conjugating enzymes of the oxidised intermediary metabolites. For thyroid hormones, the uridine diphosphate-glucuronyltransferases are responsible for glucuronidation and the phenylsulphotransferases for sulphatation. Both processes increase the solubility of the metabolites and their biliary excretion. The sulphated metabolites, particularly T_3 sulphate, are ideal substrates for deiodination, distinguishing this pathway from glucuroconjugation (VISSER 1990; VISSER et al. 1990).

The inducibility of the mixed function oxygenases varies from species to species. The rat is particularly sensitive to such drugs, while hepatic drug metabolism in primates is more resistant. Therefore, many reported effects of drugs on thyroid hormone metabolism are not, or only barely, seen in humans (KAISER et al. 1988; CURRAN and DE GROOT 1991). This is the case for the barbiturates. In the rat, phenobarbital (and to a lesser extent pentobarbital) has been shown to increase the hepatic metabolism of thyroid hormones, and the fraction of total thyroid hormone metabolism being excreted as biliary conjugates increases considerably. In normal rats this increased metabolism is compensated for by increased secretion of T_4. However, in man, early studies did not show any significant changes in thyroid hormone levels and more recent studies with sensitive TSH measurements are not available. Stronger inducers of mixed-function oxygenases have been studied in the rat. Nafenopin, for instance, markedly increases the biliary excretion of conjugated T_4 but, interestingly, it did not increase the clearance of T_3. This can be explained by the preferential sulphatation of T_3, which is not affected by inducers of mixed function oxygenases.

Antiepileptic drugs such as phenytoin and carbamazepine, both inducers of the mixed function oxygenases, are a definite source of alterations of thyroid hormone levels in man (ROOTWELT et al. 1978; SMITH and SURKS 1984; SCHRODER VAN DER ELST et al. 1996). Phenytoin-treated and, to a lesser extent, carbamazepine-treated subjects show a decrease in serum total and free T_4 and total T_3. The results on free T_3 levels are more sparse and are less clear. Knowing the difficulties in obtaining accurate measurements of free hormone levels, the mostly unchanged serum TSH levels are probably more indicative of a normal thyroid function in such patients. However, one is entitled to postulate that this occurs only at the expense of a slight increase in hormone secretion. A word of caution for phenytoin should be added since this drug also interferes in the binding of T_4 to thyroxine-binding globulin (TBG) and is possibly a weak thyroid hormone agonist.

Another well-known and potent inducer of mixed function oxygenases has been studied in man, the antituberculosis drug rifampicin (FINKE et al. 1987; CHRISTENSEN et al. 1989; OHNHAUS and STUDER 1980). Contrary to phenytoin it does not interfere in T_4 binding to TBG and its effects can therefore be considered purely the consequence of enzyme induction. The effects in normal man are significant, but not major, since serum thyroid hormone levels remain generally within the normal range. The findings are a lowering of total and free T_4 and reverse T_3 while serum T_3 levels tend to increase. The metabolism of T_4 is clearly increased but monodeiodination remains unchanged.

In conclusion, the effects of certain drugs on mixed function oxygenases are clear and important in rats, where there is substantial loss of T_4 by glucurono-conjugation. There may be some hepatobiliary recycling in rats but there is no evidence for an enterohepatic circulation of thyroid hormones in man. In primates the effects of these drugs are less marked; they are best seen with phenytoin, although the action of this drug is more complex than that of a pure inducer of mixed function oxygenases. Part of its action is still not well understood.

Hypothyroid patients treated with an inducer of hepatic mixed function oxygenases should be carefully monitored and possibly such substitution therapy should be increased (SURKS 1985). With rare exceptions, only minor adjustments are necessary. Contrary to glucuronidation, sulphatation is an integral part of monodeiodination of tri- and diiodothyronines, the sulphated compounds being better substrates for monodeiodination than the intact metabolites. However, in terms of thyroid hormone action, it is important to realise that sulphation is not an intermediary step for the conversion of T_4 to T_3.

D. Drug Effects on Cellular and Intestinal Uptake of Thyroid Hormone

Inhibition of thyroid hormone uptake by drugs may occur at the intestinal level, thereby leading to decreased serum hormone levels in T_4-replaced patients, or in other target tissues, potentially resulting in cellular hypothyroidism despite normal serum levels (see also Chap. 13, this volume). However, the physiological relevance of cellular thyroid hormone transport systems is still controversial (KRENNING and DOCTER 1986; PONTECORVI and ROBBINS 1989; DEJONG et al. 1993).

I. Cellular Uptake

Amiodarone is the best-characterised drug inhibiting cellular thyroid hormone uptake. A selective decrease in hepatic T_4 transport was demonstrated in hepatocytes and perfused rat liver, and impaired T_3 uptake was observed in an anterior pituitary cell line (NORMAN and LAVIN 1989; DE JONG et al. 1994). Benzodiazepines were also shown to inhibit cellular L-T_3 uptake, possibly due to their conformational similarity with this hormone, allowing an interaction with the hepatic iodothyronine membrane transporter at sites similar to those for the endogenous ligand (KRAGIE et al. 1994). Interestingly, hepatic and muscle L-T_3 uptake seems to be a calcium-dependent process, as has been inferred from the profound inhibition of hormone uptake by various calcium channel blockers, such as nifedipine, verapamil and diltiazem (TOPLISS et al. 1993). Finally, frusemide and some non-steroidal anti-inflammatory drugs compete for cytosolic T_3-binding sites in cultured cells (BARLOW et al. 1994). However, whether the in vitro observations for these various drugs are quantitatively relevant in vivo remains to be demonstrated.

II. Intestinal Absorption

Several drugs are known to markedly reduce the absorption of T_4 from the gut, such as colestipol, cholestyramine, sucralfate, ferrous sulphate, aluminum hydroxide, phenytoin, propranolol and activated charcoal (NORTHCUTT et al. 1969; FABER et al. 1985; LUMHOLTZ et al. 1978). While normally 80% of a 1000-μg dose of thyroxine is absorbed within 6h, this value drops to 23% when sucralfate is taken simultaneously, resulting in lower T_4 and higher TSH serum levels (SHERMAN et al. 1994). This problem can be circumvented by separating the intake of the two drugs by several hours. The malabsorption of T_4 in the presence of sucralfate may be due to either the formation of an insoluble complex or an inhibition of hormone transport by intestinal cells.

References

Barlow JW, Curtis AJ, Raggatt LE, Loidl NM, Topliss DJ, Stockigt JR (1994) Drug competition for intracellular triiodothyronine-binding sites. Eur J Endocrinology 130:417–421

Berry MJ, Banu L, Larsen PR (1991) Type I iodothyronine deiodinase is a selenocysteine-containing enzyme. Nature 349:438–440

Bourdoux P, Delange F, Gérard M, Mafuta M, Hanson A, Ermans AM (1978) Evidence that cassava ingestion increases thiocyanate formation: a possible etiologic factor in endemic goiter. J Clin Endocrinol Metab 46:613–625
Brosen K (1990) Recent developments in hepatic drug oxidation. Implications for clinical pharmacokinetics. Clin Pharmacokinet 18:220–239
Brown CG, Fowler KL, Nicholls PJ, Atterwill C (1986) Assessment of thyrotoxicity using in vitro cell culture systems. Food Chem Toxicol 24:557–562
Burgi H, Wimpfheimer C, Burger A, Zaunbauer W, Rosler H, Lemarchand-Beraud T (1976) Changes of circulating thyroxine, triiodothyronine, reverse triiodothyronine after radiographic contrast agents. J Clin Endocrinol Metab 43:1203–1210
Burman P, Titterman TH, Orberg K, Karlsson FA (1986) Thyroid autoimmunity in patients on long term therapy with leukocyte-derived interferon. J Clin Endocrinol Metab 63:1086–1090
Cavalieri RR, Castle JN, McMahon FA (1984) Effects of dexamethasone on kinetics, distribution of triiodothyronine in the rat. Endocrinology 114:215–221
Chopra IJ, Sakane S, Teco GN.C (1991) A study of the serum concentration of tumor necrosis factor-alpha in thyroidal, nonthyroidal illnesses. J Clin Endocrinol Metab 72:1113–1116
Christensen HR, Simonsen K, Hegedus L et al (1989) Influence of rifampicin on thyroid gland volume, thyroid hormones, antipyrine metabolism. Acta Endocrinol (Copenh) 121:406–410
Contempré B, Dumont JE, Denef JF, Many MC (1995) Effects of selenium deficiency on thyroid necrosis, fibrosis, proliferation: a possible role in myxoedematous cretinism. Eur J Endocrinol 133:99–109
Curran PG, De Groot LJ (1991) The effect of hepatic enzyme-inducing drugs on thyroid hormones, the thyroid gland. Endocr Rev 12:135–150
Davey JC, Becker KB, Schneider MJ, St. Germain DL, Galton VA (1995) Cloning of a cDNA for the type II iodothyronine deiodinase. J Biol Chem 270:26786–26789
de Jong M, Docter R, Van der Hoek H et al (1994) Different effects of amiodarone on transport of T_4, T_3 into the perfused rat liver. Am J Physiol 266:E44–E49
Dejong M, Visser TJ, Bernard BF et al (1993) Transport, Metabolism of iodothyronines in cultured human hepatocytes. J Clin Endocrinol Metab 77:139–143
Dumont JE, Corvilain B, Contempré B (1994) The biochemistry of endemic cretinism: roles of iodine, selenium deficiency, goitrogens. Mol Cell Endocrinol 100:163–166
Ekholm R, Engstrom G, Ericson LE, Melander A (1975) Exocytosis of protein into the thyroid follicle lumen: an early effect of TSH. Endocrinology 97:337–346
Faber J, Friis T, Kirkegaard C et al (1979) Serum T_4, T_3, reverse T_3 during treatment with propranolol in hyperthyroidism, L-T_4 treated myxedema, in normal man. Horm Metab Res 11:34–36
Faber J, Lumholtz IB, Kirkegaard C et al (1985) The effects of phenytoin (diphenylhydantoin) on the extrathyroidal turnover of thyroxine, 3,5,3′-triiodothyronine, 3,3′,5′-triiodothyronine, 3′,5′-diiodothyronine in man. J Clin Endocrinol Metab 61:1093–1099
Finke C, Juge C, Goumaz M, Kaiser O, Davies R, Burger AG (1987) Effects of rifampicin on the peripheral turnover kinetics of thyroid hormones in mice, in men. J Endocrinol Invest 10:157–162
Hegedus L, Karstrup S, Veiergang D, Jacobsen B, Skovsted L, Feldt-Rasmussen U (1985) High frequency of goitre in cigarette smokers. Clin Endocrinol (Oxf) 22:287–292
Hoekman K, von Blomberg-van der Flier BM, Wagstaff J, Drexhage HA, Pinedo HM (1991) Reversible thyroid dysfunction during treatment with GM-CSF (see comments). Lancet 338:541–542
Kaiser CA, Seydoux J, Giacobino JP, Girardier L, Burger AG (1988) Increased plasma clearance rate of thyroxine despite decreased 5′-monodeiodination: study with a peroxisome proliferator in the rat. Endocrinology 122:1087–1093

Kasuga Y, Matsubayashi S, Akasu F, Miller N, Jamieson C, Volpé R (1991) Effects of recombinant human interleukin-2, tumor necrosis factor-alpha with or without interferon-gamma on human thyroid tissues from patients with Graves' disease, from normal subjects xenografted into nude mice. J Clin Endocrinol Metab 72:1296–1301

Kragie L, Forrester ML, Cody V, Mccourt M (1994) Computer-assisted molecular modeling of benzodiazepine, thyromimetic inhibitors of the HepG2 iodothyronine membrane transporter. Mol Endocrinol 8:382–391

Kraiem Z, Sobel E, Sadeh O, Kinarty A, Lahat N (1990) Effects of gamma-interferon on DR antigen expression, growth, 3,5,3′-triiodothyronine secretion, iodide uptake, cyclic adenosine 3′,5′-monophosphate accumulation in cultured human thyroid cells. J Clin Endocrinol Metab 71:817–824

Krenning EP, Docter R (1986) Plasma membrane transport of thyroid hormone. In: Hennemann G (ed) Thyroid hormone metabolism. Dekker, New York, p 131

Liang H, Morin O, Burger AG (1993) Effect of the antioxidant TK 12627 (Irganox) on monodeiodination, on the levels of messenger ribonucleic acid of 5′-deiodinase type I, spot 14. Acta Endocrinol (Copenh) 128:451–458

LoPresti JS, Eigen A, Kaptein E, Anderson KP, Spencer CA, Nicoloff JT (1989) Alteration in 3,3′,5′-triiodothyronine metabolism in response to propylthiouracil, dexamethasone, and thyroxine administration in man. J Clin Invest 84:1650–1656

Lumholtz IB, Siersbaek-Nielsen K, Faber J, Kirkegaard C, Friis T (1978) Effect of propanolol on extrathyroidal metabolism of thyroxine, 3,3′,5-triiodothyronine evaluated by noncompartmental kinetics. J Clin Endocrinol Metab 47:587–589

Mandel SJ, Berry MJ, Kieffer JD, Harney JW, Warne RL, Larse PR (1992) Cloning, in vitro expression of the human selenoprotein, type I deiodinase. J Clin Endocrinol Metab 75:1133–1139

Melander A, Ericson LE, Ljunggren JG et al (1974) Sympathetic innervation of the normal human thyroid. J Clin Endocrinol Metab 39:713–718

Melander A, Ranklev E, Sundler F, Westgren U (1975a) $Beta_2$-adrenergic stimulation of thyroid hormone secretion. Endocrinology 97:332–336

Melander A, Sundler F, Westgren U (1975b) Sympathetic innervation of the thyroid: variation with species, with age. Endocrinology 96:102–106

Mooradian AD, Reed RL, Osterweil D, Schiffman R, Scuderi P (1990) Decreased serum triiodothyronine is associated with increased concentrations of tumor necrosis factor (TNF). J Clin Endocrinol Metab 71:1239–1242

Nogimori T, Braverman LE, Taurog A, Fang SL, Wright G, Emerson CH (1986) A new class of propylthiouracil analogs: comparison of 5′-deiodinase inhibition, antithyroid activity. Endocrinology 118:1598–1605

Norman MF, Lavin TN (1989) Antagonism of thyroid hormone action by amiodarone in rat pituitary tumor cells. J Clin Invest 83:306–313

Northcutt RC, Stiel JN, Hollifield JW, Stant EG (1969) The influence of cholestyramine on thyroxine absorption. JAMA 208:1857–1861

Ohnhaus EE, Studer H (1980) The effect of different doses of rifampicin on thyroid hormone metabolism (proceedings). Br J Clin Pharmacol 9:285–286

Palmblad J, Akerstedt T, Froberg J, Melander A, von Schenck H (1979) Thyroid, adrenomedullary reactions during sleep deprivation. Acta Endocrinol (Copenh) 90:233–239

Pontecorvi A, Robbins J (1989) The plasma membrane, thyroid hormone entry into cells. Trends Endocrinol Metab 1:90–94

Reichlin S (1993) Neuroendocrine-immune interactions. N Engl J Med 329:1246–1253

Rootwelt K, Ganes T, Johannessen SI (1978) Effect of carbamazepine, phenytoin, phenobarbitone on serum levels of thyroid hormones, thyrotropin in humans. Scand J Clin Lab Invest 38:731–736

Roti E, Robuschi G, Gardini E et al (1988) Comparison of methimazole, methimazole, sodium ipodate, methimazole, saturated solution of potassium iodide in the early treatment of hyperthyroid Graves' disease. Clin Endocrinol (Oxf) 28:305–314

Salvatore D, Low SC, Berry MJ et al (1995) Type 3 iodothyronine deiodinase: cloning, in vitro expression, functional analysis of the placental selenoenzyme. J Clin Invest 96:2421–2430

Sato K, Satoh T, Shizume K, et al (1990) Inhibition of ^{125}I organification, thyroid hormone release by interleukin-1, tumor necrosis factor-alpha, interferon-gamma in human thyrocytes in suspension culture. J Clin Endocrinol Metab 70:1735–1743

Schroder van der Elst JP, Van der Heide D, Van der Bent C, Kaptein E, Visser TJ, DiStefano JJ (1996) Effects of 5,5′-diphenylhydantoin on the thyroid status in rats. Eur J Endocrinol 134:221–224

Schwartzentruber DJ, White DE, Zweig MH, Weintraub BD, Rosenberg SA (1991) Thyroid dysfunction associated with immunotherapy for patients with cancer. Cancer 68:2384–2390

Sherman SI, Tielens ET, Ladenson PW (1994) Sucralfate causes malabsorption of L-thyroxine. Am J Med 96:531–535

Shulkin BL, Peele ME, Utiger RD (1984) Beta-adrenergic antagonist inhibition of hepatic 3,5,3′-triiodothyronine production. Endocrinology 115:858–861

Smith PJ, Surks MI (1984) Multiple effects of 5,5′-diphenylhydantoin on the thyroid hormone system. Endocr Rev 5:514–524

Surks MI (1985) Hypothyroidism, phenytoin (letter). Ann Intern Med 102:871

Thilly CH, Vanderpas JB, Bebe N et al (1992) Iodine deficiency, other trace elements, goitrogenic factors in the etiopathogeny of iodine deficiency disorders (IDD). Biol Trace Elem Res 32:229–243

Topliss DJ, Scholz GH, Kolliniatis E, Barlow JW, Stockigt JR (1993) Influence of calmodulin antagonists, calcium channel blockers on triiodothyronine uptake by rat hepatoma, myoblast cell lines. Metabolism 42:376–380

Vassilopoulou-Sellin R, Sella A, Dexeus FH, Theriault RL, Pololoff DA (1992) Acute thyroid dysfunction (thyroiditis) after therapy with interleukin-2. Horm Metab Res 24:434–438

Vialettes B, Guillerand MA, Viens P et al (1993) Incidence rate, risk factors for thyroid dysfunction during recombinant interleukin-2 therapy in advanced malignancies. Acta Endocrinol (Copenh) 129:31–38

Visser TJ, Kaplan MM, Leonard JL, Larsen PR (1983) Evidence for two pathways of iodothyronine 5′-deiodination in rat pituitary that differ in kinetics, propylthiouracil sensitivity, response to hypothyroidism. J Clin Invest 71:992–1002

Visser TJ (1990) Importance of deiodination, conjugation in the hepatic metabolism of thyroid hormone. In: Greer MA (ed) The thyroid gland. Raven, New York, p 255

Visser TJ, van Buuren JCJ, Rutgers M, Eelkman Rooda SJ, de Herder WW (1990) The role of sulfation in thyroid hormone metabolism. TEM 211–218

Yamazaki K, Kanaji Y, Shizume K, et al (1993) Reversible inhibition by interferons alpha, beta of ^{125}I incorporation, thyroid hormone release by human thyroid follicles in vitro. J Clin Endocrinol Metab 77:1439–1441

Ziegler DM (1993) Recent studies on the structure, function of multisubstrate flavin-containing monooxygenases. Annu Rev Pharmacol Toxicol 33:179–199

CHAPTER 12

Effects of Environmental Agents on Thyroid Function

E. GAITAN

A. Introduction

A large number of agents in the environment, both naturally occurring and man-made, are known to interfere with thyroid gland morphology and function, posing the danger of thyroid disease (Table 1). Thyroid enlargement or goitre is the most prominent effect of these agents. They may cause the goitrous condition by acting directly on the thyroid gland (Fig. 1), but also indirectly by altering the regulatory mechanisms of the thyroid gland and the peripheral metabolism and excretion of thyroid hormones (GAITAN 1988, 1989a, 1990).

Figure 1 illustrates the three main steps in thyroid gland function, showing the environmental agents that act directly on the gland by interfering with the process of hormone synthesis. However, the mechanism that induces the trophic changes leading to goitre formation is not well understood, because besides thyroid-stimulating hormone (TSH), other humoral, paracrine, and autocrine growth factors appear to be involved in the process (WENZEL and BOTTAZZO 1987; DUMONT et al. 1991, 1992).

These agents may enter into the food, water, and air exposure pathways, becoming important environmental antithyroid and/or goitrogenic factors in man (GAITAN 1988, 1989a, 1990). Their effects may be additive to those of iodine deficiency, making the intensity of the manifestations of goitre, hypothyroidism, and iodine deficiency disorders (cretinism, congenital hypothyroidism, and various degrees of impairment of growth and mental development) more severe. In iodine-sufficient areas, these compounds may be responsible for the development of some "sporadic" goitres or the persistence of the goitre endemia with its associated disorders, namely, autoimmune thyroiditis, hypothyroidism, hyperthyroidism, and, probably, thyroid carcinoma (GAITAN et al. 1991; GAITAN and DUNN 1992; MORENO-REYES et al. 1993).

Table 1. Environmental agents producing goitrogenic and/or antithyroid effects

Compounds	Goitrogenic/antithyroid effects		
	In vivo		In vitro
	Human	Animals	
Sulfurated organics			
Thiocyanate (SCN^-)[a]	+	+	+
Isothiocyanates	NT	+	+
L-5-Vinyl-2-thio-oxazolidone (goitrin)	+	+	+
Disulfides (R-S-S-R)	NT	+	0, + (?)[b]
Flavonoids (polyphenols)			
Glycosides	NT	+	+
Aglycones	NT	+	+
C-Ring fission metabolites (i.e., phloroglucinol, phenolic acids)	NT	+	+
Polyhydroxyphenols and phenol derivatives			
Phenol	NT	NT	+
Catechol (1,2-dihydroxybenzene)	NT	NT	+
Resorcinol (1,3-dihydroxybenzene)[a]	+	+	+
Hydroquinone (1,4-dihydroxybenzene)	NT	NT	+
m-Dihydroxyacetophenones	NT	NT	+
2-Methylresorcinol	NT	+	+
5-Methylresorcinol (orcinol)	NT	+	+
4-Methylcatechol	NT	NT	+
Pyrogallol (1,2,3-trihydroxybenzene)	NT	+	+
Phloroglucinol (1,3,5-trihydroxybenzene)	NT	+	+
4-Chlororesorcinol	NT	+	+
3-Chloro-4-hydroxybenzoic acid	NT	NT	+
2,4-Dinitrophenol	+	+	0
Pyridines			
3-Hydroxypyridine	NT	NT	+
Dihydroxypyridines	NT	+	+
Phthalate esters and metabolites			
Diisobutyl phthalate	NT	NT	0
Dioctyl phthalate	NT	+	0
o-Phthalic acid	NT	NT	0
m-Phthalic acid	NT	NT	0
3,4-Dihydroxybenzoic acid (DHBA)	NT	NT	+
3,5-Dihydroxybenzoic acid	NT	NT	+
Polychlorinated (PCB) and polybrominated (PBB) biphenyls			
PCBs (Aroclor)	NT	+	NT
PBBs and PBB oxides	+	+	NT
Other organochlorines			
Dichlorodiphenyltrichloroethane (*p,p'*-DDT)	NT	+	NT
Dichlorodiphenyldichloroethane (*p,p'*-DDE) and dieldrin	NT	+	NT
2,3,7,8-Tetrachlorodibenzo-*p*-dioxin (TCDD)	NT	+	NT
Polycyclic aromatic hydrocarbons (PAH)			
3,4-Benzpyrene (BaP)	NT	+ (?)	NT
3-Methylcholanthrene (MCA)	NT	+	NT
7,12-Dimethylbenzanthracene (DMBA)	NT	+	NT
9-Methylanthracene (MA)	NT	+	0
Inorganics			
Excess iodine[a]	+	+	+
Lithium[a]	+	+	+

+, active; 0, inactive; NT, nontested.
[a] Agents also used as medications.
[b] Inactive in TPO assay; active (?) in thyroid slices assay.

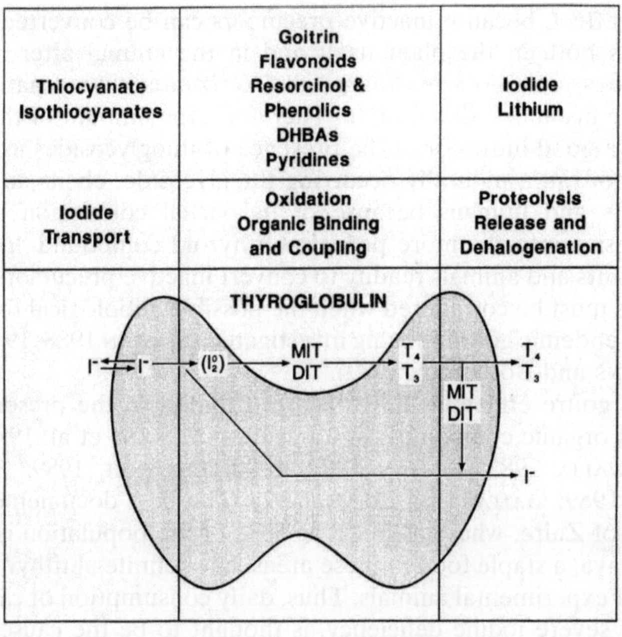

Fig. 1. Environmental antithyroid/goitrogenic compounds and their site of action in the thyroid gland. *Goitrin*, L,5-vinyl-2-thiooxazolidone; *DHBAs*, dihydroxybenzoic acids; *I*, iodide; *MIT*, monoiodotyrosine; *DIT*, diiodotyrosine; T_4, thyroxine; T_3, triiodothyronine. (Reproduced with permission, from GAITAN 1990, copyright 1990 Annual Reviews Inc.)

B. Chemical Categories, Sources, Pharmacokinetics, and Mechanism of Action

I. Sulphurated Organics

1. Thiocyanate, Isothiocyanates, and Thio-oxazolidone (Goitrin)

Thiocyanates and isothiocyanates have been demonstrated as goitrogenic principles in plants of the Cruciferae family. The potent antithyroid compound L-5-vinyl-2-thio-oxazolidone or "goitrin" was isolated from yellow turnips and from brassica seeds. Cyanogenic glycosides (thiocyanate precursors) have also been found in several staple foods (cassava, maize, bamboo shoots, sweet potatoes, lima beans) from the Third World. After ingestion these glycosides can be readily converted to thiocyanate by widespread glycosidases and the sulphur transferase enzyme. Isothiocyanates not only use the thiocyanate metabolic pathway but react with amino groups, forming derivatives with thiourea-like antithyroid effects. Thus, the actual concentration of thiocyanates or isothiocyanates in a given foodstuff may not represent its true goitrogenic potential, nor does the absence of these compounds negate a possible antithyroid effect, because inactive precursors can be converted into goitrogenic agents both in the plant itself and in the animal after its ingestion. Thioglycosides undergo a rearrangement to form isothiocyanate derivatives and, in some instances, thiocyanate. Therefore, the amount of thiocyanate in the urine is a good indicator of the presence of thioglycosides in food. Ingestion of progoitrin, a naturally occurring thioglycoside, elicits antithyroid activity in rats and humans because of its partial conversion by intestinal microorganisms into the more potent antithyroid compound "goitrin". This ability of plants and animals readily to convert inactive precursors into goitrogenic agents must be considered when the possible aetiological role of dietary elements in endemic goitre is being investigated (GAITAN 1988, 1990; DELANGE 1989; ERMANS and BOURDOUX 1989).

Several goitre endemias have been attributed to the presence of these sulphurated organic compounds in foodstuffs (ERMANS et al. 1980; DELANGE and AHLUWALIA 1983; GAITAN 1988, 1990; DELANGE 1989; ERMANS and BOURDOUX 1989; GAITAN and DUNN 1992). The best documented is that in some areas of Zaire, where as much as 60% of the population is affected by goitre. Cassava, a staple food in these areas, has definite antithyroid effects in humans and experimental animals. Thus, daily consumption of cassava, in the presence of severe iodine deficiency, is thought to be the cause of endemic goitre and cretinism in these areas of Zaire. The goitrogenic action of cassava is due to endogenous release of thiocyanate from linamarin, a cyanogenic glucoside present in cassava, particularly in the tuberous roots. Thiocyanate is also present in pearl millet (*Pennisetum leeke* [L.], also known as *typhoides* or *americanum*), the staple food of people living in iodine-deficient endemic goitre areas of western Sudan. Pearl millet is rich in C-glycosylflavones, which, in combination with thiocyanate, exert additive and complementary antithyroid and goitrogenic effects, discussed further below (GAITAN et al. 1989, 1995).

Thiocyanate is also found in high concentrations (1 g/l) in wastewater effluents of coal conversion processes, and in body fluids as a metabolite of hydrogen cyanide gas consumed while smoking (GAITAN 1988). Studies in Sweden indicate that cigarette smoking may produce goitre. Similarly, goitre and hypothyroidism were documented in patients receiving long-term thiocyanate treatment for hypertension. This goitrogenic effect of thiocyanate is more evident in the presence of iodine deficiency. Several observations suggest that thiocyanate crosses the human placenta and may cause both goitre and neonatal hypothyroidism (ROTI et al. 1983; WALFISH 1983; CHANOINE et al. 1991). The thiocyanate ion involves a linear SCN group in which the double bond character of the S–C reflects the existence of two tautomeric structures, –S–C≡N and S=C=N–. Thiocyanate, like nitrate and cyanide ions, is ambident since the negative charge can be located either on S or N. This tautomerism explains the existence of two series of covalent derivatives, the thiocyanates and isothiocyanates (ERMANS and BOURDOUX 1989).

a) Thiocyanate

Thiocyanate or thiocyanate-like compounds primarily inhibit the iodine-concentrating mechanism of the thyroid, and their goitrogenic activity can be overcome by iodine administration (Fig. 1). Thiocyanate at low concentrations inhibits iodide transport by increasing the velocity constant of iodide efflux from the thyroid gland. At high concentrations, the iodide efflux is greatly accelerated while the unidirectional iodide clearance into the gland is inhibited. Thiocyanate at these high concentrations also inhibits the incorporation of iodide into thyroglobulin by competing with iodide at the thyroid peroxidase (TPO) level, thereby preventing iodide oxidation and thyroid hormone synthesis (ERMANS and BOURDOUX 1989). Thiocyanate is rapidly converted to sulphate in the thyroid gland. Administration of TSH increases the intrathyroidal catabolism of thiocyanate and is capable of reversing the block of iodide uptake produced by this ion. TSH probably accelerates the oxidation of thiocyanate to sulphate.

b) Isothiocyanates

The isothiocyanates and cyanogenic glycosides act on the thyroid mainly by their rapid conversion to thiocyanate. However, isothiocyanates, as previously mentioned, not only use the thiocyanate metabolic pathway but also react spontaneously with amino groups to form thiourea derivatives, which produce a thiourea-like antithyroid effect. Isothiocyanates also possess intrinsic antithyroid activity as demonstrated by in vitro inhibition of iodide uptake in the case of methyl- and allyl-isothiocyanates and of both iodide uptake and organification in the case of butyl-isothiocyanate (GAITAN et al. 1983; ERMANS and BOURDOUX 1989).

c) Thio-oxazolidone (Goitrin)

The thionamide or thiourea-like goitrogens interfere in the thyroid gland with the organification of iodide and formation of the active thyroid hormones, and their action usually cannot be antagonized by iodine. Naturally occurring goitrin is representative of this category (Fig. 1). Long-term administration of goitrin to rats results in increased thyroid weight and decreased radioactive iodide uptake and hormone synthesis by the thyroid gland (ERMANS and BOURDOUX 1989). The thionamide-like antithyroid effects of goitrin have been confirmed in vitro both by marked inhibition of TPO (GAITAN et al. 1986) and iodide organification (GAITAN et al. 1983). Actually, goitrin possesses 133% of the potency of propylthiouracil in man. Goitrin is unique in that it is not degraded like thioglycosides. Additive antithyroidal effects of thiocyanate, isothiocyanate, and goitrin also occur with combinations of these naturally occurring goitrogens (ERMANS and BOURDOUX 1989).

2. Disulphides

The small aliphatic disulphides (R–S–S–R; R=methyl- ethyl-, *n*-propyl-, phenyl-), the major components of onion and garlic, exert marked thiourea-like antithyroid activity in the rat (GAITAN 1988, 1990; ERMANS and BOURDOUX 1989). *n*-Propyl disulphide also suppresses the radioactive iodine uptake by the thyroid in rats on a low-iodine diet. None of these disulphides inhibits in vitro the TPO enzyme (LINDSAY et al. 1992), but fractions with sulphur-bearing organic compounds, possibly aliphatic disulphides from the goitrogenic well supplying a Colombian district with endemic goitre, inhibited in vitro ^{125}I-organification using thyroid slices (GAITAN et al. 1969; GAITAN 1973).

Disulphides are also present in high concentration (0.3–0.5 g/l) in aqueous effluents from coal-conversion processes and they have also been identified as water contaminants in the United States (GAITAN 1988, 1990; ERMANS and BOURDOUX 1989; LINDSAY et al. 1992). The most frequently isolated compounds in the United States are dimethyl, diethyl, and diphenyl disulphides.

II. Flavonoids

Flavonoids are important stable organic constituents of a wide variety of plants. Flavonoids are universally present in vascular plants and in a large number of food plants. Because of their widespread occurrence in edible plants such as fruits, vegetables, and grains, flavonoids are an integral part of the human diet (HULSE 1980; CODY et al. 1986, 1988; GAITAN 1989a). They are present in high concentrations in polymeric (tannins) and oligomeric (pigments) forms in various staple foods of the Third World, such as millet, sorghum, beans, and groundnuts.

Flavonoids are polyhydroxyphenolic compounds with a C_6-C_3-C_6 structure (CODY et al. 1986; CODY 1989; LINDSAY et al. 1989). Mammalian organisms are unable to synthesize the flavone nucleus. Flavonoids are strictly exogenous food components of exclusively vegetable origin. They have high chemical reactivity with multiple important biological implications (CODY et al. 1986, 1988). Flavonoids are quickly metabolized in higher organisms and that is the reason why they are not found in normal tissue constituents (LINDSAY et al. 1989). Most flavonoids are present as β-glucosides which cannot be absorbed in tissues. No mammalian enzymes have been found which deglycosylate these compounds to their bioactive aglycone species.

Following ingestion by mammals, flavonoid glycosides are hydrolysed by intestinal microbial glycosidases to flavonoid aglycones. These may be absorbed and undergo metabolism by mammalian tissues or be further metabolized by intestinal microorganisms to undergo B-ring hydroxylation and middle ring fission, with production of various metabolic monomeric compounds, including phenolic acids, phloroglucinol, resorcinol, and gallic acid (LINDSAY et al. 1989). Each metabolic step is characterized by a marked increase in antithyroid effects (LINDSAY et al. 1989). Flavonoid aglycones, such as apigenin and luteolin present in Fonio millet (*Digitaria exilis*) (SARTELET et al., in press), and a variety of flavonoid metabolites (phloroglucinol, resorcinol, phenolic acids) are several times more potent than the parent glycosides glucosylvitexin, glucosylorientin and vitexin present in pearl millet (HULSE 1980; GAITAN et al. 1989), as inhibitors of TPO.

This greater inhibitory effect is further enhanced by the additive effects exerted by mixtures of flavonoid aglycones and flavonoid metabolites which are formed after ingestion of mixtures of flavonoid glycosides present in many plant foodstuffs. In addition, these metabolic products may produce adverse effects on other parameters of thyroid function not observed with the glycosides. As a result, the antithyroid effects of flavonoid glycosides in foodstuffs may be greatly enhanced by metabolic alterations after ingestion by mammals, as in the case of the flavonoids present in the pearl millet grain. Furthermore, antithyroid effects in vivo of vitexin, one of the three major flavonoids in this type of millet, have recently been demonstrated (GAITAN et al. 1995), providing direct experimental evidence that C-glycosylflavones are the goitrogens in this cereal grain and that flavonoids are an obligatory step and integral part of the biogeochemical cycle of phenolic goitrogens in nature (GAITAN 1990). It is of interest that a significant portion of the flavonoids isolated by SARTELET et al. (1996) from Fonio millet, the staple food of people living in the severely affected endemic goitre area of Guinea in west Africa, are already present as the aglycones apigenin and luteolin, with more potent antithyroid activity than their parent glycosides, as demonstrated also in their experiments using a porcine thyroid-cell bioassay system.

Flavonoids not only inhibit TPO but, acting on iodothyronine deiodinase enzymes, also inhibit the peripheral metabolism of thyroid hormones. Flavonoids in addition affect serum thyroid hormone binding and TSH regulation. Furthermore, polymers of the flavonoid phloretin interact with TSH, preventing its action at the thyroid cell (CODY et al. 1986, 1988, 1989; GAITAN 1989a). The flavonoid quercetin, an inhibitor of heat shock protein (HSP-70) mRNA, has also been shown to increase iodide uptake in rat FRTL-5 thyroid cells and the quercetin glycoside, rutin, to produce a similar effect in porcine thyroid slices (LINDSAY et al. 1989; ISOSAKI et al. 1993). The isoflavone genistein, a specific tyrosine kinase inhibitor, blocks the epidermal growth factor desensitization of TSH adenylate cyclase "cross-talk" in thyroid cells (TEZELMAN et al. 1993). Finally, SARTELET et al. (1996) found that the flavonoid luteolin depresses the cyclic AMP phosphodiesterase, implying a concomitant overproduction of the TSH-dependent nucleotide. Thus, these experimental observations indicate that this class of compounds alter thyroid hormone economy in a complex manner.

At this point, there is substantial epidemiological and experimental evidence indicating, first, that various millet species used as staple food by populations in the semiarid tropics are rich in flavonoids. Second, that flavonoids have potent and diverse antithyroid properties and, third, that under the appropriate environmental-dietary conditions of low iodine and protein-calorie intakes, which are prevalent in most countries of the Third World, flavonoids become an important aetiological determinant of endemic goitre and hypothyroidism (Osman and Fatah 1981; Eltom et al. 1985; Gaitan 1989a; Gaitan et al. 1989; Gaitan and Dunn 1992; Moreno-Reyes et al. 1993; Konde et al. 1994).

III. Polyhydroxyphenols and Phenol Derivatives

Coal is a source of a large variety of antithyroid and goitrogenic compounds, such as phenol, dihydroxyphenols (resorcinol), substituted dihydroxybenzenes, thiocyanate, disulphides, phthalic acids, pyridines, and halogenated and polycyclic aromatic hydrocarbons (PAHs) (Pitt et al. 1979; Klibanof et al. 1983; Moskowitz et al. 1985; Gaitan 1986, 1988, 1989a, 1990) (Table 1). Most of these compounds have been identified in drinking water from the iodine-sufficient goitrous areas of Kentucky in the United States and Colombia (Gaitan 1986, 1989a). Phenolics are the major organic pollutants in wastewater effluents from various types of coal treatment processes. Resorcinol, substituted resorcinols, and other antithyroid phenolic pollutants are present at levels of as much as 5 g/l in coal-derived effluents. Up to 8% of shale bitumen is also composed of phenols.

Phenol, dihydroxyphenols, trihydroxyphenols, and halogenated phenols are readily absorbed from the gastrointestinal tract and phenol, resorcinol, and catechol, in suitable preparations, are readily absorbed through human skin. Essentially all phenols, polyhydroxyphenols, and halogenated phenols are readily absorbed after injection (Lindsay and Gaitan 1989). A major route of metabolism of polyhydroxyphenols, polydroxyphenolic acids, and halogenated phenols is by conjugation to glucuronic or sulphuric acids. The pattern of conjugation varies with animal species. Although the polyhydroxyphenols and their derivatives, including halogenated dihydroxyphenols, possess more than one hydroxyl group capable of undergoing conjugation, only one group is conjugated. The major route of excretion of these compounds is the urinary tract and various amounts of the free parent compound and its monoglucuronide and monosulphate conjugates are excreted in the urine (Lindsay and Gaitan 1989).

Resorcinol, the prototype of this group of compounds, is antithyroid and goitrogenic both in man and experimental animals (Gaitan 1988, 1989a, 1990). In the early 1950s the goitrogenic effect of resorcinol was demonstrated when patients applying resorcinol ointments for the treatment of varicose ulcers developed goitre and hypothyroidism. Several observations also suggest that resorcinol crosses the human placenta and may cause both goitre and neonatal hypothyroidism (Walfish 1983). Resorcinol has been shown both in vivo and in vitro to inhibit thyroidal organification of iodide (Gaitan 1989a). A comparison of the antiperoxidase activity of resorcinol (1,3-dihydroxybenzene), catechol (1,2-dihydroxybenzene), and hydroquinone (1,4-dihydroxybenzene)

(Table 1) indicates the importance of hydroxyl groups in the meta position for maximal activity (LINDSAY et al. 1992).

Furthermore, the net anti-TPO effects of mixtures of dihydroxyphenols, as well as dihydroxyphenols and thiocyanate, also a coal derived pollutant, are equivalent to or greater than the sum of the effects produced by individual compounds, indicating that the true goitrogenic potential of the major water-soluble compounds present in coal and shales is due to the combined effects of the individual consitutents rather than to any single compound (LINDSAY et al. 1992). Recent demonstration in vivo and in vitro of antithyroid and goitrogenic activities of coal-water extracts from iodine-sufficient goitre areas (GAITAN et al. 1993) indicate that shale- and coal-derived organic pollutants appear to be a major factor contributing to the high goitre prevalence and associated disorders observed in certain areas with aquifers and watersheds rich in these organic rocks (GAITAN 1986, 1988, 1989a, 1990).

Studies of the physical state of organic goitrogens in water indicate that the active compounds form dissociable complexes and that they are part of larger organic molecules, possibly humic substances (HS) (COOKSEY et al. 1985; GAITAN 1988, 1989a, 1990). Furthermore, resorcinol and other parent antithyroid phenolic and phenolic-carboxylic compounds are degradation monomeric by-products of reduction, oxidation, and microbial degradation of HS. HS are high molecular weight complex polymeric compounds and are the principal organic components of soils and waters. More than 90% of total organic matter in water consists of HS, which are also present in coals and shales. Decaying organic matter becomes the substrate of lignin and flavonoid types of HS during the process of fossilization (or coalification). Actually, cyanidin, a naturally occurring flavonol used as the model subunit of flavonoid-type HS, yields by reductive degradation the following antithyroid compounds: resorcinol, phloroglucinol, orcinol, and 3,4-dihydroxybenzoic acid (DHBA) (GAITAN 1988) (Table 1). Demonstration in vivo and in vitro of antithyroid effects of vitexin (GAITAN et al. 1995), a major C-glucosylflavone in pearl millet, provided direct evidence that flavonoid structures are the link for phenolic goitrogens in foodstuffs (e.g., millet) and those present in coals, shales, soils, and water, all of which are an obligatory step and integral part of the biogeochemical cycle of organic-phenolic goitrogens in nature (LINDSAY and GAITAN 1989; GAITAN 1990).

Cigarette smoke, besides thiocyanate, contains a variety of goitrogenic resorcinol derivatives, flavonoids, and hydroxypyridines (GAITAN 1988).

The presence of halogenated organic compounds with known or potential harmful effects has awakened public health and environmental concerns. These compounds are produced by the chlorination of water supplies, sewage, and power plant cooling waters. Present at milligram per liter concentrations (parts per billion) in treated domestic sewage and cooling waters, 4-chlororesorcinol and 3-chloro-4-hydroxybenzoic acid possess antithyroid activities, as inhibitors of TPO and thyroidal iodide organification (GAITAN 1988;

LINDSAY and GAITAN 1989). Whether these pollutants exert additive or synergistic antithyroid effects, and/or act as "triggers" of autoimmune thyroiditis, requires investigation, particularly because more than 60 soluble chloro-organics have been identified in the primary and secondary effluents of typical domestic sewage treatment plants.

Derivatives of 2,4-dinitrophenol (DNP) are widely used in agriculture and industry. An insecticide, herbicide, and fungicide, DNP is also used in the manufacture of dyes, to preserve timber, and as an indicator; it is also a by-product of ozonization of parathion. DNP is readily absorbed through intact skin and respiratory tract. DNP causes toxicity by the uncoupling of oxidative phosphorylation in the mitochondria of cells throughout the body. Administration of 2,4-DNP to human volunteers resulted in rapid and pronounced decline of circulating thyroid hormones. A decrease in TSH secretion results in decreased synthesis and release of thyroxine (T_4) and triodothyronine (T_3), and possibly involution of the thyroid gland. The antithyroid effect of 2,4-DNP is due in part to an inhibition of pituitary TSH secretion. Once T_4 and T_3 are released into the circulation, they are instantaneously bound to serum carrier proteins. DNP also interferes with T_4 binding, further decreasing serum T_4 concentration. In addition to inhibiting TSH and interfering with T_4 binding, DNP also accelerates the disappearance of T_4 from the circulation, and thus the serum concentration is lowered even more (GAITAN 1988; LINDSAY and GAITAN 1989). The public health impact of this pollutant on the thyroid is still unknown.

IV. Pyridines

Hydroxypyridines also occur in aqueous effluents from coal conversion processes, as well as in cigarette smoke (PITT et al. 1979; KLIBANOF et al. 1983; MOSKOWITZ et al. 1985; GAITAN 1986, 1988, 1990; LINDSAY 1989; LINDSAY et al. 1992). Dihydroxypyridines and 3-hydroxypyridine are potent inhibitors of TPO, producing effects comparable to or greater than those of propylthiouracil (LINDSAY et al. 1992). After ingestion, mimosine, a naturally occurring amino acid in the seeds and foliage of the tropical legume *Leucaena leucocephala*, is metabolized to 3,4-dihydroxypyridine (3,4-DHP), a potent antithyroid agent that produces goitre in mice, rats, sheep, and cattle (GAITAN 1988, 1990; LINDSAY 1989). 3,4-DHP crosses the placental barrier, producing goitrous offspring. The phenolic properties of the 3-hydroxy group in various hydroxypyridines are reflected in the metabolism of these compounds in vivo. 3-Hydroxypyridine fed to rabbits is converted to ethereal glucuronide and sulphate conjugates. 3,4-DHP glucuronide and sulphate conjugates account for the majority of 3,4-DHP in the blood of cattle grazing on *Leucaena*. The ring structure of dihydroxypyridines does not appear to be broken down in the body and also appears to be relatively resistant to bacterial degradation (LINDSAY 1989).

V. Phthalate Esters and Metabolites

Phthalic acid esters, or phthalates, are ubiquitous in their distribution and have been frequently identified as water pollutants (PEAKALL 1975; PROCEEDINGS 1982; GAITAN 1988, 1989b, 1990). Dibutyl (DBP) and dioctyl phthalates (DOP) have been isolated from water-supplying areas of endemic goitre in western Colombia and eastern Kentucky in the United States (GAITAN 1986, 1988, 1989a, 1990). Although phthalate esters are most commonly the result of industrial pollution, they also appear naturally in shale, crude oil, petroleum, plants, and fungal metabolites, and as emission pollutants from coal liquefaction plants (PITT et al. 1979; KLIBANOF et al. 1983; MOSKOWITZ et al. 1985; GAITAN 1986, 1988, 1989b, 1990).

Phthalate esters are well absorbed from the gastrointestinal tract. Prior to intestinal absorption there is hydrolysis to the corresponding monoester metabolite. This is particularly true of the longer chain derivatives such as DOP. Phthalates are widely distributed in the body, the liver being the major, initial repository. Clearance from the body is rapid. Short-chain phthalates can be excreted unchanged or following complete hydrolysis to phthalic acid. Prior to excretion most longer-chain compounds are converted, by oxidative metabolism, to polar derivatives of the monoesters. The major route of phthalate esters elimination from the body is urinary excretion (PEAKALL 1975; PROCEEDINGS 1982; GAITAN 1989b).

Phthalate esters are commonly used as plasticizers to impart flexibility to plastics, particularly polyvinylchloride polymers (PVC), which have a wide variety of biomedical and others uses: building and construction, home furnishings, cars, clothing, food wrappings, etc. A small fraction of phthalate esters are used as non-plasticizers for pesticide carriers, oils, and insect repellents. Phthalates may be present in concentrations of up to 40% of the weight of the plastic (PEAKALL 1975; PROCEEDINGS 1982).

Phthalate esters are known to leach out from finished PVC products into blood and physiological solutions. The entry of these plasticizers into a patient's bloodstream during blood transfusion, intravenous fluid administration, or haemodialysis has become a matter of concern among public health officials and the medical community (PEAKALL 1975; PROCEEDINGS 1982; GAITAN 1988, 1989b). A high incidence of goitre in patients receiving maintenance haemodialysis has been reported. Whether phthalate ester metabolites, contaminants in the water entering the patient's bloodstream, or middle molecules (e.g., hydroxybenzoic and vanillic acids), which accumulate in uraemic serum and are poorly removed by haemodialysis, are responsible for this condition remains to be determined (GAITAN 1988, 1989b).

Although phthalate esters and phthalic acids do not possess intrinsic antithyroid activity (Table 1), they undergo degradation by gram-negative bacteria to form DHBA (GAITAN 1988, 1989b, 1990). DHBAs are known to possess antithyroid properties (COOKSEY et al. 1985; GAITAN 1988, 1989b)

(Table 1). The 3,4- and 3,5-DHBAs also inhibit in vitro TPO and the incorporation of iodide into thyroid hormones. The proven effective role of gram-negative bacteria in phthalate biodegradation may explain in part the relationship established between frequency of goitre and bacterial contamination of water supplies (GAITAN et al. 1980; GAITAN 1988, 1989a, 1990). Furthermore, marked ultrastructural changes of the thyroid gland, similar to those seen after administration of TSH, and decreased serum T_4 concentration, have been observed in rats treated with phthalic acid esters (HINTON et al. 1986). Thus, phthalates may become goitrogenic under appropriate conditions; they are also actively concentrated and metabolized by several species of fish. Whether these widely distributed pollutants exert deleterious effects on the thyroids of humans has not been investigated.

VI. Polychlorinated and Polybrominated Biphenyls

Polychlorinated (PCB) and polybrominated (PBB) biphenyls are aromatic compounds containing two benzene nuclei with two or more substituent chlorine or bromine atoms. They have a wide variety of industrial applications, including electric transformers, capacitors, and heat transformers (BUCKLEY 1982; GAITAN 1988; BARSANO 1989).

There is growing evidence that atmospheric transport is the primary mode of global distribution of PCBs from sites of use and disposal (BUCKLEY 1982). Plant foliage accumulates the vapor of PCBs from the atmosphere. In addition to their occurrence in surface water (rivers, lakes, etc.), PCBs have also been detected in drinking water (SAFE DRINKING WATER COMMITTEE 1980). Perhaps the most significant human exposures are limited to individuals consuming freshwater fish from contaminated streams and lakes, and to occupational exposure of industrial workers. PCBs can also be found in the milk of nursing mothers who have eaten large amounts of sport fish or who have been occupationally exposed (SAFE DRINKING WATER COMMITTEE 1980; GAITAN 1988; BARSANO 1989).

PCBs and PBBs have high lipid solubility and resistance to physical degradation. They are slowly metabolized, and their excretion is limited. Long-term low-level exposure to the organohalides results in their gradual accumulation in fat, including the fat of breast milk. PCBs have been found in the adipose tissue of 30%–45% of the general population (SAFE DRINKING WATER COMMITTEE 1980; BARSANO 1989; GAITAN 1992).

The biological and toxicological properties of PCB mixtures may vary depending on their isomeric composition. Oral administration of PCBs to various mammals results in rapid and almost complete (90%) intestinal absorption. The degradation and elimination of PCBs depend on the hepatic microsomal enzyme system (SAFE DRINKING WATER COMMITTEE 1980). The excretion of PCBs is related to the extent of their metabolism. Those with greater chlorine content have a correspondingly longer biological half-life in mammals. This resistance to metabolism is reflected in their deposition in adipose tissue. The PCBs, however, have very low acute toxicity in all animal species tested, and PBBs have biological properties similar to PCBs.

Despite the lack of evidence that dietary PCBs and PBBs have any deleterious effects on health, there is a growing concern and uncertainty about the long-range effects of bioaccumulation and contamination of our ecosystem with these chemicals. The uncertainty extends to the potential harmful effect of these pollutants on the thyroid. For instance, an increased prevalence of primary hypothyroidism (11%) was documented among workers from a plant that manufactured PBBs and PBB oxides (BAHN et al. 1980). These subjects had elevated titres of TPO-microsomal antibodies, indicating that hypothyroidism was probably a manifestation of lymphocytic autoimmune thyroiditis, perhaps a PBB-induced pathogenic autoimmune response or exacerbation of underlying subclinical disease.

PCBs are potent hepatic microsomal enzyme inducers (SAFE DRINKING WATER COMMITTEE 1980; GAITAN 1988; BARSANO 1989). Rats exposed to PCBs exhibit a greatly enhanced biliary excretion of circulating T_4. The T_4 is excreted as a glucuronide which is then lost in the faeces (GAITAN 1988; BARSANO 1989). This response is probably secondary to induction of hepatic microsomal T_4-uridine diphosphate-glucuronyl tranferase. The enhanced peripheral metabolism and reduced binding of T_4 to serum proteins in PCB-treated animals results in markedly decreased serum T_4 concentrations. These low levels stimulate the pituitary-thyroid axis and this eventually results in goitre formation. Although PCB-treated animals exhibit decreased serum T_4, their T_3 levels are unchanged. The relative iodine deficiency brought about by the accelerated metabolism of T_4 may induce increased thyroidal T_3 secretion as well as increased peripheral deiodination of T_4 to T_3. PBBs appear to act similarly to PCBs. There is, however, some indication that they may also interfere directly with the process of hormonal synthesis in the thyroid gland (GAITAN 1988).

VII. Other Organochlorines

DDT (2,2-bis-(*p*-chlorophenyl)-1,1,1-trichloroethane) is polychlorinated and non-degradable. The substance is practically insoluble in water and resistant to destruction by light and oxidation. Its stability has created difficulties in residue removal from water, soil, and foodstuffs. The dominant degradative reaction of DDT is dehydrochlorination to form DDE (2,2-bis-(*p*-chlorophenyl)-1,1-di-chloroethylene), which, like its precursor, has the same low solubility in water and high lipid-water partitioning. This substance is almost undegradable, both biologically and environmentally (SAFE DRINKING WATER COMMITTEE 1977). Dieldrin is one of the cyclodiene insecticides. It is almost insoluble in water and, like DDT and DDE, is very stable, both environmentally and biologically (SAFE DRINKING WATER COMMITTEE 1977).

DDT has been used extensively, both in malaria control and in agriculture, all over the world. Because of biomagnification and persistence, DDT and its breakdown products, DDE and DDD (dichlorodiphenyldichloroethane), are ubiquitous contaminants of water and of virtually every food product. For example, most of the fish from Lake Michigan in North America contain DDT residues. The substance is also present in milk; man is at the top of the food pyramid, so human milk is especially contaminated. The situation is basically similar for dieldrin, which is found in surface waters virtually everywhere. Dieldrin is heavily bioconcentrated in the lipids of terrestrial and aquatic wildlife, humans, and foods, especially animal fats and milk. Global distribution of high concentrations of organochlorines including DDT, DDE, DDD, and dieldrin, were recently found not only in developing countries but also in industrialized countries, which continue to be highly contaminated even though the use of many of these compounds is restricted (SIMONICH and HITES 1995).

DDT is reductively dechlorinated in biological systems to form DDE and DDD. DDE, the predominant residue stored in tissues, reaching about 70% in humans, is much less toxic than DDT. DDE is slowly eliminated from the body; little is known about its degradation pathway. DDT is also slowly eliminated from the human body through reduction to DDD and other more water-soluble derivatives (SAFE DRINKING WATER COMMITTEE 1977; GAITAN 1992).

DDT is known to cause marked alterations in thyroid gland structure, such as thyroid enlargement, follicular epithelial cell hyperplasia, and progressive loss of colloid in birds, and DDD causes goitre and increased hepatobiliary excretion of thyroid hormones in rats (BARSANO 1989). All these compounds (DDT, DDE, DDD, and dieldrin) induce microsomal enzyme activity that may affect thyroid hormone metabolism in a similar way to that of the polyhalogenated biphenyls and PAH (ROGAN et al. 1980; GAITAN 1988). The impact of these pollutants on the human thyroid is unknown.

Dioxin (tetrachlorodibenzodioxin – TCDD), one of the most toxic small organic molecules, is a contaminant in the manufacturing process of several pesticides and herbicides, including Agent Orange. Also a potent inducer of hepatic microsomal enzymes, TCDD markedly enhances the metabolism and biliary excretion of T_4-glucuronide (GAITAN 1988; BARSANO 1989). Rats treated with TCDD concomitantly develop hypothyroxinaemia, increased serum TSH concentrations, and goitre, probably as a result of T_4 loss in the bile (GAITAN 1988). The impact on the thyroid of humans exposed to this agent is unknown, and evaluation of thyroid gland function and studies of thyroid hormone metabolism are necessary in those affected.

VIII. Polycyclic Aromatic Hydrocarbons

Polycyclic aromatic hydrocarbons (PAHs) have been found repeatedly in food and domestic water supplies, and in industrial and municipal waste effluents (SAFE DRINKING WATER COMMITTEE 1977; GAITAN 1988, 1990; BARSANO 1989). They also occur naturally in coal, soils, ground water and surface water, and in their sediments and biota. One of the most potent of the carcinogenic PAH compounds, 3,4-benzpyrene (BaP), is widely distributed and, as in the case of other PAHs, is not efficiently removed by conventional water treatment processes.

The PAH carcinogens, BaP and 3-methylcolanthrene (MCA), accelerate T_4 metabolism and excretion of T_4-glucuronide by enhancement of hepatic UDP-glucuronyltransferase and glucuronidation, resulting in decreased serum T_4 concentrations, activation of the pituitary-thyroid axis, and eventually goitre formation (GAITAN 1988, 1990; BARSANO 1989). There is also indication that MCA interferes directly with the process of hormonal synthesis in the thyroid gland. Furthermore, MCA, as well as 7,12-dimethylbenzanthracene, also induces goitrous thyroiditis in the BUF strain rat (WEETMAN and MCGREGOR 1994). Thus, MCA exerts its deleterious effects on the thyroid gland by at least three different mechanisms. Finally, the coal-derived PAH methylanthracene (MA), which has been identified in drinking water from the goitrous coal-rich district of eastern Kentucky in the United States (GAITAN 1986, 1989a, 1990), was found to produce goitre in the BUF rat without alteration of hormone synthesis or lymphocytic infiltration of the thyroid gland (GAITAN 1990).

References

Bahn AK, Mills JL, Synder PJ, Gann PH, Houten L, Bialik O, Hollmann L, Utiger RD (1980) Hypothyroidism in workers exposed to polybrominated biphenyls. N Engl J Med 302:31–33

Barsano CP (1989) Polyhalogenated and polycyclic aromatic hydrocarbons. In: Gaitan E (ed) Environmental goitrogenesis. CRC, Boca Raton, p 115

Buckley EH (1982) Accumulation of airborne polychlorinated biphenyls in foliage. Science 216:520–522

Chanoine JP, Toppet V, Bourdoux P, Spehl M, Delange F (1991) Smoking during pregnancy: a significant cause of neonatal thyroid enlargement. Br J Obstet Gynaecol 98:65–68

Cody V (1989) Physical and conformational properties of flavonoids. In: Gaitan E (ed) Environmental goitrogenesis. CRC, Boca Raton, p 35

Cody V, Middleton E Jr, Harborne JB (eds) (1986) Plant flavonoids in biology and medicine: biochemical, pharmacological and structure-activity relationships. Liss, New York

Cody V, Middleton E Jr, Harborne JB, Beretz A (eds) (1988) Plant flavonoids in biology and medicine II: biochemical, cellular and medicinal properties. Liss, New York

Cody V, Koehrle J, Hesch RD (1989) Structure-activity relationships of flavonoids as inhibitors of iodothyronine deiodinase. In: Gaitan E (ed) Environmental goitrogenesis. CRC, Boca Raton, p 57

Cooksey RC, Gaitan E, Lindsay RH, Hill JB, Kelly K (1985) Humic substances: a possible source of environmental goitrogens. Org Geochem 8:77–80

Delange R, Ahluwalia R (eds) (1983) Cassava toxicity and thyroid: research and public health issues. IDRC-207e. International Development Research Centre, Ottawa

Delange F (1989) Cassava and the thyroid. In: Gaitan E (ed) Environmental goitrogenesis. CRC, Boca Raton, p 173

Dumont JE, Maenhaut C, Pirson I, Baptist M, Roger PP (1991) Growth factors controlling the thyroid gland. Balliere Clin Endocrinol Metab 5:727–754
Dumont JE, Lamy F, Roger P, Maenhaut C (1992) Physiological and pathological regulation of thyroid cell proliferation and differentiation by thyrotropin and other factors. Physiol Rev 72:667–697
Eltom M, Salih MAM, Bastrom H, Dahlberg PA (1985) Differences in aetiology and thyroid function in endemic goitre between rural and urban areas of the Darfur region of the Sudan. Acta Endocrinol (Copenh) 108:356–360
Ermans AM, Bourdoux P (1989) Antithyroid sulfurated compounds. In: Gaitan E (ed) Environmental goitrogenesis. CRC, Boca Raton, p 15
Ermans AM, Mbulamoko NB, Delange F, Ahluwalia R (eds) (1980) Role of cassava in the etiology of endemic goiter and cretinism, IDRC-136e. International Development Research Centre, Ottawa
Gaitan E (1973) Water-borne goitrogens and their role in the etiology of endemic goiter. World Rev Nutr Diet 17:53–90
Gaitan E (1986) Thyroid disorders: possible role of environmental pollutants and naturally occurring agents. Am Chem Soc Div Environ Chem 26:58–85
Gaitan E (1988) Goitrogens. Bailliere Clin Endocrinol Metab 2:683–702
Gaitan E (ed) (1989a) Environmental goitrogenesis. CRC, Boca Raton
Gaitan E (1989b) Phthalate esters and phthalic acid derivatives. In: Gaitan E (ed) Environmental goitrogenesis. CRC, Boca Raton, p 107
Gaitan E (1990) Goitrogens in food and water. Annu Rev Nutr 10:21–39
Gaitan E (1992) Disorders of the thyroid. In: Tarcher AB (ed) Principles and practice of environmental medicine. Plenum Medical Book, New York, pp 371–387
Gaitan E, Dunn JT (1992) Epidemiology of iodine deficiency. Trends Endocrinol Metab 3:170–175
Gaitan E, Island DP, Liddle GW (1969) Identification of a naturally occurring goitrogen in water. Trans Assoc Am Physicians 82:141–152
Gaitan E, Medina, P, DeRouen TA, Zia MS (1980) Goiter prevalence and bacterial contamination of water supplies. J Clin Endocrinol Metab 51:957–961
Gaitan E, Cooksey RC, Matthews D, Presson R (1983) In vitro measurement of antithyroid compounds and environmental goitrogens. J Clin Endocrinol Metab 56:767–773
Gaitan E, Cooksey RC, Lindsay RH (1986) Factors other than iodine deficiency in endemic goiter: goitrogens and protein calorie malnutrition. In: Dunn JT, Pretell EA, Daza CH, Viteri FE (eds) Towards the eradication of endemic goiter, cretinism and iodine deficiency. Pan Am Health Org (Wash) 502:28–45
Gaitan E, Lindsay RH, Reichert RD, Ingbar SH, Cooksey RC, Legan J, Meydrech EF, Hill J, Kubota K (1989) Antithyroid and goitrogenic effects of millet: role of C-glycosylflavones. J Clin Endocrinol Metab 68:707–714
Gaitan E, Nelson NC, Poole GV (1991) Endemic goiter and endemic thyroid disorders. World J Surg 15:205–215
Gaitan E, Cooksey RC, Legan K, Cruse JM, Lindsay RH, Hill J (1993) Antithyroid and goitrogenic effects of coal-water extracts from iodine-sufficient goiter areas. Thyroid 3:49–53
Gaitan E, Cooksey RC, Legan J, Lindsay RH (1995) Antithyroid effects in vivo and in vitro of vitexin: a C-glucosylflavone in millet. J Clin Endocrinol Metab 80:1144–1147
Hinton RH, Mitchell FE, Mann A, Chescoe D, Price SC (1986) Effects of phthalic acid ester on liver and thyroid. Environ Health Perspect 70:195–210
Hulse JH (ed) (1980) Polyphenols in cereals and legumes. IDRC-145e, Int Dev Res Cent, Ottawa
Isozaki O, Emoto N, Miyakawa M, Sato Y et al (1993) Heat shock protein (HSP) regulation of iodide uptake in rat FRTL-5 thyroid cells. Thyroid [Suppl] 3:T-78
Klibanof AM, Tu T, Scott KP (1983) Peroxidase-catalyzed removal of phenols from coal conversion waste waters. Science 221:259–261

Konde M, Ingenbleek Y, Daffe M, Sylla B, Barry O, Diallo S (1994) Goitrous endemic in Guinea. Lancet 344:1675–1678
Lindsay RH (1989) Hydroxypyridines. In: Gaitan E (ed) Environmental goitrogenesis. CRC, Boca Raton, p 97
Lindsay RH, Gaitan E (1989) Polyhydroxyphenols and phenol derivatives. In: Gaitan E (ed) Environmental goitrogenesis. CRC, Boca Raton, p 73
Lindsay RH, Gaitan E, Cooksey RC (1989) Pharmacokinetics and intrathyroidal effects of flavonoids. In: Gaitan E (ed) Environmental goitrogenesis. CRC, Boca Raton, p 43
Lindsay RH, Hill JB, Gaitan E, Cooksey RC, Jolley RL (1992) Antithyroid effects of coal-derived pollutants. J Toxicol Environ Health 37:467–481
Moreno-Reyes R, Boelaert M, El Badwi S, Eltom M, Vanderpas JB (1993) Endemic juvenile hypothyroidism in a severe endemic goitre area of Sudan. Clin Endocrinol (Oxf) 38:19–24
Moskowitz PD, Morris SC, Fisher H, Thode HD Jr, Hamilton LD (1985) Synthetic fuel plants: potential tumor risks to public health. Risk Anal 5:181–193
Osman AK, Fatah AA (1981) Factors other than iodine deficiency contributing to the endemicity of goitre in Darfur province (Sudan). J Hum Nutr 35:302–309
Peakall DB (1975) Phthalate esters: occurrence and biological effects. Residue Rev 54:1–41
Pitt WW, Jolley RL, Jones G (1979) Characterization of organics in aqueous effluents of coal-conversion plants. Environ Int 2:167–171
Kluwe WM (1982) Proceedings of the conference on phthalates, Washington DC, June 9–11, 1981. Environ Health Perspect 45:1–156
Rogan WJ, Bagniewska A, Damstra T (1980) Pollutants in breast milk. N Engl J Med 30:1450–1453
Roti E, Grundi A, Braverman, LE (1983) The placental transport, synthesis and metabolism of hormones and drugs which affect thyroid function. Endocr Rev 4:131–149
Safe Drinking Water Committee (1977) Drinking water and health. National Academy Press, Washington DC
Safe Drinking Water Committee (1980) Drinking water and health, vol 3. National Academy Press, Washington DC
Sartelet H, Serghat S, Lobstein A, Ingenbleek Y, Anton R, Petitfrere E, Aguie-Aguie G, Martin L, Haye B (1996) Flavonoids extracted from Fonio millet (Digitaria exilis) reveal potent antithyroid properties. Nutrition 12:100–106
Simonich SL, Hites RA (1995) Global distribution of persistent organochlorine compounds. Science 269:1851–1854
Tezelman S, Siperstein AE, Duh QY, Clark OH (1993) Crosstalk between epidermal growth factor and thyrotropin induced desensitization of adenylate cyclase in human neoplastic thyroid cells, Thyroid [Suppl] 3:T-79
Walfish PG (1983) Drug and environmentally induced neonatal hypothyroidism. In: Dussault JH, Walker P (eds) Congenital hypothyroidism. Dekker, New York, pp 303–316
Weetman AP, McGregor AM (1994) Autoimmune thyroid disease: further developments in our understanding. Endocr Rev 15:788–830
Wenzel BE, Bottazzo GF (eds) (1987) Advances in thyroidology: cell and immunobiological aspects: thyroid cell growth. Acta Endocrinol (Copenh) [Suppl] 281: 215–301

CHAPTER 13

Thyroid Hormone Antagonism

J.W. BARLOW, T.C. CROWE, and D.J. TOPLISS

A. Introduction

The development of hormone antagonists, or compounds which can reverse the physiological effects of hormone hypersecretion, has been a desirable and achievable goal for many small molecular weight hormones. The spectacular successes achieved with hormone antagonists such as spironolactone, RU-486 and cimetidine have stimulated pharmacologists and pharmaceutical companies to use similar strategies in the search for an antagonist to thyroid hormone. For the most part the development of steroid hormone antagonists followed a classical chemical synthetic route; systematic modifications either to the ring structure or to side chains of the steroid were carried out, the new compounds were tested in a hormone bioassay ultimately leading to clinical trials, and subsequently effective compounds were applied in clinical practice. Consequently, there is now a range of compounds which are safely able to inhibit the actions of mineralocorticoids, glucocorticoids, androgens and progestagens and which have extensive clinical utility. These compounds are also remarkably useful tools which can be used to understand the molecular mechanisms of steroid hormone action in the laboratory.

In marked contrast, the same approach for thyroid hormone (T_3) has been almost entirely unsuccessful. Despite the design and synthesis of a large variety of compounds structurally analogous to T_3, few of them are able to modulate the activity of the parent compound and none has yet had clinical application or is a useful tool for in vitro analysis.

There are two main reasons for this lack of success. First, the mechanism of action of T_3 is not the same as that of steroid hormones. Even though T_3 induces changes in gene transcription in a manner which is broadly similar to that for steroids, there are some fundamental differences in the interactions of T_3 with cell-associated proteins in comparison with steroids. Second, T_3 does not have a unique action. While most hormones have a range of cellular effects, their initial discovery and characterisation historically occurred because of induction of a primary recognisable cellular response. T_3, however, probably affects every tissue in the body at some stage between embryogenesis and senescence and for many tissues it induces multiple and apparently contrasting responses. In hypothyroid rat liver, for example, as many as 20 mRNAs have been shown to respond to T_3 administration (SEELIG et al.

1981). Responses can be positive, negative or biphasic and none has yet been defined as uniquely associated with this hormone.

In the absence of a T_3 antagonist, current treatment of thyroid hormone hypersecretion is targeted at the gland rather than at the peripheral tissue level (WARTOFSKY 1993). This treatment is often less than optimal, with many patients progressing to surgery. Accordingly, the development of a new class of compounds with anti-T_3 activity or compounds which can modulate hormone activity is a desirable, if elusive, goal. The potential sites of action of such compounds are distributed throughout the cell although the most likely areas are those concerned with intracellular transport and regulation of transcription. These include plasma membrane uptake mechanisms, cytoplasmic binding proteins and hormone receptors. In this review we will consider each of these sites and the possibilities that physiological or pharmacological manipulations of each of them could lead to modulation of T_3 responsiveness.

B. Inhibition of Uptake

I. Mechanisms of Cell Entry

Given the heterogeneity of responses to T_3, perhaps the ideal T_3 antagonist would be one which can prevent access of T_3 to the transcriptional machinery by blocking entry of the hormone into cells. However, the mechanism of cellular entry of thyroid hormones is still the subject of some controversy and while the view that hormone entry is by simple diffusion (WEISIGER et al. 1992) has largely been superseded by the concept of specific uptake mechanisms, detailed understanding of the exact nature of these mechanisms has remained obscure.

Carrier-mediated uptake systems for thyroid hormones have been clearly demonstrated using a perfused isolated rat liver model (for review see KRENNING and DOCTOR 1986), which can differentiate between transport into the liver and subsequent metabolism. Transport can be reduced by reduction of hepatic ATP with fructose, an effect which can be reversed by addition of insulin and glucose, suggesting that cell entry is an energy-dependent process (DE JONG et al. 1992). Other experiments in primary hepatocytes (KRENNING et al. 1981) or thymocytes (CENTANNI et al. 1991) suggest uptake is not only energy dependent but is also sodium dependent, sensitive to metabolic inhibitors such as potassium cyanide and to the concentration of extracellular sodium. Others have found uptake to be energy sensitive but have not been able to confirm sensitivity to extracellular sodium concentrations. For example, the substitution of *N*-methyl glucamine for sodium did not affect uptake in primary (BLONDEAU et al. 1988) or cultured rat liver cells (TOPLISS et al. 1989). Similar sodium independent uptake has also been observed in erythrocytes (OSTY et al. 1988a), astrocytes (BLONDEAU et al. 1993) and choriocarcinoma cells (MITCHELL et al. 1992a,b).

These differences in uptake may relate to cell type or cell culture conditions or they may reflect the heterogeneous nature of T_3 entry into cells. In thymocytes, sodium increased uptake of T_3, but not T_4, by about 40%, suggesting a degree of heterogeneity in the uptake site. Part of the problem is that the majority of studies have assumed that membrane uptake shows a specificity for T_3 rather than T_4. Certainly, cell culture experiments suggest this to be the case, although differential studies of a separate T_4 uptake site using sodium sensitivity to diminish the involvement of T_3 uptake have not been pursued. In erythrocytes, T_3 uptake is closely related to the system T amino acid uptake system (ZHOU et al. 1992) but in astrocytes (BLONDEAU et al. 1993) and neuroblastoma cells (LAKSHMANAN et al. 1990) system L amino acids inhibit uptake. Some of the characteristics of sodium-independent thyroid hormone uptake sites are summarised in Table 1. In essence, T_3 is taken up by cells by a mechanism which exhibits low affinity and which cross-reacts with amino acid uptake. Both of these features are compatible with a generalised uptake system which has broad specificity for a range of cellular regulatory factors. Sodium-dependent uptake, demonstrated in liver (KRENNING et al. 1981), muscle (CENTANNI and ROBBINS 1987) and pituitary cells (EVERTS et al. 1993), is less well defined although it may bind more hormone at lower T_3 concentrations than the sodium-independent site (EVERTS et al. 1993).

II. Purification of Membrane-Binding Sites

A major stumbling block in the definitive characterisation of the mechanism of cell entry of T_3 has been the inability to purify the uptake site by conventional techniques. Affinity labelling studies suggest that membrane-associated proteins which bind T_4 or T_3 are less heterogeneous than either cytosolic or nuclear proteins and are of the order of 44–64 kDa in molecular size (DOZIN et al. 1985; ANGEL et al. 1990). While there appears to be no relationship between

Table 1. Characteristics of sodium-independent T_3 uptake systems in primary and cultured mammalian cells. The affinity, expressed as K_t, is the concentration of T_3 required for half-maximal uptake over a given period of time

Tissue	Molecular weight	Affinity, K_t	Amino acid cross-reactivity	References
Rat erythrocytes	50, 65	130 nM, 220 pM, 36 pM	System T	ZHOU et al. 1992 ANGEL et al. 1990 OSTY et al. 1988
Rat hepatocytes	30, 44, 70	680 nM, 340 nM	System T	TOPLISS et al. 1989 BLONDEAU et al. 1988 DOZIN et al. 1986
Rat astrocytes		~2 μM	System L	BLONDEAU et al. 1993
Mouse neuroblastoma cells	48, 53, 58	136 nM, 119 pM	System L	LAKSHMANAN et al. 1990 GONCALVES et al. 1990
Human choriocarcinoma cells		586–755 nM	Neither system L nor system T	PRASAD et al. 1994 MITCHELL et al. 1992a,b

proteins in these three compartments in liver (DOZIN et al. 1985), the cellular distribution of these proteins may be cell specific. Antibodies raised against a predominantly plasma membrane fraction from A431 cells localised a 55-kDa protein to the endoplasmic reticulum and nuclear envelope rather than the plasma membrane (CHENG et al. 1986). Furthermore, hormone-binding profiles of membrane-bound proteins either in the crude (BARLOW et al. 1991) or semipurified (GONCALVES et al. 1990; ANGEL et al. 1990) states show poor reproducibility and are not consistent with a single class of saturable binding sites.

Even without purification and detailed biochemical characterisation of a plasma membrane T_3-binding site, hormone uptake is a critical physiological event and can be inhibited by a range of compounds.

III. Inhibition of Uptake

Uptake of $[^{125}I]T_3$ can be inhibited by hormone analogues with a clear preference being shown for unlabelled T_3. Triac, T_4 and a range of other analogues are approximately 10- to 100-fold less potent (BLONDEAU et al. 1988; TOPLISS et al. 1989). A surprising array of other compounds is also able to inhibit uptake (Table 2). Some of these compounds give clues as to the nature of the uptake site, particularly with regard to uptake inhibition by amino acids. Other compounds, such as the inhibitor of glucose transport, phloretin, probably inhibit uptake because of structural similarities to T_3, rather than through inhibition of glucose transport (MOVIUS et al. 1989).

Table 2. Some chemical inhibitors of T_3 uptake in mammalian cells (from BLONDEAU et al. 1988, 1993; KRAGIE and DOYLE 1992; LAKSHMANAN et al. 1990; MOVIUS et al. 1989; PRASAD et al. 1994; TOPLISS et al. 1989, 1993; ZHOU et al. 1992)

Amino acids	**Naphthalene sulphonamides (calmodulin antagonists)**
Leucine	Calmidazolium
Phenylalanine	Trifluoperazine
Tryptophan	W7, W12, W13
Benzodiazepines	**Non-bile acid cholephils**
Lormetazepam	Bromosulphthalein
Triazolam	Iopanoic acid
Ro5 4864	Indocyanine green
Diazepam	**Non-steroidal anti-inflammatory drugs**
Calcium channel blockers	Diclofenac
Diltiazem	Fenclofenac
Nifedipine	Flufenamic acid
Verapamil	Meclofenamic acid
Inhibitors of receptor-mediated endocytosis	Mefenamic acid
Chloroquine	**Other**
Monodansylcadaverine	Phenytoin
	Phloretin

Similarly, benzodiazepines are able to inhibit uptake because of structural homology to T_3 and independently of benzodiazepine receptors (KRAGIE and DOYLE 1992).

Uptake may involve calcium. Benzodiazepines affect mitochondrial calcium dynamics and T_3 uptake can be blocked by calcium channel blockers and by calmodulin antagonists (TOPLISS et al. 1993). Studies with the rat hepatoma cell line H4 also showed that compounds such as non-bile acid cholephils inhibited T_3 uptake, with almost complete inhibition being achieved with iopanoic acid or indocyanine green at 0.1 m*M* (TOPLISS et al. 1988). Phenytoin inhibits uptake at concentrations similar to those found therapeutically. These studies were performed in serum-free medium, but since this drug is extensively bound to serum proteins the pharmacological significance of the membrane interaction is yet to be established.

Surprisingly, non-steroidal anti-inflammatory drugs (NSAIDs) are also potent inhibitors of uptake and although the same serum binding considerations for phenytoin apply to this class of drug, they can be used to define the characteristics of the ligand which determine cell entry. For this study we used a series of synthetic phenylanthranilic acids, and found that inhibition of uptake was highly dependent on hydrophobicity of the ligand. There was a parabolic relationship between uptake and the calculated ethanol-water partition coefficient, which was independent of size and position of substitution (CHALMERS et al. 1993). These studies included the clinically important NSAIDs flufenamic acid, meclofenamic acid and mefenamic acid, and potentially may lead to the design of compounds with higher affinity for the uptake site.

IV. Uptake Inhibition and Hormone Responsiveness

It is not yet clear whether inhibition of uptake leads to alterations in hormone responsiveness. Impaired T_3 production by perfused livers from fasted rats is associated with diminished T_4 uptake (JENNINGS et al. 1979) but caloric restriction also reduces 5′-deodinase activity (DOCTOR et al. 1993). Which effect predominates is unclear. Good evidence that agents which block uptake also prevent intracellular accumulation of the hormone comes from studies using hepatocytes and human serum taken from individuals with non-thyroidal illness. In experiments which carefully preserved the correct ligand-serum binding relationship, LIM et al. (1993a) showed that uptake was inhibited up to 42% by sera from critically ill patients. These sera contained elevated concentrations of bilirubin, oleic acid, a furan fatty acid or indoxyl sulphate. Importantly, uptake measured in terms of iodide production was also inhibited when these compounds were added to normal serum, which suggests that exposure of T_4 to the intracellular deiodinase was prevented (LIM et al. 1993b). Thus, compounds which decrease uptake also decrease intracellular accumulation although whether hormone responsiveness is also influenced is not known.

C. Cytoplasmic Binding

I. Role of Cytoplasmic Binding

Thyroid hormone-binding proteins (CTBPs) in the cytoplasm of mammalian cells have been observed for almost 40 years, but as yet there is no consensus concerning their identity or their role in mediating thyroid hormone responsiveness. The simplest interpretation is that CTBPs are the intracellular equivalent of serum-binding proteins and have a pivotal role in hormone transport. Given that T_3 partitions into phospholipid membranes in preference to aqueous media by about 20000 to 1 (HILLIER 1970), CTBPs must have at least some role in keeping T_3 and T_4 in the aqueous phase, thereby maintaining intracellular free hormone concentrations. Whether they have other functions and whether blocking these functions has an effect on a thyroid response is largely unknown.

Multiple forms of CTBP have been identified in cytosols of liver (DOZIN et al. 1985), heart (OSTY et al. 1988b), kidney (HASHIZUME et al. 1989a,b), brain (LENNON 1992) erythrocytes (FANJUL and FARIAS 1991) and a number of cultured cell lines. Photoaffinity labelling studies have shown that these proteins, at least in liver, are different from membrane or nuclear binding sites and have molecular weights between 30 and 70kDa (DOZIN et al. 1985).

Of all the cellular proteins which bind thyroid hormones, those localised between the membrane and nucleus seem to be the most heterogeneous, and their hormone-binding capacity is perhaps secondary to their primary role. Thus, binding has been observed to protein disulphide isomerase (OBATA et al. 1988), pyruvate kinase (KATO et al. 1989), glutathione-*S*-transferases (ISHIGAKI et al. 1989) and haemoglobin (SAKATA et al. 1990). In addition, binding may be regulated by cofactors in vitro which may influence responsiveness in vivo. For example, in rat kidney, a 58-kDa protein binds T_3 with moderate affinity and acts as a hormone reservoir in the presence of NADPH to prevent nuclear binding (HASHIZUME et al. 1989b). Upon addition of NADP, the protein facilitates the uptake of T_3 from cytoplasm to nucleus in vitro in cell culture (HASHIZUME et al. 1989c). Whether the ratio of NADPH to NADP subsequently affects T_3-induced gene transcription has not been tested.

In human epidermoid carcinoma A431 cells, a similar 58-kDa binding protein has been observed which is a monomer of pyruvate kinase subtype M_2 (KATO et al. 1989; PARKISON et al. 1991). This enzyme exists in two forms, either as a monomeric protein designated as p58-M_2 or as a tetrameric form called PKM_2. It is attractive as a cytosolic binding protein because of its wide tissue distribution (ASHIZAWA et al. 1991). It is an important glycolytic enzyme and its activity is affected by fructose 1,6-bisphosphate, which causes monomeric p-58M_2 to form tetrameric PKM_2. Monomeric p-58M_2 binds T_3 whereas the tetrameric form does not. ASHIZAWA and CHENG (1992) found that the response to T_3 of a reporter gene construct was in inverse proportion to the intracellular concentration of monomeric p-58M_2 (Fig. 1). They hypothesised

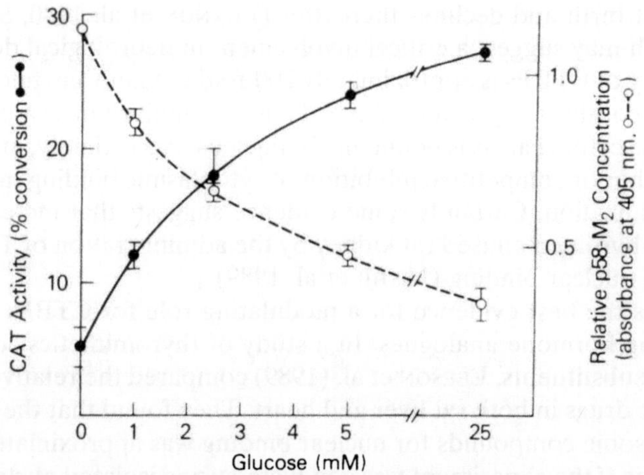

Fig. 1. Reciprocal relationship between p58-M_2 (*open circles*) and T_3-dependent transcription (*closed circles*) in JEG-3 cells. The intracellular concentration of monomeric p58-M_2, which binds T_3, was depleted with fructose 1,6-bisphosphate via addition of glucose. As a result the intracellular binding protein was reduced, allowing intracellular free T_3 to increase. Accordingly, transcriptional activation by T_3 also increased. (From Ashizawa and Cheng 1992b, with permission)

that by increasing levels of monomeric p-58M_2, intracellular binding increases, resulting in a reduction in intracellular free T_3 concentrations, rendering the hormone less available to nuclear receptors (Ashizawa and Cheng 1992). The hypothesis is supported by the observation that pyruvate kinase subtype R fulfils a similar role in human erythrocytes but that the ratio of monomer to tetramer is controlled by ATP in addition to fructose 1,6-bisphosphate (Fanjul and Farias 1993).

Interestingly, reduced transcription of the reporter gene by raised cytoplasmic concentrations of pyruvate kinase monomer could be overcome by very high concentrations of T_3, consistent with the role of CTBPs as a storage or transport protein. Furthermore, reporter gene responsiveness to Triac was not influenced by factors which altered monomer concentrations, suggesting the involvement of multiple CTBPs, some of which are sensitive to the ratio of monomer to tetramer, but some of which are not.

II. Cytoplasmic Binding and Hormone Responsiveness

Despite these observations in cultured cells, it is not yet known whether CTBPs have a role in mammalian tissues or whether physiological or pharmacological manipulations can influence a hormone response. The cellular concentration of the NADPH-dependent form corresponds approximately with tissue responsiveness to thyroid hormone, being highest in tissues such as heart, liver and kidney and lowest in testis and spleen (Suzuki et al. 1991). Levels tend to be low at birth and rise with age, although in the brain, binding is highest at birth and declines thereafter (Lennon et al. 1980; Suzuki et al. 1991), which may suggest a critical involvement in neurological development. The capacity of CTBPs is approximately 200-fold greater than nuclear binding sites and of considerably lower affinity. Thus, at equilibrium as much T_3 will be bound in the cytoplasm as is bound in the nucleus. Accordingly, modulation of CTBP number or competitive inhibition of cytoplasmic binding may influence nuclear localization. Certainly some evidence suggests that increasing CTBP number in thyroidectomised rat kidney by the administration of T_4 results in a decrease in nuclear binding (Nishii et al. 1989).

Perhaps the best evidence for a modulating role for CTBPs comes from studies using hormone analogues. In a study of thyromimetics containing 3′-arylmethyl substituents, Leeson et al. (1989) compared the relative potency of 33 synthetic drugs in both rat liver and heart. They found that the competitive potency of some compounds for nuclear binding was approximately the same in each tissue if the experiment was conducted using isolated nuclei. However, when the potency of these compounds was assessed in vivo after intramuscular injection, they were at least tenfold more potent in liver than in heart. One compound in particular, SKF-94901, was about 50% as active as T_3 in liver nuclear receptor binding in vivo but only 1% as active in vitro and had nearly 200 times more enzyme-inducing activity in liver than in heart (Fig. 2; Underwood et al. 1986). The difference between in vitro and in vivo activity can be adequately explained by the fact that SKF 94901 has a low affinity for

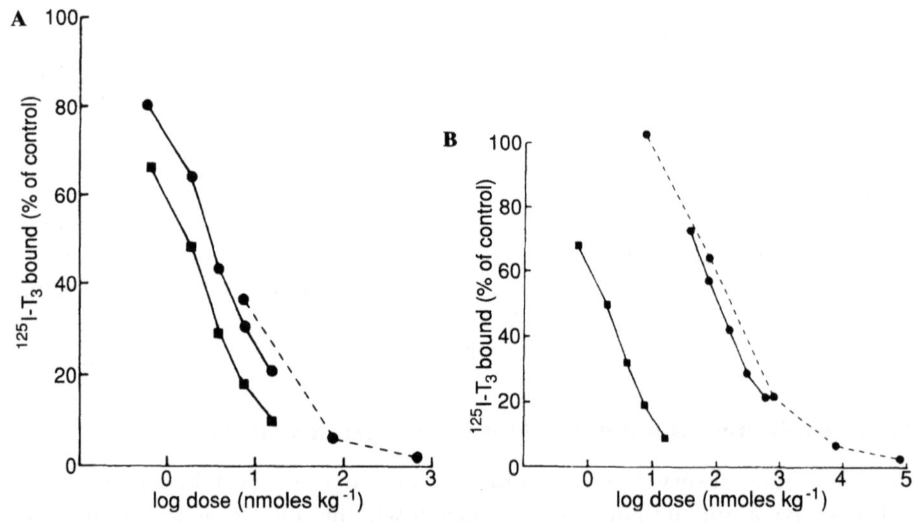

Fig. 2A,B. Competition of T_3 and the analogue SKF-94901 with [^{125}I]T_3 for occupation of nuclear receptors in vivo in hepatic nuclei (*left panel*) or cardiac nuclei (*right panel*). Potency of unlabelled T_3 was approximately the same in each tissue but SKF-94901 was at least 30-fold less potent in cardiac nuclei than in hepatic nuclei, despite being equipotent in competition studies in vitro. (From Underwood et al. 1986, with permission)

serum proteins, which results in a free fraction of approximately 4% (Barlow et al. 1989).

Despite the fact that different forms of T_3 receptors are expressed in liver and heart, the selectively of SKF-94901 appears not to depend on receptor recognition but rather on penetration or access to the nucleus in vivo (Underwood et al. 1986; Leeson et al. 1989). This conclusion is supported by studies using cultured cells in which the apparent competitive potency of SKF-94901 for nuclear binding sites was greater in nuclear extract than in whole cells studied under identical conditions (Barlow et al. 1989). To determine which cellular compartment is responsible for this affinity difference in normal tissues, the competitive potency of SKF-94901 was examined in three tissue extracts: membranes, cytosol and nuclei, from mammalian heart and liver. While no difference in relative potency was found with membrane preparations or nuclear extracts between the two tissues, SKF-94901 was tenfold more potent in relation to T_3 in cytoplasmic extracts from liver than from heart (Barlow et al. 1991). These binding studies are entirely consistent with the concept that tissue selectivity of these analogues is conferred at an extranuclear site, probably in the cytoplasm. On the basis of their selective activity, these analogues have been proposed as agents which could be used therapeutically to lower cholesterol without having adverse thyromimetic effects (Underwood et al. 1986).

III. Pharmacological Antagonism of Cytoplasmic Binding

While the foregoing information suggests a pivotal role for CTBP in tissue-specific transport of T_3 to the nucleus, there are as yet no descriptions of pharmacological interference with these sites resulting in antagonism of a T_3 effect. In an extension of earlier serum binding studies in which we examined a range of compounds for binding to thyroxine-binding globulin and transthyretin, we studied the same compounds for their competitive potency at the cytoplasmic level. The drugs were chosen as representative of non-steroidal anti-inflammatory agents, non-esterified fatty acids and non-bile acid cholephils and amiodarone, frusemide and EMD 21388.

None of the drugs was of sufficient potency to be considered as a T_3 antagonist, however, one agent, diclofenac, was considerably more potent as a cytoplasmic competitor than as a nuclear competitor. Subsequently, we tested this compound for its ability to influence a T_3-induced response. In human hepatoma cells, diclofenac promoted the efflux of T_3 from pre-labelled cells and inhibited T_3 stimulation of the mRNA of an endogenous gene (Barlow et al. 1996).

While the results with diclofenac are encouraging, the effect was only achieved at free drug concentrations which were suprapharmacological and although the use of the drug may indicate a mechanism, the concentrations needed to achieve an effect preclude any clinical utility. The other potential cytoplasmic antagonist, SKF-94901, has wide-ranging and probably lethal ef-

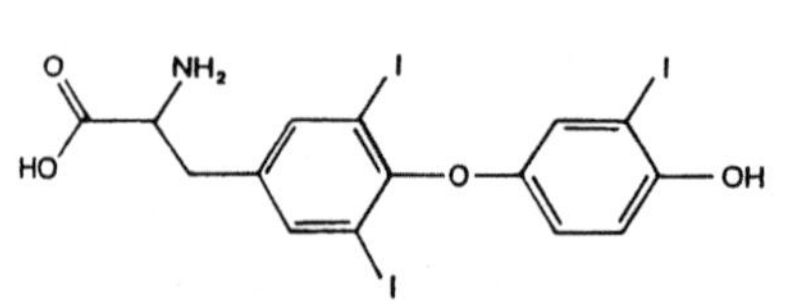

1.

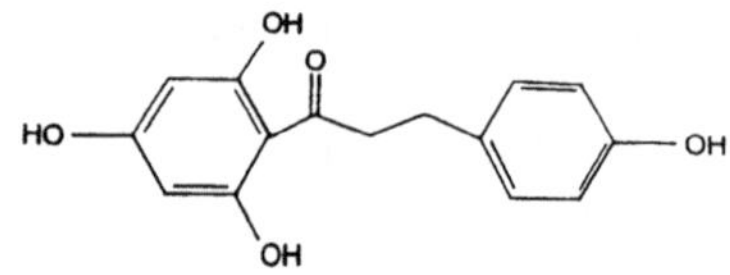

4.

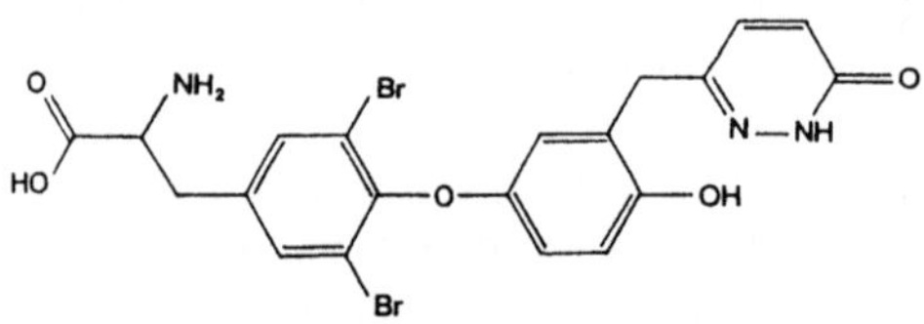

2.

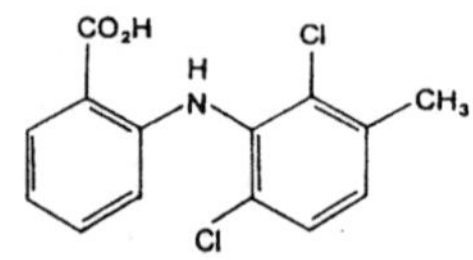

5.

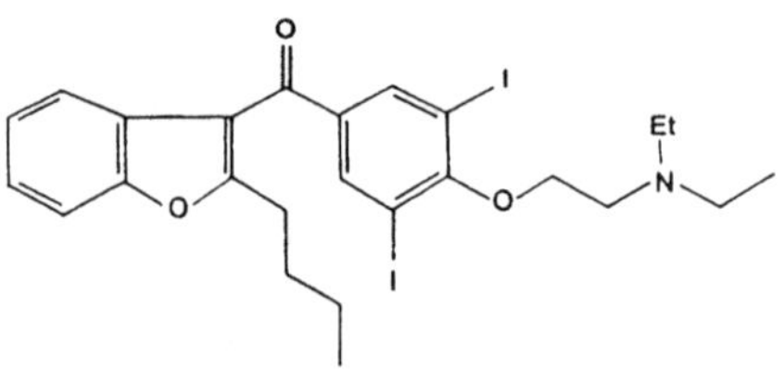

3.

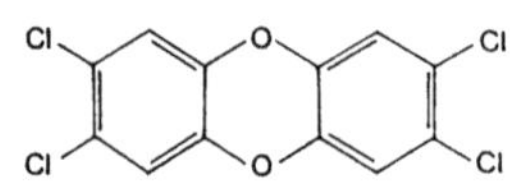

6.

Fig. 3. Structures of: *1*, T_3 and some non-thyroidal drugs which show competitive potency for intracellular T_3-binding sites; *2*, SKF-94901; *3*, amidarone; *4*, phloretin; *5*, flufenamic acid, a phenylanthranilic acid. The toxin dioxin, which is structurally related to phenylanthranilic acid, is shown in *6*

fects on liver and kidney. Other competitors developed as potential tools for NMR studies of hormone-binding sites which may have antagonist activity, bear a structural resemblance to the low molecular weight poison dioxin (2, 3, 6, 7-tetrachlorodibenzo dioxin; CHALMERS et al. 1993). Some of these structures are illustrated in Fig. 3. A considerably greater understanding of CTBPs and the nature of their binding sites is required before antagonism by these or similar compounds at this site will be possible.

D. Antagonism at the Receptor Level

I. Thyroid Hormone Receptors and the Receptor Superfamily

The possibility of developing a receptor antagonist depends on a complete understanding of receptor structure and function, which are reviewed in Chap. 6, this volume. Receptors for T_3 are members of a nuclear receptor superfamily which includes receptors for steroids, thyroid hormones and retinoids, as well as a large number of related proteins for which regulatory ligands have not been identified (LAUDET 1992; ZHANG and PFAHL 1993).

These receptors regulate the transcription of complex networks of genes and thus control diverse aspects of growth, development and homeostasis. They bind to specific DNA sequences within particular genes that are targets for regulation. Understanding the mechanisms that underlie gene-specific recognition therefore forms a central problem in understanding how various members of the nuclear receptor superfamily function to regulate gene expression differentially.

The members of the steroid hormone receptor family act as ligand-responsive transcriptional factors that activate or repress expression of hormone-responsive genes. These transcriptional regulators are characterised by a highly conserved, cysteine-rich, zinc finger DNA-binding domain and a less well conserved ligand-binding domain which confers specificity for a given hormone (Evans 1988; Freedman and Luisi 1993).

There are two major and fundamental differences between T_3 receptors and steroid hormone receptors. First, classical steroid receptors undergo an activation step and dissociation from a heat shock protein complex upon activation by hormone binding. In contrast, T_3 receptors (TRs) do not normally associate with heat shock proteins (Dalman et al. 1990). Second, in the unliganded state, TRs are bound to DNA and can directly repress gene transcription (Damm et al. 1989; Yen and Chin 1994). There is also increasing evidence that these receptors can interact with another member of the receptor superfamily, the retinoid X receptor (RXR), which has been shown to have a potentiating effect on binding and function of TR and on the highly homologous retinoic acid and vitamin D receptors (Williams and Brent 1992; Zhang and Pfahl 1993).

By virtue of sequence homology with other members of the steroid family, TRs share a similar domain organisation, including a central DNA-binding domain containing two "zinc fingers" composed of cysteine residues formed into a loop structure and chelated with a zinc atom, and a carboxy-terminal ligand-binding domain. Protein-DNA interactions are mediated by the highly conserved DNA-binding domain while protein-protein interactions are mediated by the extensive C-terminal dimerisation interface that is contained within the ligand-binding domain (Evans 1988; Beato 1989; Glass 1994).

II. Heterogeneity Among Thyroid Hormone Receptors

There are two major TR isoforms, ranging in size from 400 to slightly over 500 amino acids, which mediate T_3-regulated gene expression. These isoforms are designated α and β, and are encoded on human chromosomes 17 and 3, respectively (Evans 1988; Lazar 1993). TR diversity is further increased by the generation of additional isoforms from the α and β genes. There is a high degree of homology between the critical DNA and ligand-binding domains of these receptor isoforms.

Heterogeneity among TRα isoforms arises as a consequence of alternative splicing of a common mRNA precursor leading to the generation of two mature mRNAs that are each translated into two proteins, TRα_1 and TRα_2 (LAZAR 1993). These proteins are identical for the first 370 amino acid residues but their respective sequences diverge markedly thereafter. TRα_2 contains a 122-amino-acid carboxy terminus that replaces the region in TRα_1 that is necessary for hormone binding, and thus TRα_2 cannot bind T_3. Additionally, TRα_2 binds weakly to DNA and cannot transactivate thyroid hormone-responsive genes. Accordingly, only TRα_1 is regarded as an authentic thyroid hormone receptor.

The function of TRα_2 is unknown but it may inhibit thyroid hormone action by competing for DNA binding in vitro (KATZ and LAZAR 1993) and in vivo (HODIN et al. 1990). Recent evidence suggests that dephosphorylation of TRα_2 increases its affinity for DNA and its ability to inhibit responses mediated by TRα_1 in vitro (KATZ et al. 1995). This suggests that phosphorylation may provide a mechanism for modulation of the expression of T_3-responsive genes. TRα_2 is widely expressed in tissues, particularly the brain, and conceivably regulation of this isoform in vivo may lead to TRα_1 antagonism. Further exploration of this possibility rests upon the identification of factors controlling expression and/or phosphorylation of TRα_2 or of a ligand for this receptor.

Similarly the protein encoded by the virus responsible for avian erythroblastosis (v-*erb*A) functions as an antagonist of TRα_1 in vitro (DAMM et al. 1989). This study suggests that v-*erb*A contributes to cellular transformation by inhibiting the function of its normal endogenous counterpart. While this does not exclude the use of v-*erb*A as an antagonist in vivo, a more detailed understanding of the outcome of this antagonism and of the factors controlling this virus is required before the observation has application.

There are also two TRs encoded by the TRβ gene (HODIN et al. 1989). There are two promoter regions in this gene, each of which is essential for the transcription of an mRNA coding for a distinctive protein. Alternative promoter choice and/or RNA splicing selects one or both of the coding mRNAs, with their translated products designated as TRβ_1 and TRβ_2. Both are bona fide receptors by virtue of their abilities to bind DNA and thyroid hormone with high affinity and specificity as well as their ability to transactivate thyroid hormone-responsive genes.

Another important aspect of transcriptional activation by T_3 is that of the role of non-receptor cofactors. TRs, in contrast to other steroid receptors, actively repress transcription in the absence of ligand. This repression is thought to occur through a corepressor protein which binds to TRβ_1 in the absence of ligand and is released on hormone binding (BANIAHMAD et al. 1995). A candidate corepresser has recently been identified. It is a 2453 amino acid protein which interacts with the hinge region between the ligand and DNA-binding domains of TRβ_1 and is thought to be released upon binding of T_3 to the receptor (HÖRLEIN et al. 1995; CHEN and EVANS 1995). Other transcription factors may also act as repressors by distinct mechanisms (BANIAHMAD et al. 1993). A detailed understanding of the function and regulation of these corepressors may allow the design of protocols or techniques which use the inhibitory activity of these molecules to control gene expression especially in the presence of high circulating concentrations of ligand.

III. Tissue Distribution of Receptors

An important consideration in the search for ways to influence T_3 response through its receptors is their tissue distribution. When expressed per gram of tissue, the most highly abundant TR isoform is TRβ_2, but expression of this isoform is confined mainly to the pituitary and hypothalamus (HODIN et al. 1989). Messenger RNAs encoding the TRα_1, α_2 and β_1 isoforms are expressed in virtually all tissues, although they have characteristic distributions. For example, TRα_1 is in highest abundance in skeletal muscle and brown fat whereas α_2 mRNA expression is extremely prominent in the brain (BRADLEY et al. 1992). TRβ_1 is more homogeneously distributed, but higher in brain, liver and kidney (HODIN et al. 1990).

Even within a tissue there is a differential expression of TR subtypes; for example, there is region-specific expression of TRα and β in the brain (BRADLEY et al. 1992). Recent studies of the expression of TR mRNAs have revealed a dissociation between T_3-binding activity and the levels of the mRNAs that code the functional TRs in some tissues. The liver, which contains high levels of TR, as measured by T_3-binding assay (SCHWARTZ et al. 1992; TAGAMI et al. 1993), contains surprisingly low levels of mRNAs coding for functional receptors TRα_1 and β_1 (HODIN et al. 1989, 1990). In contrast, the brain expresses relatively high levels of TRα_1 and β_1 mRNA (MURRAY et al. 1988; HODIN et al. 1989, 1990; TAGAMI et al. 1993) despite much lower T_3-binding capacity (SCHWARTZ et al. 1992).

These results draw attention to the need for careful interpretation of the physiological significance of changes in TR mRNA. The fact that certain tissues have variable amounts of TR mRNA and functional protein suggests that tissue-specific regulation at both the pre- and post-translational levels plays important roles in gene regulation by thyroid hormones and its modulation.

IV. Receptor Regulation of Tissue Responsiveness

A number of factors influence the expression of TR mRNA and tissue TR concentrations, particularly T_3. For example, in amphibians, the expression of TRβ mRNA increases exponentially immediately before metamorphosis, as thyroid hormone becomes available and thyroid hormone-regulated genes are first detected (CHATTERJEE and TATA 1992).

In rats, injection of T_3 increases the concentration of TRβ_1 mRNA and decreases the concentration of TRβ_2 in the pituitary while also decreasing the concentrations of TRα_1 and TRα_2 mRNA in the heart, kidney and pituitary (HODIN et al. 1990; WILLIAMS et al. 1991). In cultured rat pituitary cells, TRβ_2 mRNA levels were downregulated by T_3 at the level of gene transcription in accordance with in vivo studies (Hodin et al. 1990; Davis and Lazar 1992).

The physiological purpose of the hormonal regulation of TRβ_2 is unclear. It has been suggested that TRβ_2 may be particularly important for pituitary T_3-responsiveness (Lazar 1993). The expression of TRβ_2 mRNA in the pituitary is greatest in thyrotrophs and somatotrophs, cells that express genes regulated by T_3. Experimentally induced hypothyroidism alters the relative expression of TRβ_2 mRNA in these pituitary cells, with thyrotrophs increasing production and somatotrophs decreasing production (Childs et al. 1991). The divergent effects of the removal of T_3 on expression of TRβ_2 mRNA by thyrotrophs and somatotrophs indicate that the receptor may subserve different functions in these two cell populations.

Receptor levels are also profoundly influenced by short-chain fatty acids, particularly sodium butyrate. Sodium butyrate produces a wide variety of effects on cells in culture: proliferation, differentiation and specific gene expression. It increases the level of histone acetylation by inhibition of deacetylation (Ortiz-Caro et al. 1986). In GH1 cells, sodium butyrate reduces levels of the 47-kDa receptor (presumably TRα_1) by reducing its half-life but increases levels of TRβ_2 (Casanova et al. 1984). Similar responses were seen in another pituitary cell line, GH3 cells, in which butyrate decreased receptor concentrations and virtually abolished T_3 responsiveness (Cattini et al. 1988). Sodium butyrate has also been reported to reduce receptor levels in rat liver cells and human skin fibroblasts (Mitsuhashi et al. 1987; Ichikawa et al. 1992) although it causes an increase in receptor number in cultured glial cells (Ortiz-Caro et al. 1986). It is highly likely that modulating histone acetylation has opposite effects on the predominant receptor isoforms TRα_1 and TRα_2, thus limiting the utility of short-chain fatty acids to in vitro studies only.

Other factors also reduce receptor number, particularly those associated with illness or reduced caloric intake. Fasting reduces TRβ_1 and TRα_1 concentrations in rat liver to 43% and 32% of the fed state, respectively. Total protein is also reduced but receptor mRNA levels are unchanged (Lane et al. 1991). The reduction in receptor levels probably arises from a calorie-sparing mechanism although why the mRNA levels are preserved is not understood. Mediators of the acute inflammatory responses in critical illness such as interleukin-1β, interleukin-6 and tumour necrosis factor reduce nuclear receptor number in human HepG2 cells by up to 30% in vitro (Wolf et al. 1994). This study contrasts with a clinical study by Williams et al. 1989), who found that both TRα and TRβ mRNAs were increased in chronic illness. They proposed that increased receptor number compensates for the low hormone levels associated with severe illness. Given that unoccupied TRs are gene repressors, an increase in receptor number is unlikely to compensate for reduced availability of hormone by increasing gene transcription.

Special mention needs to be made of the relationship between T_3 and retinoids. An amelioration of response to thyroid hormone by co-administration of vitamin A was first noted nearly 50 years ago (Sadhu and

Brody 1947), but detailed study of thyroid-retinoid interactions did not begin until structural homology between thyroid and retinoid receptors was recognised by Giguere et al. in 1987.

For the most part, studies of transcriptional regulation by T_3, and the effect of retinoids and vice versa, have been restricted to artificial gene constructs transfected together with receptor genes into receptor negative cell lines. These studies have shown that there are no general rules for the reaction that occurs between TRs and retinoid receptors at the level of the gene. Rather, the data suggest that changes in gene expression depend on the subtypes of the TR and retinoid receptors present, the structure of the response element located within the regulatory part of the gene, and the context of the gene in terms of cell function.

It is likely that TRs form dimers with other nuclear factors to mediate transcription by T_3 (Yen and Chin 1994) and that the principal dimerising partner is the retinoid X receptor, although it is not yet clear whether the RXR ligand, 9-*cis* RA, plays a pivotal role in this process (Sugawara et al. 1994a). If TRs and RXRs are bound to DNA in the absence of ligand, the most likely role of the RXR is to localise and orient the TR at the appropriate position on a responsive gene (Zhang and Pfahl 1993). Addition of T_3 may then allow removal of a corepressor, receptor phosphorylation (Sugawara et al. 1994b) and activation of transcription.

It is tempting to infer that modulation of RXR levels should therefore modulate T_3 responsiveness. While such a scenario is entirely possible in vitro (Hsu et al. 1995), the ubiquitous nature of RXRs makes this phenomenon unlikely to be of any practical benefit in vivo. RXRs probably serve a similar role in mediating responses to vitamin D, retinoic acid (RA) and the peroxisome proliferator activators, so that changes in RXR levels may also influence responses to these hormones. Even so, this approach may be applicable to other factors which are not yet completely defined but which are involved in T_3 responsiveness (Lee et al. 1995) and which may be responsible for some of the observed interplay between T_3 and RA.

For example, T_3 and RA both increase the expression of growth hormone mRNA and their combined effects are additive. In contrast, RA is without effect on $TR\beta_2$ mRNA but completely reverses the inhibitory effect of T_3 on this gene. Furthermore, RA does not influence, positively or negatively, the effect of T_3 on $TR\beta_1$ mRNA (Davis and Lazar 1992). Similarly, T_3 has been shown to block the ability of RA to induce ornithine amino transferase mRNA in rat liver but not kidney (Shull et al. 1995). Blocking effects have also been observed in vitro on the alcohol dehydrogenase gene in Hep G2 cells (Harding and Duester 1992), although in HL-60 cells T_3 enhanced the ability of RA to induce differentiation (Miyoshi et al. 1994).

We also found an interrelationship between T_3 and RA in Hep G2 cells. Using increased secretion of sex-hormone-binding globulin (SHBG) as a response parameter, we found that T_3 induced a doubling of SHBG concentration in Hep G2 cell supernatants. RA was able to reduce the maximal response to T_3 without altering the effective half-maximal T_3 concentration. It was of interest that a different response in the same cell was not influenced by T_3. Levels of thyroxine-binding globulin (TBG), the secretion of which is reduced by T_3 (CROWE et al. 1995) in the same cell supernatant, were not affected by RA (Fig. 4).

Other cell culture experiments provide further evidence that RA can enhance, inhibit or not change T_3 responsiveness (HIGUERET et al. 1992; ELFAHIME et al. 1994; GERRELLI et al. 1994; SATYANARAYANA et al. 1994). These studies suggest that the interplay between thyroid and retinoid responses arises in part because of the overlapping actions of their respective receptors but also that the heterogeneous nature of these responses makes the interrelationship unpredictable for a given gene. A more detailed understanding of the control of TR, RAR and RXR isoforms and their associated cofactors in all tissue will be required before their modulation can be used to influence hormone responsiveness.

V. Drug Interactions at the Ligand-Binding Site

The final, and perhaps preferred, option in the development of a T_3 antagonist is to design an analogue which binds to the TR-binding site but which does not activate transcription.

The structure of the binding site is not known. On the basis of the competitive potencies of a range of analogues to mutant $TR\beta_1$ receptors derived from cases of thyroid hormone resistance, CHENG et al. (1994) have defined the

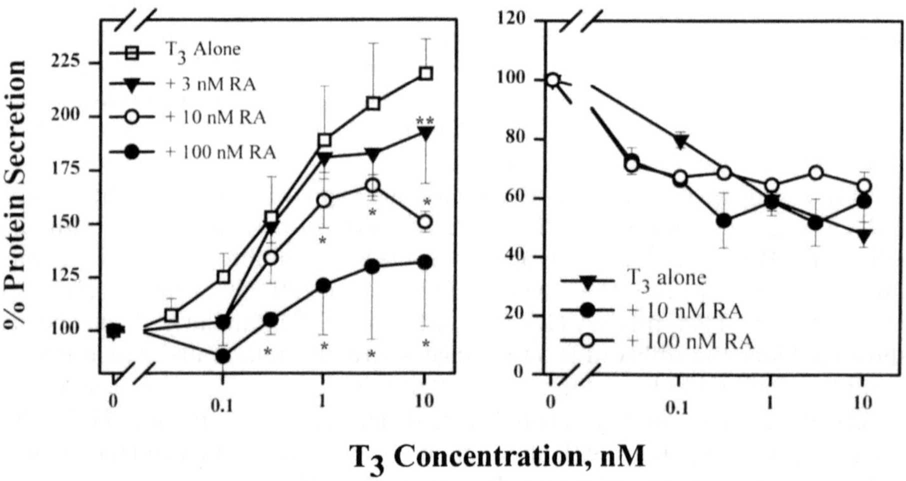

Fig. 4. Differential effects of retinoic acid on T_3 responsiveness within the one cell line. HepG2 cells were incubated for 4 days with a range of concentrations of T_3 and retinoic acid. Retinoic acid had a significant, dose-responsive downregulating effect on T_3-induced stimulation of SHBG secretion (*left panel*) but no effect on T_3-induced reduction in TBG secretion (*right panel*). (From CROWE et al. 1996, with permission)

binding site for T_3 as an eightfold α/β barrel with one extra α-helix. The ligand-binding site is adjacent to the DNA-binding domain, which putatively allows regulation of the DNA-binding properties of the receptor. Steroid hormone receptors which have a similar ligand-binding site (GOLDSTEIN et al. 1993) are thought to activate transcription via a co-activator which acts as a communication link between the occupied receptor and the transcription initation complex (NORDEEN et al. 1993). Antagonists fail to activate this co-activator and, by competition at the ligand-binding site, prevent activation by agonists.

For thyroid hormone receptors, the communication link is probably a corepressor (HÖRLEIN et al. 1995; CHEN and EVANS 1995) but how ligand binding relieves this repression is unknown. Indeed, analogue studies suggest that binding alone is sufficient to relieve repression and promote responsiveness, the response being proportional to the affinity of the ligand for the receptor.

A range of compounds has been shown to interact with the TR. These include non-esterified fatty acids (VAN DER KLIS et al. 1991; MAZZACHI et al. 1992), protease inhibitors (BRTKO et al. 1993) and non-steroidal anti-inflammatory agents (BARLOW et al. 1994). The concentrations required for receptor binding are in the pathophysiological range, and in those studies where activity has been examined no compound demonstrates agonist or antagonist properties with regard to T_3 responsiveness.

The only compound which has ever been reported to have T_3 antagonist activity is the antiarrhythmic agent amiodarone (NORMAN and LAVIN 1989). Amiodarone is an iodinated benzofuran derivative which has a number of pharmacological activities suggesting T_3 antagonism (see Chap. 10, this volume). These include bradycardia, depression of myocardial oxygen consumption and lengthening of the cardiac action potential (MASON 1987). It also inhibits conversion of 5′-deiodination of thyroxine but this effect is unrelated to its putative antagonist activity (SCHRÖDER-VAN DER ELST and VAN DER HEIDE 1990). In tissue extracts, amiodarone is a weak competitor for solubilised nuclear receptors, with a potency 3000–40000 less than that of T_3. In cell culture experiments it is able to inhibit the T_3-induced accumulation of growth hormone mRNA in GC cells in parallel with its ligand-displacing activity (NORMAN and LAVIN 1989). Both in vivo and in vitro evidence has confirmed this finding. Amiodarone antagonises the T_3 effect on β-adrenoreceptors in chicken cardiac myocytes (YIN et al. 1994), and reversal of hypothyroidism with T_3 in rats is prevented by administration of amiodarone (PARADIS et al. 1991).

However, the mechanism of the antithyroid effects of amiodarone are more complex than competitive displacement of T_3 from nuclear receptor sites. Recent evidence suggests that amiodarone reduced the mRNAs for $TR\alpha_1$, β_1 and β_2 in cardiomyocytes after a catecholamine stress (DRVOTA et al. 1995). In addition, in rats treated with amiodarone, the maximum binding capacity of cardiac nuclear receptors was reduced (GOTZSCHE and ORSKOV 1994). These data suggest that amiodarone may act by inducing a state of thyroid hormone resistance by depletion of receptor number. Alternatively, in some cell types amiodarone has no effect on receptor binding but rather inhibition of T_3 occurs with the major metabolite of the drug, desethylamiodarone (BAKKER et al. 1994; GOTZSCHE 1993). Curiously, the inhibition of T_3 binding to purified TRβ_1 by desethylamiodarone is non-competitive (BAKKER et al. 1994), a finding which is consistent with the reduction in receptor number in cardiac cells in vivo and in vitro but at variance with the original observation in GC cells.

Two other factors may limit the use of this drug as a T_3 antagonist: limited solubility in aqueous media (BARLOW et al. 1994) and cytotoxicity, particularly with regard to thyroid cells (CHIOVATO et al. 1994). Amiodarone or one of its derivatives will only be useful as an antagonist when we have a thorough understanding of the ligand-binding site of the receptor, the mechanisms of ligand binding and the transcriptional sequelae that follow ligand-receptor interaction.

References

Angel RC, Botta JA, Morero RD Farias RN (1990) Solubilization and purification of a membrane-associated 3,3′,5-tri-iodo-L-thyronine-binding protein from rat erythrocytes. Biochem J 270:577–582

Ashizawa K, Willingham MC, Liang C-M, Cheng S-Y (1991) In vivo regulation of monomer-tetramer conversion of pyruvate kinase subtype M_2 by glucose is mediated via fructose 1,6-biphosphate. J Biol Chem 266:16842–16846

Ashizawa K, Cheng S-Y (1992) Regulation of thyroid hormone receptor-mediated transcription by a cytosol protein. Proc Natl Acad Sci USA 89:9277–9281

Bakker O, van Beeren HC, Wiersinga WM (1994) Desethylamiodarone is a noncompetitive inhibitor of the binding of thyroid hormone to the thyroid hormone β_1-receptor protein. Endocrinology 134:1665–1670

Baniahmad A, Ha I, Reinberg D, Tsai S, Tsai M-J, O'Malley BW (1993) Interaction of human thyroid hormone receptor β with transcription factor TFIIB may mediate target gene derepression and activation by thyroid hormone. Proc Natl Acad Sci USA 90:8832–8836

Baniahmad A, Leng X, Burris TP, Tsai SY, Tsai M-J, O'Malley BW (1995) The τ_4 activation domain of the thyroid hormone receptor is required for release of a putative co-repressor(s) necessary for transcriptional silencing. Mol Cell Biol 15:76–86

Barlow JW, Raggatt LE, Lim C-F, Munro SL, Topliss DJ, Stockigt JR (1989) The thyroid hormone analogue SKF L-94901: nuclear occupancy and serum binding studies. Clin Sci 76:495–501

Barlow JW, Raggatt LE, Lim C-F, Kolliniatis E, Topliss DJ, Stockigt JR (1991) The thyroid hormone analogue SKF-94901 and iodothyronine binding sites in mammalian tissues: Differences in cytoplasmic binding between liver and heart. Acta Endocrinol (Copenh) 124:37–44

Barlow JW, Curtis AJ, Raggatt LE, Loidl NM, Topliss DJ, Stockigt JR (1994) Drug competition for intracellular triiodothyronine-binding sites. Eur J Endocrinol 130:417–421

Barlow JW, Raggatt LE, Scholz GH, Loidl NM, Blok RB, Topliss DJ, Stockigt JR (1996) Preferential inhibition of cytoplasmic T_3 binding is associated with reduced nuclear binding in cultured cells. Thyroid 6:47–51

Beato M (1989) Gene regulation by steroid hormones. Cell 56:335–344

Blondeau J-P, Osty J, Francon J (1988) Characterization of the thyroid hormone transport system of isolated hepatocytes. J Biol Chem 263:2685–2692
Blondeau J-P, Beslin A, Chantoux F, Francon J (1993) Triiodothyronine is a high-affinity inhibitor of amino acid transport system L_1 in cultured astrocytes. J Neurochem 60:1407–1413
Bradley D, Towle H, Young W (1992) Spatial and temporal expression of α- and β-thyroid hormone receptor mRNAs, including the β_2-subtype, in the developing mammalian nervous system. J Neurosci 12:2288–22302
Brtko J, Knopp J, Baker ME (1993) Inhibition of 3,5,3′-triiodothyronine binding to its receptor in rat liver by protease inhibitors and substrates. Mol Cell Endocrinol 93:81–86
Casanova J, Horowitz ZD, Copp RP, McIntyre WR, Pascaul A, Samuels HH (1984) Photoaffinity labeling of thyroid hormone nuclear receptors. J Biol Chem 259:12084–12091
Cattini PA, Kardami E, Eberhardt NL (1988) Effect of butyrate on thyroid hormone-mediated gene expression in rat pituitary tumour cells. Mol Cell Endocrinol 56:263–270
Centanni M, Robbins J (1987) Role of sodium in thyroid hormone uptake by rat skeletal muscle. J Clin Invest 80:1068–1072
Centanni M, Sapone A, Taglienti A, Andreoli M (1991) Effect of extracellular sodium on thyroid hormone uptake by mouse thymocytes. Endocrinology 129:2175–2179
Chalmers DK, Scholz GH, Topliss DJ, Kolliniatis E, Munro SL, Craik DJ, Iskander MN, Stockigt JR (1993) Thyroid hormone uptake by hepatocytes: structure-activity relationships of phenylanthranilic acids with inhibitory activity. J Med Chem 36:1272–1277
Chatterjee VK, Tata JR (1992) Thyroid hormone receptors and their role in development. Cancer Surv 14:147–167
Chen JD, Evans RM (1995) A transcriptional co-repressor that interacts with nuclear hormone receptors. Nature 377:454–457
Cheng S-Y, Hasumura S, Willingham MC, Pastan I (1986) Purification and characterization of a membrane-associated 3,3′,5-triiodo-L-thyronine binding protein from a human carcinoma cell line. Proc Natl Acad Sci USA 83:947–951
Cheng S-Y, Ransom SC, McPhie P, Bhat MK, Mixson AJ, Weintraub BD (1994) Analysis of the binding of 3,3′,5-triiodo-L-thyronine and its analogues to mutant human β_1 thyroid hormone receptors: a model of the hormone binding site. Biochemistry 33:4319–4326
Childs GV, Taub K, Jones KE, Chin WW (1991) Triiodothyronone receptor β-2 messenger RNA expression by somatotrophs and thyrotropes: effect of propylthiouracil-induced hypothyroidism in rats. Endocrinology 129:2767–2773
Chiovato L, Martino E, Tonacchera M, Santini F, Lapi P, Mammoli C, Braverman LE, Pinchera A (1994) Studies on the in vitro cytotoxic effect of amiodarone. Endocrinology 134:2277–2282
Crowe TC, Cowen NL, Loidl NM, Topliss DJ, Stockigt JR, Barlow JW (1995) Down-regulation of thyroxine-binding globulin messenger ribonucleic acid by 3,5,3′-triiodothyronine in human hepatoblastoma cells. J Clin Endocrinol Metab 80: 2233–2237
Crowe TC, Loidl NM, Payne KL, Topliss DJ, Stockigt JR, Barlow JW (1996) Differential modulation of thyroid hormone responsiveness by retinoids in a human cell line. Endocrinology 137:3187–3192
Dalman FC, Koenig RJ, Perdew GH, Massa E, Pratt WB (1990) In contrast to the glucocorticoid receptor, the thyroid hormone receptor is translated in the DNA binding state and is not associated with hsp90. J Biol Chem 265:3615–3618
Damm K, Thompson CC, Evans RM (1989) Protein encoded by v-erbA functions as a thyroid-hormone receptor antagonist. Nature 339:593–597
Davis KD, Lazar MA (1992) Selective antagonism of thyroid hormone action by retinoic acid. J Biol Chem 267:3185–3189

Docter R, Krenning EP, de Jong M, Hennemann G (1993) The sick euthyroid syndrome: changes in thyroid hormone serum parameters and hormone metabolism. Clin Endocrinol (Oxf) 39:499–518

Dozin B, Cahnmann HJ, Nikodem VM (1985) Comparative characterization of thyroid hormone receptors and binding proteins in rat liver nucleus, plasma membrane, and cytosol by photoaffinity labeling with L-thyroxine. Biochemistry 24:5203–5208

Drvota V, Bronnegard M, Hagglad J, Barkhem T, Sylven C (1995) Downregulation of thyroid hormone receptor subtype mRNA levels by amiodarone during catecholamine stress in vitro. Biochem Biophys Res Comm 211:991–996

Elfahime EL, Felix JM, Koch B (1994) Antagonistic effects of retinoic acid and triiodothyronine in the expression of corticoid-binding globulin (CBG) by cultured fetal hepatocytes. J Steroid Biochem Molec Biol 48:467–474

Evans RM (1988) The steroid and thyroid hormone receptor superfamily. Science 240:889–895

Everts ME, Docter R, van Buuren JCJ, van Koetsveld PM, Hofland LJ, de Jong M, Krenning EP, Hennemann G (1993) Evidence for carrier-mediated uptake of triiodothyronine in cultured anterior pituitary cells of euthyroid rats. Endocrinology 132:1278–1285

Everts ME, Visser TJ, Moerings EPCM, Tempelaars AMP, van Toor H, Docter R, de Jong M, Krenning EP, Hennemann G (1995) Uptake of 3,3′,5,5′-tetraiodothyroacetic acid and 3,3′,5′-triiodothyronine in cultured rat anterior pituitary cells and their effects on thyrotropin secretion. Endocrinology 136:4454–4461

Fanjul AN, Farias RN (1991) Novel cold-sensitive cytosolic 3,5,3′-triiodo-L-thyronine-binding proteins in human red blood cell. J Biol Chem 266:16415–16419

Fanjul AN, Farias RN (1993) Cold-sensitive cytosolic 3,5,3′-triiodo-L-thyronine-binding protein and pyruvate kinase from human erythrocytes share similar regulatory properties of hormone binding by glycolytic intermediates. J Biol Chem 268:175–179

Freedman LP, Luisi BF (1993) On the mechanism of DNA binding by nuclear hormone receptors: a structural and functional perspective. J Cell Biochem 51:140–150

Gerrelli D, Huntriss JD, Latchman DS (1994) Antagonistic effects of retinoic acid and thyroid hormone on the expression of the tissue-specific splicing protein SmN in a clonal cell line derived from rat heart. J Mol Cell Cardiol 26:713–719

Giguere V, Ong ES, Segui P, Evans RM (1987) Identification of a receptor for the morphogen retinoic acid. Nature 330:624–629

Glass C (1994) Differential recognition of target genes by nuclear receptor monomers, dimers, and heterodimers. Endocr Rev 15:391–407

Goldstein RA, Katzenellenbogen JA, Luthey-Schultzen ZA, Seielstad DA, Wolynes PG (1993) Three-dimensional model for the hormone binding domain of steroid receptors. Proc Natl Acad Sci USA 90:9949–9953

Gotzsche LB (1993) Beta-adrenergic receptors, voltage-operated Ca^{2+}-channels, nuclear triiodothyronine receptors and triiodothyronine concentration in pig myocardium after long-term low-dose amiodarone treatment. Acta Endocrinologica (Copenh) 129:337–347

Gotzsche LB, Orskov H (1994) Cardiac triiodothyronine nuclear receptor binding capacities in amiodarone-treated, hypo- and hyperthyroid rats. Eur J Endocrinol 130:281–290

Gonçalves E, Lakshmanan M, Cahnmann HJ, Robbins J (1990) High-affinity binding of thyroid hormones to neuroblastoma plasma membranes. Biochim Biophys Acta 1055:151–156

Harding PP, Duester G (1992) Retinoic acid activation and thyroid hormone repression of the human alcohol dehydrogenase gene ADH3. J Biol Chem 20:14145–14150

Hashizume K, Miyamoto T, Ichikawa K, Yamauchi K, Kobayashi M, Sakurai A, Ohtsuka H, Nishii Y, Yamada T (1989a) Purification and characterization of

NADPH-dependent cytosolic 3,5,3′-triiodo-L-thyronine binding protein in rat kidney. J Biol Chem 264:4857–4863
Hashizume K, Miyamoto T, Ichikawa K, Yamauchi K, Sakurai A, Ohtsuka H, Kobayashi M, Nishii Y, Yamada T (1989b) Evidence for the presence of two active forms of cytosolic 3,5,3′-triiodo-L-thyronine (T_3)-binding protein (CTBP) in rat kidney. J Biol Chem 264:4864–4871
Hashizume K, Miyamoto T, Yamauchi K, Ichikawa K, Kobayashi M, Ohtsuka H, Sakurai A, Suzuki S, Yamada T (1989c) Counterregulation of nuclear 3,5,3′-triiodo-L-thyronine (T_3) binding by oxidised and reduced-nicotinamide adenine dinucleotide phosphates in the presence of cytosolic T_3-binding protein in vitro. Endocrinology 124:1678–1683
Higueret P, Pallet V, Coustaut M, Audouin I, Begueret J, Garcin H (1992) Retinoic acid decreases retinoic acid and triiodothyronine nuclear receptor expression in the liver of hyperthyroidic rats. FEBS Lett 310:101–105
Hillier AP (1970) The binding of thyroid hormones to phospholipid membranes. J Physiol 211:585–597
Hodin RA, Lazar MA, Wintman BI, Darling DS, Koenig RJ, Larsen PR, Moore DD, Chin WW (1989) Identification of a thyroid hormone receptor that is pituitary-specific. Science 244:76–79
Hodin RA, Lazar MA, Chin WW (1990) Differential and tissue-specific regulation of the multiple rat c-erbA messenger RNA species by thyroid hormone. J Clin Invest 85:101–105
Hörlein AJ, Näär AM, Heinzel T, Torchia J, Gloss B, Kurokawa R, Ryan A, Kamei Y, Söderström M, Glass CK, Rosenfeld MG (1995) Ligand-independent repression by the thyroid hormone receptor mediated by a nuclear receptor co-repressor. Nature 377:397–404
Hsu J-H, Zavacki AM, Harney JW, Brent GA (1995) Retinoid-X receptor (RXR) differentially augments thyroid hormone response in cell lines as a function of the response element and endogenous RXR content. Endocrinology 136:421–430
Ichikawa K, Hashizume K, Kobayashi M, Nishii Y, Ohtsuka H, Suzuki S, Takeda T, Yamada T (1992) Heat shock decreases nuclear transport of 3,5,3′-triiodo-L-thyronine in clone 9 cells. Endocrinology 130:2317–2324
Ishigaki S, Abramovitz M, Listowsky I (1989) Glutathione-S-transferases are major cytosolic thyroid hormone binding proteins. Arch Biiochem Biophys 273:265–272
Jennings AS, Ferguson DC, Utiger RD (1979) Regulation of the conversion of thyroxine to triiodothyronine in the perfused rat liver. J Clin Invest 64:1614–1623
de Jong M, Docter R, van der Hoek HJ, Vos RA, Krenning EP, Hennemann G (1992) Transport of 3,5,3′-triiodothyronine into the perfused rat liver and subsequent metabolism are inhibited by fasting. Endocrinology 131:463–470
Kato H, Fukuda T, Parkison C, McPhie P, Cheng S-Y (1989) Cytosolic thyroid hormone-binding protein is a monomer of pyruvate kinase. Proc Natl Acad Sci USA 86:7861–7865
Katz D, Lazar MA (1993) Dominant negative activity of an endogenous thyroid hormone receptor variant (α_2) is due to competition for binding sites on target genes. J Biol Chem 268:20904–20910
Katz D, Reginato MJ, Lazar MA (1995) Functional regulation of thyroid hormone receptor variant TRα_2 by phosphorylation. Mol Cell Biol 15:2341–2348
van der Klis FRM, Nijenhuis AA, Wiersinga WM (1991) Inhibition of nuclear T_3 binding by fatty acids liberated from nuclear membranes via phospholipase C. Int J Biochem 23:1031–1034
Kragie L, Doyle D (1992) Benzodiazepines inhibit temperature-dependent L-[^{125}I] triiodothyronine accumulation into human liver, human neuroblast, and rat pituitary cell lines. Endocrinology 130:1211–1216
Krenning EP, Docter R, Bernard HF, Visser RJ, Hennemann G (1981) Characteristics of active transport of thyroid hormone into rat hepatocytes. Biochem Biophys Acta 676:314–320

Krenning EP, Docter R (1986) Plasma membrane transport of thyroid hormone. In: Henneman G (ed) Thyroid hormone metabolism. Dekker, New York, pp 107–131
Lakshmanan M, Gonçalves E, Lessly G, Foti D, Robbins J (1990) The transport of thyroxine into mouse neuroblastoma cells, NB41A3: the effect of L-system amino acids. Endocrinology 126:3245–3250
Lane JT, Godbole M, Strait KA, Schwartz HL, Oppenheimer JH (1991) Prolonged fasting reduces rat hepatic β1 thyroid hormone receptor protein without changing the level of its messenger ribonucleic acid. Endocrinology 129:2881–2885
Laudet V, Hanni C, Coll J, Catzeflis F, Stehelin D (1992) Evolution of the nuclear receptor gene superfamily. EMBO J 11:1003–1013
Lazar MA (1993) Thyroid hormone receptors: multiple forms, multiple possibilities. Endocr Rev 14:184–193
Lee JW, Choi H-S, Gyuris J, Brent R, Moore DD (1995) Two classes of proteins dependent on either the presence or absence of thyroid hormone for interaction with the thyroid hormone receptor. Mol Endocrinol 9:243–254
Leeson PD, Emmett JC, Shah VP, Showell GA, Novelli R, Prain HD, Benson MG, Ellis D, Pearce NJ, Underwood AH (1989) Selective thyromimetics. Cardiac-sparing thyroid hormone analogues containing 3′-arylmethyl substituents. J Med Chem 32:320–336
Lennon AM, Osty J, Nunez J (1980) Cytosolic thyroxine-binding protein and brain development. Mol Cell Endocrinol 18:201–214
Lennon AM (1992) Purification and characterization of rat brain cytosolic 3,5,3′-triiodo-L-thyronine-binding protein. Eur J Biochem 210:79–85
Lim C-F, Bernard BF, de Jong M, Docter R, Krenning EP, Hennemann G (1993a) A furan fatty acid and indoxyl sulfate are the putative inhibitors of thyroxine hepatocyte transport in uremia. J Clin Endocrinol Metab 76:318–324
Lim C-F, Docter R, Visser TJ, Krenning EP, Bernard B, van Toor H, de Jong M, Hennemann G (1993b) Inhibition of thyroxine transport into cultured rat hepatocytes by serum of non-uremic critically-ill patients, bilirubin and non-esterified fatty acids. J Clin Endocrinol Metab 76:1165–1172
Mason JW (1987) Amiodarone. N Engl J Med 316:455–466
Mazzachi BC, Kennedy JA, Wellby ML, Edwards AM (1992) Effect of fatty acids on rat liver nuclear T_3-receptor binding. Metabolism 41:788–792
Mitchell AM, Manley SW, Mortimer RH (1992a) Uptake of L-tri-iodothyronine by human cultured trophoblast cells. J Endocrinol 133:483–486
Mitchell AM, Manley SW, Mortimer RH (1992b) Membrane transport of thyroid hormone in the human choriocarcinoma cell line, JAR. Mol Cell Endocrinol 87:139–145
Mitsuhashi T, Uchimura H, Takaku F (1987) n-Butyrate increases the level of thyroid hormone nuclear receptor in non-pituitary cultured cells. J Biol Chem 262:3993–3999
Miyoshi Y, Nakamura H, Tagami T, Sasaki S, Nakao K (1994) 3,5,3′-Triiodothyronine stimulates retinoic acid-induced differentiation in HL-60 cells. Mol Cell Endocrinol 103:119–123
Movius EG, Phyillaier MM, Robbins J (1989) Phloretin inhibits cellular uptake and nuclear receptor binding of triiodothyronine in human Hep G2 hepatocarcinoma cells. Endocrinology 124:1988–1997
Murray MB, Zilz ND, McCreary NL, MacDonald MJ, Towle HC (1988) Isolation and characterisation of rat cDNA clones for two distinct thyroid hormone receptors. J Biol Chem 263:12770–12777
Nishii Y, Hashizume K, Ichikawa K, Miyamoto T, Suzuki S, Takeda T, Yamauchi K, Kobayashi M, Yamada T (1989) Changes in cytosolic 3,5,3′-triiodo-L-thyronine (T_3) binding activity during administration of L-thyroxine to thyroidectomised rats: cytosolic T_3-binding protein and its activator act as intracellular regulators for nuclear T_3 binding. J Endocrinol 123:99–104

Nordeen SK, Bona BJ, Moyer ML (1993) Latent agonist activity of the steroid antagonist, RU486, is unmasked in cells treated with activators of protein kinase A. Mol Endocrinol 7:731–742

Norman MF, Lavin TN (1989) Antagonism of thyroid hormone action by amiodarone in rat pituitary tumor cells. J Clin Invest 83:306–313

Obata T, Kitagawa S, Gong Q-H, Pastan I, Cheng S-Y (1988) Thyroid hormone down-regulates p55, a thyroid hormone-binding protein that is homologous to protein disulfide isomerase and the β-subunit of prolyl-4-hydroxylase. J Biol Chem 263: 782–785

Ortiz-Caro J, Montiel F, Pascual A, Aranda A (1986) Modulation of thyroid hormone nuclear receptors by short-chain fatty acids in glial C6 cells. J Biol Chem 261: 13997–14004

Osty J, Jego L, Francon J, Blondeau J-P (1988a) Characterization of triiodothyronine transport and accumulation in rat erythrocytes. Endocrinology 123:2303–2311

Osty J, Rappaport L, Samuel JL, Lennon AM (1988b) Characterization of a cytosolic triiodothyronine binding protein in atrium and ventricle of rat heart with different sensitivity toward thyroid hormone levels. Endocrinology 122:1027–1033

Paradis P, Lambert C, Rouleau J (1991) Amiodarone antagonises the effects of T_3 at the receptor level: an additional mechanism for its in vivo hypothyroid-like effects. Can J Physiol Pharmacol 69:865–870

Parkison C, Ashizawa K, McPhie P, Lin K-H, Cheng S-Y (1991) The monomer of pyruvate kinase, subtype M_1, is both a kinase and a cytosolic thyroid hormone binding protein. Biochem Biophys Res Comm 179:668–674

Prasad PD, Leibach FH, Mahesh VB, Ganapathy V (1994) Relationship between thyroid hormone transport and neutral amino acid transport in JAR human choriocarcinoma cells. Endocrinology 134:574–581

Sadhu DP, Brody S (1947) Excess vitamin A ingestion, thyroid size and energy metabolism. Am J Physiol 149:400–403

Sakata S, Komaki T, Nakamura S, Ohshima M, Sagisaka K, Yoshioka N, Atassi MZ, Miura K (1990) Binding of thyroid hormones to human hemoglobin and localization of the binding site. J Protein Chem 9:743–750

Satyanarayana M, Sarvesh A, Khadeer MA, Ved HS, Robert Soprano D, Rajeswari MR, Pieringer RA (1994) Regulation of neuronal thyroid hormone receptor α_1 mRNA by hydrocortisone, thyroid hormone and retinoic acid. Dev Neurosci 16:255–259

Schröder-van der Elst JP, van der Heide D (1990) Thyroxine, 3,5,3′-triiodothyronine, and 3,3′,5-triiodothyronine concentrations in several tissues of the rat: effects of amiodarone and desethylamiodarone on thyroid hormone metabolism. Endocrinology 127:1656–1664

Schwartz HL, Strait KA, Ling NC, Oppenheimer JH (1992) Quantitation of rat tissue thyroid hormone binding receptor isoforms by immunoprecipitation of nuclear triiodothyronine binding capacity. J Biol Chem 267:11794–11799

Seelig S, Law C, Towle HC, Oppenheimer JH (1981) Thyroid hormone attenuates and augments hepatic gene expression at a pretranslational level. Proc Natl Acad Sci USA 78:4733–4737

Shull JD, Pennington KL, Gurr JA, Ross AC (1995) Cell-type specific interactions between retinoic acid and thyroid hormone in the regulation of expression of the gene encoding ornithine aminotransferase. Endocrinology 136:2120–2126

Sugawara A, Yen PM, Chin WW (1994a) 9-cis Retinoic acid regulation of rat growth hormone gene expression: potential roles of multiple nuclear hormone receptors. Endocrinology 135:1956–1962

Sugawara A, Yen PM, Apriletti JW, Ribeiro RCJ, Sacks DB, Baxter JD, Chin WW (1994b) Phosphorylation selectively increases triiodothyronine receptor homodimer binding to DNA. J Biol Chem 269:433–437

Suzuki S, Hashizume K, Ichikawa K, Takeda T (1991) Ontogenesis of the high affinity NADPH-dependent cytosolic 3,5,3′-triiodo-L-thyronine-binding protein in rat. Endocrinology 129:2571–2574

Tagami T, Nakamura H, Sasaki S, Miyoshi Y, Imura H (1993) Estimation of the protein content of thyroid hormone receptor α_1 and β_1 in rat tissues by western blotting. Endocrinology 132:275–279

Topliss DJ, Kolliniatis E, Barlow JW, Lim C-F, Stockigt JR (1989) Uptake of 3,5,3′-triiodothyronine by cultured rat hepatoma cells is inhibitable by nonbile acid cholephils, diphenylhydantoin, and nonsteroidal antiinflammatory drugs. Endocrinology 124:980–986

Topliss DJ, Scholz GH, Kolliniatis E, Barlow JW, Stockigt JR (1993) Influence of calmodulin antagonists and calcium channel blockers on triiodothyronine uptake by rat hepatoma and myoblast cell lines. Metabolism 42:376–380

Underwood AH, Emmett JC, Ellis D, Flynn SB, Leeson PD, Benson GM, Novelli R, Pearce NJ, Shah VP (1986) A thyromimetic that decreases plasma cholesterol levels without increasing cardiac activity. Nature 324:425–429

Wartofsky L (1993) Has the use of antithyroid drugs for Graves' disease become obsolete? Thyroid 3:335–344

Weisiger RA, Luxon BA, Cavalieri RR (1992) Hepatic uptake of 3,5,3′-triiodothyronine: electrochemical driving forces. Am J Physiol 262:G1104–G1112

Williams GR, Franklyn JA, Neuberger J, Sheppard MC (1989) Thyroid hormone receptor expression in the "sick" euthyroid syndrome. Lancet 2:1477–1481

Williams GR, Franklyn JA, Sheppard MC (1991) Thyroid hormone and glucocorticoid regulation of receptor and target gene mRNAs in pituitary GH_3 cells. Mol Cell Endocrinol 80:127–138

Willams GR, Brent GA (1992) Specificity of nuclear hormone receptor action: who conducts the orchestra? J Endocrinol 135:191–194

Wolf M, Hansen N, Greten H (1994) Interleukin 1β, tumor necrosis factor-α and interleukin 6 decrease nuclear thyroid hormone receptor capacity in a liver cell line. Eur J Endocrinol 131:307–312

Yen PM, Chin WW (1994) New advances in understanding the molecular mechanisms of thyroid hormone action. Trends Endocrinol Metab 5:65–72

Yin Y, Vassy R, Nicolas P, Perret GY, Laurent S (1994) Antagonism between T_3 and amiodarone on the contractility and the density of beta-adrenoceptors of chicken cardiac myocytes. Eur J Pharmacol 261:97–104

Zhang X-K, Pfahl M (1993) Regulation of retinoid and thyroid hormone action through homodimeric and heterodimeric receptors. Trends Endocrinol Metab 4:156–162

Zhou Y, Samson M, Francon J, Blondeau J-P (1992) Thyroid hormone concentrative uptake in rat erythrocytes. Biochem J 281:81–86

CHAPTER 14

Immunomodulatory Agents in Autoimmune Thyroid Disease

A.P. WEETMAN

A. Introduction

The term autoimmune thyroid disease encompasses several common disorders: Hashimoto's thyroiditis, primary myxoedema, Graves' disease and postpartum thyroiditis, as well as the subclinical forms of these disorders. The basis for these disorders has been reviewed extensively (WEETMAN and MCGREGOR 1994); this chapter will concentrate on the effect of immunomodulatory agents, beginning in each section with the results from animal models of experimental autoimmune thyroiditis (EAT). The close relationship between thyroid-associated ophthalmopathy (TAO) and autoimmune thyroid disease suggests a common pathogenesis. This autoimmune eye disorder may be disfiguring and a threat to vision. Since developments in immunotherapy are likely to have their greatest impact in this condition, because present agents have major side effects and a suboptimal effect, immunomodulation in TAO is considered separately, at the end of the chapter.

B. Hormones and Autoimmune Thyroid Disease

I. Sex Hormones

A female preponderance is found in susceptibility in several models of EAT and in human autoimmune thyroiditis, in which the ratio of women to men is around 10:1. There is good evidence that sex hormones are responsible for this effect. Castration or oestrogen increases thyroglobulin (TG) antibody levels in male mice immunised with TG plus adjuvant (OKAYASU et al. 1981). This effect was reversed by continuous administration of testosterone. EAT can also be induced by neonatal thymectomy and sublethal irradiation (Tx – X) of genetically susceptible strains of rats, and in this model, oestrogen led to suppression of both TG antibody levels and the severity of thyroiditis in castrated male or female animals; progesterone exacerbated both indices of EAT (ANSAR AHMED et al. 1983). Oestrogen may have a dual action, low doses enhancing autoimmunity and high levels inhibiting it, particularly in sublethally irradiated animals.

A third type of spontaneously developing autoimmune thyroiditis (SAT) occurs in certain genetically predisposed animal strains. Thyroiditis in the OS (obese strain) chicken closely resembles Hashimoto's thyroiditis and results in irreversible hypothyroidism. Testosterone administered shortly after birth reduced the severity of thyroiditis and was associated with changes in thymic development and T cell regulation (GAUSE and MARSH 1986).

There is no direct evidence for a role of sex hormone in human autoimmune thyroiditis, but the change at puberty from a previously equal sex ratio to one of female excess is clearly suggestive. Autoimmune thyroid diseases usually become less severe in pregnancy, as shown by a decline in thyroid autoantibody levels, and this is succeeded by an exacerbation in the postpartum period (in subclinical patients this causes postpartum thyroiditis). Elevation of progesterone and oestrogen levels during pregnancy and their subsequent fall to subnormal levels may be responsible in part for these changes (WILDER 1995). Enhanced production of prolactin may also play a role; hyperprolactinaemia has been associated with an increase in thyroid autoantibodies (FERRARI et al. 1983). If anything, there is a decrease in thyroid autoimmunity with oral contraceptive use (FRANK and RAY 1978).

II. Glucocorticoids

Immune responses in general are subject to complex neuroendocrine regulation in which the hypothalamo-pituitary-adrenal axis plays a key role. Stress, as the result of an array of physical and psychological changes, activates this axis and there is increasing evidence that failure to produce adequate endogenous glucocorticoids exacerbates autoimmunity (REICHLIN 1993). OS chickens have a genetically determined elevation in corticosteroid binding globulin, decreased free corticosterone and an impaired glucocorticoid response to the cytokine interleukin-1 (IL-1), as reviewed extensively elsewhere (WICK et al. 1993). There is also some evidence for increased resistance of OS thymic lymphocytes to apoptosis induced by glucocorticoids (WICK et al. 1994).

Autoimmune thyroid disease has been observed after excess cortisol production due to Cushing's syndrome is corrected (TAKASU et al. 1990), indicating that endogenous glucocorticoids are also important in man. High concentrations of exogenous glucocorticoid are widely used to suppress immunological and inflammatory disorders. They have been used in Graves' disease with some success (WERNER and PLATMAN 1965) but the well-known side effects of excess glucocorticoids prevent their adoption for the treatment of this relatively benign autoimmune condition. The use of steroids in TAO is considered below.

III. Thyroid Hormones

There is clear evidence that EAT is suppressed by excess thyroid hormones. Thyroxine (T_4) administration, sufficient to raise serum T_4 levels, decreased TG antibody levels and reduced the severity of thyroiditis in rats immunised with TG plus adjuvant (Hassman et al. 1985a). These effects were associated with thymic and splenic hypertrophy and suppressed lymphocyte proliferation after in vitro mitogen stimulation. In SAT in the BB strain of rat, T_4 at doses sufficient to suppress the level of thyroid stimulating hormone (TSH) also reduced the severity of thyroiditis and reduced TG antibody levels (Banovac et al. 1988; Reinhardt et al. 1988). Thyroid hormone receptors are found in lymphocytes and thyroid hormones may also modulate immune responses via their effects on other hormones (Wilder 1995).

Besides these generalised immunomodulatory effects of thyroid hormones, the severity of EAT may be affected via feedback effects on TSH. The level of circulating TG is critical to the development of thyroiditis (although not necessarily TG antibodies), and an increase in TG levels, produced either by administration of exogenous TG or by TSH to raise endogenous TG levels, has been shown to reduce thyroiditis severity (Lewis et al. 1987). This suppressive effect is transferable and mediated by $CD4^+$ T cells (Fuller et al. 1993), although tolerance might also be induced at the B cell level (Parish et al. 1988). Suppression of TSH by excessive thyroid hormone would therefore be expected to exacerbate EAT through a decrease in TG levels, but low TSH levels may have a number of other beneficial effects, for instance by reducing TG below a critical level to drive the autoimmune process or by inducing thyrocyte inactivity or "rest", thus reducing the participation of thyroid cells in a number of immunological interactions in thyroiditis (Weetman 1994).

Short-term administration of triiodothyronine has no effect on normal human lymphocyte function (Weetman et al. 1984a), but sustained thyrotoxicosis of any cause is associated with elevated levels of circulating soluble IL-2 receptor (Koukkou et al. 1991). A number of other effects have been ascribed to excessive thyroid hormones in Graves' disease, particularly alterations of circulating lymphocyte subsets (reviewed by Volpé 1994), but it is not clear whether these changes may be the result of the underlying autoimmune process. Administration of T_4 after stopping antithyroid drug treatment for Graves' disease has been shown to decrease TSH-receptor antibody levels and improve remission rates (Hashizume et al. 1991), which again could be the result of thyroid cell rest. However, other studies have not demonstrated such an effect (Alexander et al. 1970; Tamai et al. 1995) and the reason for these differences is unclear.

Spontaneous remission of Hashimoto's thyroiditis and primary myxoedema has been reported after several years of treatment with thyroxine (Takasu et al. 1992; Comtois et al. 1995). This outcome seems particularly likely in patients with TSH-receptor (TSH-R) blocking antibodies which fall during T_4 administration. Thyroid peroxidase (TPO) antibodies and the size of the goitre also decrease (Chiovato et al. 1986). These observations suggest that T_4 has a direct or indirect (via reduction in TSH levels) effect on the autoimmune process.

C. Toxins and Autoimmune Thyroid Disease

Many compounds have been identified as goitrogens but a role for toxins in thyroid autoimmunity is largely unexplored. The best example is the Buffalo strain rat, which has a low prevalence of SAT that is increased by 3-methylcholanthrene (REUBER and GLOVER 1968). This compound is a polycyclic aromatic hydrocarbon found in exhaust emissions, cigarette smoke and charcoal-broiled food; such hydrocarbons are carcinogenic and have T cell immunosuppressive properties (GHONEUM et al. 1987). Subcutaneous or oral administration of 3-methylcholanthrene induces an irreversible lymphocytic thyroiditis (with weak or absent production of TG antibodies) in up to 80% of female and 20% of male rats (GLOVER et al. 1968; SILVERMAN and ROSE 1975; COHEN and WEETMAN 1987). Only this strain of rat is susceptible to thyroiditis after 3-methylcholanthrene, and because neonatal Tx also increases the prevalence of thyroiditis, it is possible that the effects are mediated via an alteration in the regulation of thyroid-autoreactive T cells.

Carbon tetrachloride and trypan blue given by injection, and 7,12-dimethylbenzanthracene given orally, also produce chronic thyroiditis in Buffalo strain rats (GLOVER and REUBER 1967; REUBER 1969; REUBER and GLOVER 1969), showing that the autoimmune response to thyroid antigens is readily disturbed by a variety of agents in this strain of rat. The immunohistochemical features of thyroiditis induced by trypan blue and 3-methylcholanthrene differ from SAT, there being more dendritic cells and macrophages but fewer T cells in the induced disease (COHEN and WEETMAN 1987). This raises the possibility of thyroid toxicity with release of thyroid antigens as an alternative cause for the thyroiditis.

It is unknown whether environmental toxins affect thyroid autoimmunity in man, although there is clearly scope for this. For instance, TAO and to a lesser extent Graves' disease are associated with smoking (SHINE et al. 1990; PRUMMEL and WIERSINGA 1993), conceivably as a result of polycyclic aromatic hydrocarbon exposure.

D. Trace Elements and Autoimmune Thyroiditis

The role of iodine in thyroid physiology is considered in detail in Chap. 7. There is a considerable body of evidence showing that excess iodine intake, either in the diet or via drugs (including contrast medium), exacerbates thyroid autoimmunity. The prevalence of SAT in the OS chicken and in the BB and Buffalo strains of rat is increased by additional dietary iodine (ALLEN et al. 1986; COHEN and WEETMAN 1988). Indeed, iodine is essential for the development of SAT in OS chickens (BROWN et al. 1991) and this may be because a critical epitope on TG is iodine dependent. In other strains of rat, paradoxically, a low iodine diet may induce signs of thyroid autoimmunity, including an increase in intrathyroidal dendritic cells and T cells and the production of colloid autoantibodies (MOOIJ et al. 1993). Thus, it seems to be the balance of iodine intake for the individual animal, and probably rapid changes in level, which determine effects on thyroid autoimmunity.

Epidemiological evidence supports an effect of iodine on autoimmune thyroiditis in man (Weetman and McGregor 1994). Iodine in cough medicines produces goitre and half of these patients have thyroid antibodies (Hall et al. 1966). Amiodarone contains 75 mg iodine per 200 mg and has a number of important effects on thyroid function (Chap. 10). In one study there was enhanced production of thyroid antibodies in patients treated with amiodarone (Monteiro et al. 1986) but this has not been confirmed subsequently (Weetman et al. 1988; Machado et al. 1992).

Selenium deficiency aggravates the thyroid cell damage produced by the sudden introduction of a high dietary dose of iodine in previously iodine-deficient rats (Contempre et al. 1993). There is also an increase in thyroid cell inflammatory infiltrate. Whilst of most interest to the pathogenesis of myxoedematous cretinism, it is possible that these effects could also play a role in autoimmunity within the gland.

Lithium is used in the treatment of manic depression and is associated with the development of goitre and hypothyroidism in up to 30% of patients (Chap. 9). These two complications are mainly the result of adenylate cyclase inhibition within the thyroid, but in addition a high prevalence of thyroid antibodies has been reported in patients receiving lithium (Lazarus et al. 1981). Complex effects on thyroid antibody formation in EAT have been reported, depending on the dose and stage of disease at which lithium was administered (Hassman et al. 1985b). The incidence of Graves' disease may be increased by lithium therapy (Barclay et al. 1994) and since the biochemical action of lithium is to decrease thyroid hormone production, this paradoxical side effect is further indirect evidence for an enhancing action of lithium on thyroid autoimmune mechanisms.

E. Drugs and Autoimmune Thyroid Disease

Apart from lithium and iodine-containing medications, drugs are not thought to induce autoimmune thyroid disease in man. A recent report has shown that alimemazine, a phenothiazine, induces major histocompatibility complex class II molecule expression on murine thyroid follicular cells and allows them to serve as antigen presenting cells for TG (Takorabet et al. 1995). It will be of interest to see whether phenothiazine-treated patients have an excess of thyroid autoimmunity, based on this report.

The evidence that thionamides have immunomodulatory effects is discussed in detail in Chap. 8, this volume. They cause a reduction in the aetiologically important TSH-R antibodies in Graves' disease, and also lessen the severity of the thyroidal lymphocytic infiltration (Weetman 1995). This reduction in antibodies is accompanied by a fall in serum markers of complement activation (Fig. 1). However, non-thyroid autoantibodies, such as those

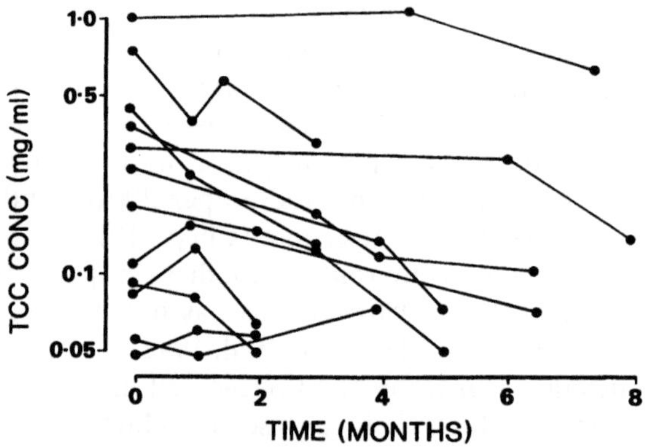

Fig. 1. Serial measures of circulating terminal complement complexes (*TCC*) in patients with Graves' disease treated for 6 months (from time 0) with carbimazole; TCC concentrations provide an indirect measure of the formation of membrane attack complexes of complement

against gastric parietal cells, are not reduced and this is most likely because the drugs must be concentrated within the thyroid to achieve their immunomodulatory effect. The reduction seen in the production of cytokines and reactive oxygen metabolites by thyroid cells when cultured with antithyroid drugs may explain the specificity of this effect, as shown in Fig. 2 (WEETMAN et al. 1992).

Perchlorate also reduces the level of TSH-R antibodies when given to patients with Graves' disease (WENZEL and LENTE 1984). This agent reduces thyroid hormone production by inhibiting iodine uptake, which could, in addition, interefere with thyroid cell-lymphocyte interactions critical to the autoimmune process. Perchlorate reduces mitogen-stimulated immunoglobulin synthesis by lymphocytes in vitro (WEETMAN et al. 1984b), thus having a similar effect to thionamides. It also diminishes TG antibody synthesis in EAT (Fig. 3).

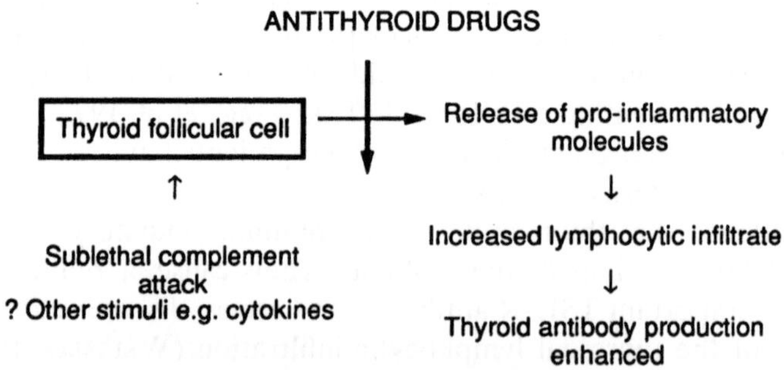

Fig. 2. Possible role of antithyroid drugs in suppressing the autoimmune response in Graves' disease. (From WEETMAN 1995, with permission)

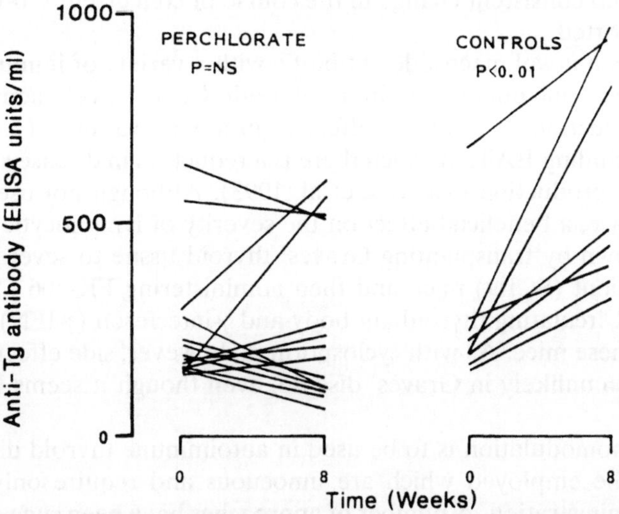

Fig. 3. Effect of perchlorate (4 mg/rat per day) given in the drinking water of Buffalo rats with experimental autoimmune thyroiditis induced by neonatal thymectomy; the normal rise in thyroglobulin (*Tg*) antibodies with time is not seen. *NS*, not significant

More conventional immunosuppressive drugs have not been used in thyroid autoimmunity in man, as their side effects outweigh potential benefits. However, a modest effect of the fungal metabolite cyclosporin A has been demonstrated in the Tx-X model of EAT in rats (HASSMAN et al. 1985c). There was a reduction in thyroiditis severity but disease was not prevented, and long-term administration was required to achieve even this. Cyclosporin A had no effect on SAT in OS chickens (WICK et al. 1982), but decreased TG antibody formation and the severity of thyroiditis in mice immunised with TG in adjuvant (VLADUTIU 1983). The timing of cyclosporin A administration is critical, as treatment early in life exacerbates SAT and EAT, presumably by altering the developing T cell repertoire (WICK et al. 1982; SAKAGUCHI and SAKAGUCHI 1989).

In view of the dose-dependent nephrotoxicity and hepatotoxicity of cyclosporin A, attempts have been made to use low-dose cyclosporin A with other immunosuppressive agents. In Tx-induced EAT in Buffalo strain rats, low-dose cyclosporin A (1.5 mg/kg per day) had no effect but prevented the development of thyroiditis when given with subtherapeutic concentrations of an IL-2 receptor monoclonal antibody (COHEN et al. 1989). Similarly, 1,25-dihydroxyvitamin D has weak immunosuppressive properties, insufficient to affect EAT, but when given with cyclosporin A (at suboptimal dose) there was a significant decrease in the prevalence of thyroiditis in mice immunised with TG plus adjuvant (FOURNIER et al. 1990). Cyclosporin A has been used for the treatment of TAO but, although there is some improvement in this condition (see below), no consistent change in the course of concurrent Graves' disease has been reported.

FK-506 is a novel macrolide antibiotic with a variety of immunosuppressive properties, including inhibition of both $CD4^+$ T cell activation and cytokine production. It has been effective in a wide variety of autoimmune disorders, including EAT, in which there is a reduction in disease severity and TG antibody production (TAMURA et al. 1993). Although not used so far in Graves' disease, a beneficial effect on the severity of lymphocytic infiltration has been shown by transplanting Graves' thyroid tissue to severe combined immunodeficient (SCID) mice and then administering FK-506 (YOSHIKAWA et al. 1994). Circulating thyroid antibody and γ-interferon (γ-IFN) levels also declined in these mice. As with cyclosporin A, however, side effects make the use of FK-506 unlikely in Graves' disease, even though it seems likely to be beneficial.

If immunomodulation is to be used in autoimmune thyroid disease, strategies must be employed which are innocuous and require only a limited period of administration. A number of approaches have been suggested by the characterisation of the critical molecules involved in antigen presentation and T cell activation (Fig. 4) but these have yet to find a clear place in human autoimune disorders (SINHA et al. 1990; WEINER 1994; LINSLEY 1995; KRENSKY and CLAYBERGER 1995). Administration of monoclonal antibodies against $CD4^+$ but not $CD8^+$ T cells reduced the severity of EAT in a murine adoptive transfer model (FLYNN et al. 1989). Another broad approach has been the in vivo use of monoclonal antibodies against the adhesion molecules LFA-1 (lymphocyte function associated antigen-1) and its ligand CD54 (ICAM-1). Both reduced the severity of EAT induced by rats by immunisation with TG and adjuvant, but a lowering of TG antibodies was only found with LFA-1 antibody treatment (METCALFE et al. 1993).

These non-specific effects seem unlikely to be refined enough for safe usage in human thyroid autoimmunity. Thyroid-specific therapy is possible and more appealing. For instance, protection from immunisation-induced EAT in mice has been described after administration of a monoclonal antibody to a T cell receptor from a TG-specific cytotoxic T cell hybridoma (TEXIER et al. 1992). Also, modulation of suppressor T cells using appropriate concentrations of TG is effective in diminishing EAT (LEWIS et al. 1987). More recently, oral tolerance to a variety of autoantigens has been effective in experimental autoimmune disease and it has been shown that oral TG reduces (but does not abolish) the induction of immunisation-induced EAT in mice (GUIMARAES et al. 1995). Both T and B cell responses were affected in a specific manner, probably by anergy induction in the T cell compartment. However, it is not yet clear whether this approach will be successful after the initiation phase of autoimmune thyroiditis. Moreover, the T cell response to thyroid autoantigens is heterogeneous by the time disease is clinically apparent, in terms of T cell receptor usage, the number of autoantigens involved and their epitopes stimulating autoreactivity (WEETMAN and MCGREGOR 1994).

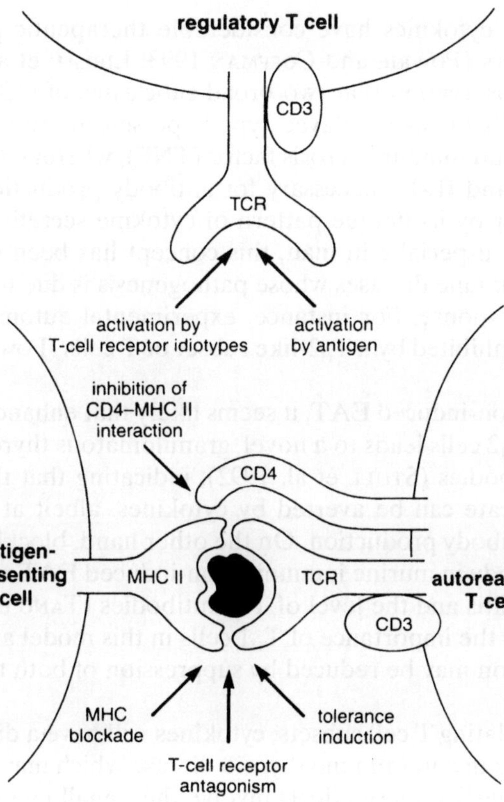

Fig. 4. Potential sites for immunomodulatory treatment in the interaction between T cells and antigen presenting cells. (From ADORINI et al. 1993, with permission)

This makes any approach along the lines shown in Fig. 4 difficult to contemplate at present, although presumably there is restriction early on in disease which could be utilised therapeutically if individuals at risk were identified.

F. Cytokines and Autoimmune Thyroid Disease

The use of a variety of cytokines in the treatment of malignancies or hepatitis has been associated with exacerbation of underlying autoimmune thyroiditis, as well as other autoimmune disorders, in genetically predisposed individuals. Leucocyte-derived and recombinant α-IFN induce reversible hypothyroidism and the appearance of thyroid antibodies is around 20% of patients over a period of months (BURMAN et al. 1986; RONNBLOM et al. 1991; GISSLINGER et al. 1992). Similar effects have been seen with IL-2 or granulocyte-macrophage colony stimulating factor (VAN LIESSUM et al. 1989; HOEKMAN et al. 1991) but γ-IFN has no apparent effect (KUNG et al. 1990).

Paradoxically, cytokines have considerable therapeutic potential in autoimmune disorders (POWRIE and COFFMAN 1993; LIBLAU et al. 1995). This is founded on the observation that two broad subclasses of $CD4^+$ ("helper") T cells exist. T_H1 cells mediate delayed type hypersensitivity reactions and secrete γ-IFN, IL-2 and tumour necrosis factor (TNF), whereas T_H2 cells provide B cells with IL-4 and IL-13, necessary for antibody production. Each subset regulates the other by its unique pattern of cytokine secretion. Although an oversimplification, especially in man, this concept has been exploited in experimental autoimmune diseases whose pathogenesis is due to a delayed type hypersensitivity response. For instance, experimental autoimmune diabetes mellitus in rats is inhibited by a T_H2-like subset of T cells (FOWELL and MASON 1993).

In immunisation-induced EAT, it seems likely that enhanced activation of thyroid-specific T_H2 cells leads to a novel, granulomatous thyroiditis with high levels of TG antibodies (STULL et al. 1992), indicating that the more typical lymphocytic infiltrate can be averted by cytokines, albeit at the expense of enhanced autoantibody production. On the other hand, blocking γ-IFN with a monoclonal antibody in murine immunisation-induced EAT reduced both the severity of thyroiditis and the level of TG antibodies (TANG et al. 1993). This is compatible with the importance of T_H1 cells in this model and suggests that antibody production may be reduced by suppression of both the T_H1 and T_H2 population.

Besides modulating T cell subsets, cytokines will have a diversity of direct and indirect effects in autoimmune thyroid disease which may be amenable to treatment, particularly if these effects involve the signalling between lymphocytes and thyroid cells (WEETMAN 1994). IL-1 is a pleiotropic cytokine and has divergent effects in EAT, which may depend on the complex interrelationships between its immunological, metabolic and endocrine actions. High-dose IL-1 induces goitre development, severe lymphocytic thyroiditis and hypothyroidism in the BB rat (WILSON et al. 1990). In contrast, low-dose IL-1 reduces the incidence of SAT. High-dose IL-1 exacerbates murine EAT and lower doses interfere with the induction of suppression (NABOZNY and KONG 1992). Thus, IL-1 antagonists could have a beneficial effect in human autoimmune thyroid disease, but could also be harmful depending on the overall effects of IL-1 in vivo in this setting. IL-10 is another cytokine which could have immunotherapeutic potential as IL-10 reduced the severity of murine EAT by enhancing activation-induced apoptosis of T cells (MIGNON-GODEFROY et al. 1995) but, as with IL-1 modulation, such effects could also interfere with beneficial immune reponses to microorganisms.

Considerable work will, therefore, be needed before cytokine modulation could be considered in autoimmune thyroid disease, but its application to those patients with severe, congestive ophthalmopathy seems likely in the near future, as there is a large body evidence for a central role of cytokines (especially γ-IFN, TNF and IL-1) in pathogenesis (BAHN and HEUFELDER 1993). In this setting, trials of already available monoclonal antibodies against TNF would provide unique insights into the disease process in TAO, as well as a novel approach to this serious medical problem.

G. Immunomodulatory Agents in TAO

In the majority of patients with TAO, the signs and symptoms are mild to moderate and require only reassurance or local measures, while surgery is appropriate for residual burnt-out disease, topics which are considered elsewhere (FELLS 1991). The place of immunomodulatory agents currently is for severe TAO, where congestive changes, including optic nerve compression, are progressive and debilitating. The aims of treatment are to (1) improve visual acuity, (2) correct diplopia, (3) reduce proptosis, (4) improve appearance and (5) relieve pain (WIERSINGA 1992). The risk-benefit ratio of current treatments has reduced their application to less severe cases of TAO but the introduction of safe and relatively specific immunotherapy (e.g. via cytokine modulation as discussed above) is eagerly anticipated and would have a more extensive application.

I. Glucocorticoids

High-dose prednisone has been widely used in congestive ophthalmopathy. Around two-thirds of patients respond with improvement but disease recurs if steroids are discontinued too soon; at least 6 months treatment is associated with an improved outcome (BURCH and WARTOFSKY 1993). As a result, side effects frequently limit steroid use. Intravenous methylprednisolone pulse therapy has been advocated by some authors (NAGAYAMA et al. 1987; KENDALL-TAYLOR et al. 1988; KOSHIYAMA et al. 1994) but the benefits of this over oral prednisone remain unclear. Used alone in pulses, sustained remission is unlikely with methylprednisolone and the outcome when followed by oral steroids seems similar to that with high-dose oral prednisone alone. Others have advocated modest doses of prednisone prophylactically when radioiodine is given to Graves' patients with TAO, who are possibly at risk of having an exacerbation of their eye disease (BARTALENA et al. 1989). The exact importance of this is also uncertain, as the long-term outcome in those patients not receiving steroids remains unevaluated, and it is possible that any worsening prevented by steroids could be temporary and reversible.

II. Other Immunosuppressive Drugs

Azathioprine has been used in some patients but proved ineffective in a controlled trial; the same is true of ciamexone (PERROS et al. 1990; KAHALY et al. 1990). Cyclophosphamide improved diplopia and visual acuity, as well as soft tissue changes, in uncontrolled trials (BIGOS et al.1979), but the toxicity of this drug has presumably prevented further trials. Cyclosporin A similarly produced improvement in severe TAO in open trials, but controlled trials have shown only a modest effect. During a 12-week treatment period with 7.5 mg cyclosporin A/kg daily, there was a 22% response rate, judged by a decrease in extraocular muscle enlargement and proptosis, improved visual acuity and a decrease in a scoring system for signs and symptoms (PRUMMEL et al. 1989). By contrast, 61% of patients treated with prednisone showed improvement. However, five of the nine patients who failed to respond to prednisone improved when the two agents were used together. This effectiveness was underlined by a comparison of prednisone versus prednisone plus cyclosporin A (5–7.5 mg/kg per day initially); sustained improvement was seen in 60% of the patients treated with prednisone alone, compared to 95% of those receiving both drugs (KAHALY et al. 1986). Thus cyclosporin A may be useful as a steroid sparing agent, although its nephrotoxic side effects and potential to cause lymphomas remain a concern. The lowest effective dose in combination treatment has not been established but some patients appear to have a benefit with 2 mg/kg per day, which may be associated with fewer side effects.

III. Other Treatments

Plasmapheresis has been tried in TAO, although the rationale for this is rather unclear as there is no secure evidence that circulating antibodies or immune complexes play a role in pathogenesis, in contrast to myasthenia gravis or antiglomerular basement membrane disease (Goodpasture's syndrome), in which plasmapheresis has some established benefit. Uncontrolled studies have shown an apparent beneficial effect of this procedure. In the most extensive, there was a rapid improvement in eight of nine patients, even though seven of these had previously had orbital decompression, steroids or azathioprine (GLINOER et al. 1986). This improvement preceded the introduction of conventional immunosuppressive drugs but sustained improvement was dependent on the use of these agents after plasmapheresis. Without controlled trials, the exact place of this treatment remains obscure. Any benefit conferred may be mechanical (by reducing plasma viscosity and thus improving perfusion of orbital tissue) rather than immunological, but this too requires evaluation.

Intravenous immunoglobulin infusions have been reported to give the same response rate in patients with TAO as prednisone in an uncontrolled trial (ANTONELLI et al. 1992). This is a very expensive treatment and its exact place requires further study. Any beneficial effect may be due to the activity of soluble immunomodulatory molecules, such as CD4, CD8 and HLA, in the immunoglobulin-preparation, rather than the action of putative anti-idiotypic antibodies (BLASCZYK et al. 1993). Uncontrolled studies with the long-acting somatostatin analogue, octreotide, have shown a beneficial effect in both TAO and pretibial myxoedema, possibly by interfering with local insulin-like growth factor-1 synthesis, which could cause the fibroblast activation typical of these conditions (CHANG et al. 1992).

Finally, radiotherapy, usually given as a ten fractionated doses of 2 Gy over a 2-week period, appears in uncontrolled trials to give the same response rate in TAO as steroids (Petersen et al. 1990). Although the long-term side effects of this treatment remain unclear, it appears so far to be safe. Radiation retinopathy leading to blindness is the most important adverse affect but may be the result of miscalculated dosage; diabetes and previous chemotherapy also increase the risk of this complication and are, therefore, contraindications. Combined therapy with intravenous methylprednisone and irradiation is superior to methylprednisone alone (Bartalena et al. 1983), but in this trial the benefits of irradiation alone were not assessed. A double-blind randomised trial of irradiation versus prednisone showed that these treatments were equally effective in moderately severe ophthalmopathy but, predictably, side effects were greater with steroids (Prummel et al. 1993). Presumably, irradiation is effective because it destroys the radiosensitive infiltrating lymphocytes in the orbit, thereby ameliorating cytokine release and other pathogenic mechanisms.

The foregoing summary emphasises the difficulties of treating TAO and predicting the response of any individual patient is impossible due to the complex natural history of this disorder and our incomplete understanding of its pathogenesis. Establishing markers for those patients at risk, in whom early intervention could prevent progression, has some appeal but there has been little success in this direction to date. This is a key area for new developments in the field of immunomodulatory agents in thyroid autoimmunity.

References

Adorini L et al (1993) Selective immunosuppression. Immunol Today 14:285–289

Alexander WD, McLarty DG, Robertson J, Shimmins J, Brownlie BEW, McG Harden R, Patel AR (1970) Prediction of the long-term results of antithyroid drug therapy for thyrotoxicosis. J Clin Endocrinol Metab 30:540–543

Allen EM, Appel MC, Braverman LE (1986) The effect of iodine ingestion on the development of spontaneous lymphocytic thyroiditis in the diabetes prone BB/W rat. Endocrinology 118:1977–1981

Ansar Ahmed S, Young PR, Penhale WJ (1983) The effects of female sex steroids on the development of autoimmune thyroiditis in thymectomized and irradiated rats. Clin Exp Immunol 54:351–358

Antonelli A, Saracino A, Alberti B (1992) High-dose intravenous immunoglobulin treatment in Graves' ophthalmopathy. Acta Endocrinol (Copenh) 126:13–23

Bahn RS, Heufelder AE (1993) Pathogenesis of Graves' ophthalmopathy. N Engl J Med 329:1468–1475

Banovac K, Ghandur-Mnaymneh L, Zakarija M, Rabinovitch A, McKenzie JM (1988) The effect of thyroxine on spontaneous thyroiditis in BB/W rats. Int Arch Allergy Appl Immunol 87:301–305

Barclay ML, Brownlie BEW, Turner JG, Wells JE (1994) Lithium associated thyrotoxicosis: a report of 14 cases, with statistical analysis of incidence. Clin Endocrinol (Oxf) 40:759–764

Bartalena L, Marcocci C, Chiovato L, Laddaga M, Lepri G, Andreani D, Cavallaci G, Baschieri L, Pinchera A (1983) Orbital cobalt irradiation combined with systemic corticosteroids for Graves' ophthalmopathy: comparison with systemic corticosteroids alone. J Clin Endocrinol Metab 56:1139–1144

Bartalena L, Marcocci C, Bogazzi F, Panicucci M, Lepri A, Pinchera A (1989) Use of corticosteroids to prevent progression of Graves' ophthalmopathy after radioiodine therapy for hyperthyroidism. N Engl J Med 321:1349–1352
Bigos ST, Nisula BC, Daniels GH, Eastman RC, Johnston HH, Kohler PO (1979) Cyclophosphamide in the management of advanced Graves' ophthalmopathy. Ann Intern Med 90:921–923
Blasczyk R, Westhoff U, Gross-Wilde H (1993) Soluble CD4, CD8, and HLA molecules in commercial immunoglobulin preparations. Lancet 341:789–790
Brown TR, Sundick RS, Dhar A, Sheth D, Bagchi N (1991) Uptake and metabolism of iodine is crucial for the development of thyroiditis in Obese strain chickens. J Clin Invest 88:106–111
Burch HB, Wartofsky L (1993) Graves' ophthalmopathy: current concepts regarding pathogenesis and management. Endocr Rev 14:747–793
Burman P, Töttermann TH, Oberg K, Karlsson FA (1986) Thyroid autoimmunity in patients on long-term therapy with leukocyte-derived interferon. J Clin Endocrinol Metab 63:1086–1090
Chang TC, Kao SCS, Huang KM (1992) Octreotide and Graves' ophthalmopathy and pretibial myxoedema. Br Med J 304:158
Chiovato L, Marcocci C, Mariotti S, Mori A, Pinchera A (1986) L-thyroxine therapy induces a fall of microsomal and thyroglobulin antibodies in idiopathic myxedema and in hypothyroid, but not in euthyroid Hashimoto's thyroiditis. J Endocrinol Invest 9:299–305
Cohen SB, Weetman AP (1987) Characterization of different types of experimental autoimmune thyroiditis in the Buffalo strain rat. Clin Exp Immunol 69:25–32
Cohen SB, Weetman AP (1988) The effect of iodine depletion and supplementation in the Buffalo strain rat. J Endocrinol Invest 11:625–627
Cohen SB, Diamantstein T, Weetman AP (1989) The effect of T cell subset depletion on autoimmune thyroiditis in the Buffalo strain rat. Immunol Lett 23:263–268
Comtois R, Faucher L, Laflèche L (1995) Outcome of hypothyroidism caused by Hashimoto's thyroiditis. Arch Intern Med 155:1404–1408
Contempre B, Denef J-F, Dumont JE, Many M-C (1993) Selenium deficiency aggravates the necrotizing effects of a high iodide dose in iodine deficient rats. Endocrinology 132:1866–1867
Fells P (1991) Thyroid-associated eye disease: clinical management. Lancet 338:29–32
Ferrari C, Boghen M, Paracchi A, Rampini P, Raiteri F, Benco R, Romussi M, Codecasa F, Mucci M, Bianco M (1983) Thyroid autoimmunity in hyperprolactinaemic disorders. Acta Endocrinol (Oxf) 104:35–41
Flynn JC, Conaway DH, Cobbold S, Waldmann H, Kong Y-C M (1989) Depletion of $L3T4^+$ and $Lyt\text{-}2^+$ cells by rat monoclonal antibodies alters the development of adoptively transferred experimental autoimmune thyroiditis. Cell Immunol 122:377–390
Founier C, Gepner P, Sadouk MB, Charreire J (1990) In vivo beneficial effects of cyclosporin A and 1,25-dihydroxyvitamin D_3 on the induction of experimental autoimmune thyroiditis. Clin Immunol Immunopathol 54:53–63
Fowell D, Mason D (1993) Evidence that the T cell repertoire of normal rats contains cells with the potential to cause diabetes. Characterization of the $CD4^+$ T cell subset that inhibits this autoimmune potential. J Exp Med 177:627–636
Frank P, Kay CR (1978) Incidence of thyroid disease associated with oral contraceptives. Br Med J ii:1531
Fuller BE, Okayasu I, Simon LL, Giraldo AA, Kong Y-C M (1993) Characterization of resistance to murine experimental autoimmune thyroiditis: duration and afferent action of thyroglobulin- and TSH-induced suppression. Clin Immunol Immunopathol 69:60–68
Gause WC, Marsh JA (1986) Effect of testosterone treatments for varying periods on autoimmune development and on specific infiltrating leukocyte populations in the thyroid gland of Obese strain chickens. Clin Immunol Immunopathol 39:464–478

Ghoneum M, Wojdani A, Alfred L (1987) Effect of methylcholanthrene on human natural killer cytotoxicity and lymphokine production in vitro. Immunopharmacology 14:27–33

Gisslinger H, Gilly B, Woloszczuk W, Mayr WR, Havelec L, Linkesch W, Weissel M (1992) Thyroid autoimmunity and hypothyroidism during long-term treatment with recombinant interferon-alpha. Clin Exp Immunol 90:363–367

Glinoer D, Etienne-Decerf J, Schrooyen M, Sand G, Hoyoux P, Mahieu P, Winand R (1986) Beneficial effects of intensive plasma exchange followed by immunosuppressive therapy in severe Graves' ophthalmopathy. Acta Endocrinol (Oxf) 111:30–38

Glover EL, Reuber MD (1967) Chronic thyroiditis in Buffalo rats with carbon tetrachloride-induced cirrhosis. Endocrinology 80:361–364

Glover EL, Reuber MD, Grollman S (1968) Influence of age and sex on thyroiditis in rats injected subcutaneously with 3-methylcholanthrene. Pathol Microbiol 32:314–320

Guimaraes VC, Quintans J, Fisfalen M-E, Straus FH, Wilhelm K, Madeiros-Neto GA, DeGroot LJ (1995) Suppression of development of experimental autoimmune thyroiditis by oral administration of thyroglobulin. Endocrinology 136:3353–3359

Hall R, Turner-Warwick H, Doniach D (1966) Autoantibodies in iodide goitre and asthma. Clin Exp Immunol 1:285–296

Hashizume K, Ichikawa K, Sakurai A, Suzuki S, Takeda T, Kobayashi M, Miyamoto T, Arai M, Nagasawa T (1991) Effects on the level of antibodies to thyroid-stimulating hormone receptors and on the risk of recurrence of hyperthyroidism. N Engl J Med 324:947–953

Hassman R, Weetman AP, Gunn C, Stringer BMJ, Wynford-Thomas D, Hall R, McGregor AM (1985a) The effects of hyperthyroidism on experimental autoimmune thyroiditis in the rat. Endocrinology 116:1253–1258

Hassman R, Lazarus JH, Dieguez C, Weetman AP, Hall R, McGregor AM (1985b) The influence of lithium chloride on experimental autoimmune thyroid disease. Clin Exp Immunol 61:49–57

Hassman R, Dieguez C, Rennie DP, Weetman AP, Hall R, McGregor AM (1985c) The influence of cyclosporin A on the induction of experimental autoimmune thyroid disease in the PVG/c rat. Clin Exp Immunol 59:10–16

Hoekman K, von Blomberg-Van Der Flier BME, Wagstaff J, Drexhage HA, Pinedo HM (1991) Reversible thyroid dysfunction during treatment with GM-CSF. Lancet 338:541–542

Kahaly G, Schrezenmeir J, Krause U, Schweikert B, Meuer S, Muller W, Dennebaum R, Beyer J (1986) Cyclosporin and prednisone v. prednisone in treatment of Graves' ophthalmopathy: a controlled, randomized and prospective study. Eur J Clin Invest 16:415–422

Kahaly G, Lieb W, Muller-Forell W (1990) Ciamexone in endocrine orbitopathy. A randomized double-blind placebo-controlled study. Acta Endocrinol (Oxf) 122: 13–21

Kendall-Taylor P, Crombie AL, Stephenson AM, Hardwick M, Hall K (1988) Intravenous methylprednisolone in the treatment of Graves' ophthalmopathy. Br Med J 297:1574–1578

Koshiyama H, Koh T, Fujiwara K, Hayakawa K, Shimbo S-I, Misaki T (1994) Therapy of Graves' ophthalmopathy with intravenous high-dose steroid followed by orbital irradiation. Thyroid 4:409–412

Koukkou E, Panayiotidis P, Alevizou-Terzaki V, Thalassinos N (1991) High levels of serum soluble interleukin-2 receptors in hyperthyroid patients: correlation with serum thyroid hormones and independence from the etiology of the hyperthyroidism. J Clin Endocrinol Metab 73:771–776

Krezsky AM, Clayberger (1995) HLA-derived peptides as novel immunotherapeutics. Clin Immunol Immunopathol 75:112–116

Kung AWC, Jones BM, Lai CL (1990) Effects of interferon-γ therapy on thyroid function, T-lymphocyte subpopulations and induction of autoantibodies. J Clin Endocrinol Metab 71:1230–1234
Lazarus J, John R, Bennie E, Chalmers R, Crocket G (1981) Lithium therapy of thyroid function. Psychol Med 11:85
Lewis M, Giraldo AA, Kong YM (1987) Resistance to experimental autoimmune thyroiditis induced by physiologic manipulation of thyroglobulin level. Clin Immunol Immunopathol 45:92–104
Liblau RS, Singer SM, McDevitt HO (1995) Th1 and Th2 CD4+ T cells in the pathogenesis of organ-specific autoimmune diseases. Immunol Today 16:34–38
Linsley PS (1995) The CD28/CTLA-4: B7 receptor system in experimental autoimmune encephalomyelitis. J Clin Invest 95:2429–2430
Machado BB, de Silva MEP, Pinho B (1992) Long-term amiodarone therapy and antithyroid antibodies. Am J Cardiol 69:971–972
Metcalfe RA, Tandon N, Tamatani T, Miyasaka M, Weetman AP (1993) Adhesion molecule monoclonal antibodies inhibit experimental autoimmune thyroiditis. Immunology 80:493–497
Mignon-Godefroy K, Rott O, Brazillet M-P, Charreire J (1995) Curative and protective effects of IL-10 in experimental autoimmune thyroiditis (EAT). J Immunol 154:6634–6643
Monteiro E, Galvao-Teles A, Santos ML, Mourao L, Correia MJ, Lopo Tuna J, Ribeiro C (1986) Antithyroid antibodies as an early marker for thyroid disease induced by amiodarone. Br Med J 292:227–292
Mooij P, De Wit HJ, Bloot AM, Wilders-Truschnig MM, Drexhage HA (1993) Iodine deficiency induces thyroid autoimmune reactivity in Wistar rats. Endocrinology 133:1197–1204
Nabozny GH, Kong Y-C M (1992) Circumvention of the induction of resistance in murine experimental autoimmune thyroiditis by recombinant IL-1β. J Immunol 149:1086–1092
Nagayama Y, Izumi M, Kiriyama T, Yokoyama N, Morita S, Kakezono F, Ohtakara S, Morimoto I, Okamoto S, Nagataki S (1987) Treatment of Graves' ophthalmopathy with high-dose intravenous methylprednisolone pulse therapy. Acta Endocrinol (Oxf) 116:513–518
Okayasu I, Kong Y-C M, Rose NR (1981) Effect of castration and sex hormones on experimental autoimmune thyroiditis. Clin Immunol Immunopathol 20:240–245
Parish NM, Rayner D, Cooke A, Roitt IM (1988) An investigation of the nature of induced suppression to experimental autoimmune thyroiditis. Immunology 63: 199–203
Perros P, Weightman DR, Crombie AL, Kendall-Taylor P (1990) Azathioprine in the treatment of thyroid-associated ophthalmopathy. Acta Endocrinol (Oxf) 122:8–12
Petersen IA, Kriss JP, McDougall IR, Donaldson SS (1990) Prognostic factors in the radiotherapy of Graves' ophthalmopathy. Int J Radiat Oncol Biol 19:259–264
Powrie F, Coffman RL (1993) Cytokine regulation of T-cell function: potential for therapeutic intervention. Immunol Today 14:270–274
Prummel MF, Wiersinga WM (1993) Smoking and risk of Graves' disease. JAMA 269:479–482
Prummel MF, Mourits M, Berghout A, Krenning EP, van der Gaag R, Koornneef L, Wiersinga WM (1989) Prednisone and cyclosporine in the treatment of severe Graves' ophthalmopathy. N Engl J Med 321:1353–1359
Prummel MF, Mourits M, Blank L, Berghout A, Koornneef L, Wiersinga WM (1993) Randomised double-blind trial of prednisone versus radiotherapy in Graves' ophthalmopathy. Lancet 342:949–954
Reichlin S (1993) Neuroendocrine-immune interactions. N Engl J Med 329:1246–1253
Reinhardt W, Paul TL, Allen EM, Alex S, Yang Y-N, Appel MC, Braverman LE (1988) Effect of L-thyroxine administration on the incidence of iodine induced and spontaneous lymphocytic thyroiditis in the BB/WOR rat. Endocrinology 122: 1179–1181

Reuber MD (1969) Thyroiditis in rats given subcutaneous injections of trypan blue. Toxicol Appl Pharmacol 14:108–113
Reuber MD, Glover EL (1968) Thyroiditis in rats injected subcutaneously with 3-methylcholanthrene. Proc Exp Biol 129:509–511
Reuber MD, Glover EL (1969) Thyroiditis in Buffalo strain rats ingesting 7,12-dimethylbenz(A)anthracene. Experientia 25:753
Ronnblom LE, Alm BV, Oberg KE (1991) Autoimmunity after alpha-interferon therapy for malignant carcinoid tumours. Ann Intern Med 115:178–183
Sakaguchi S, Sakaguchi N (1989) Organ-specific disease induced in mice by elimination of T cell subsets. J Immunol 142:471–480
Shine B, Fells P, Edwards OM, Weetman AP (1990) Association of Graves' ophthalmopathy and smoking. Lancet i:1261–1263
Silverman DA, Rose NR (1975) The incidence and severity of the disease, and the genetics of susceptibility. J Immunol 114:145–147
Sinha AA, Lopez T, McDevitt HO (1990) Autoimmune diseases: the failure of self tolerance. Science 248:1380–1388
Stull SJ, Sharp GC, Kyriakos M, Bickel JT, Braley-Mullen H (1992) Induction of granulomatous experimental autoimmune thyroiditis in mice with in vitro activated effector T cells and anti-IFN-γ antibody. J Immunol 149:2219–2226
Takasu N, Komiya I, Nagasawa Y, Asawa T, Yamada T (1990) Exacerbation of autoimmune thyroid dysfunction after unilateral adrenalectomy in patients with Cushing's syndrome due to an adrenocortical adenoma. N Engl J Med 322:1708–1712
Takasu N, Yamada T, Takasu M, Komiya I, Nagasawa Y, Asawa T, Shinoda T, Aizawa T, Koizumi Y (1992) Disappearance of thyrotropin-blocking antibodies and spontaneous recovery from hypothyroidism in autoimmune thyroiditis. N Engl J Med 326:513–518
Takorabet L, Ropars A, Raby C, Charreire J (1995) Phenothiazine induces de novo MHC class II antigen expression on thyroid epithelial cells. J Immunol 154:3593–3602
Tamai H, Hayaki I, Kawai K, Komaki G, Matsubayashi S, Kuma K, Kumagai LF, Nagataki S (1995) Lack of effect of thyroxine administration on elevated thyroid stimulating hormone receptor antibody levels in treated Graves' disease patients. J Clin Endocrinol Metab 80:1481–1484
Tamura K, Woo J, Murase N, Carrieri G, Nalesnik MA, Thomson AW (1993) Suppression of autoimmune thyroid disease by FK 506: influence on thyroid-infiltrating cells, adhesion molecule expression and anti-thyroglobulin antibody production. Clin Exp Immunol 91:368–375
Tang H, Mignon-Godefroy K, Meroni PL, Garotta G, Charriere J, Nicoletti F (1993) The effects of a monoclonal antibody to interferon-γon experimental autoimmune thyroiditis (EAT): prevention of disease and decrease of EAT-specific T cells. Eur J Immunol 23:275–278
Texier B, Bedin C, Roubaty C, Brezin C, Charriere J (1992) Protection from experimental autoimmune thyroiditis conferred by a monoclonal antibody to T cell receptor from a cytotoxic hybridoma specific for thyroglobulin. J Immunol 148: 439–444
Van Liessum PA, De Mulder PHM, Mattijssen EJM, Corstens FHM, Wagener DJT (1989) Hypothyroidism and goitre during interleukin-2 therapy without LAK cells. Lancet i:224
Vladutiu A (1983) Effect of cyclosporine on experimental autoimmune thyroiditis in mice. Transplantation 35:518–520
Volpé R (1994) Evidence that the immunosuppressive effects of antithyroid drugs are mediated through actions on the thyroid cell, modulating thyrocyte-immunocyte signalling: a review. Thyroid 4:217–223
Weetman AP (1994) The potential immunological role of the thyroid cell in autoimmune thyroid disease. Thyroid 4:493–499

Weetman AP (1995) The effect of treatment on autoimmune thyroid disease. In: Rayner D (ed) Thyroid autoimmunity. Landes, Towata, pp 171–198
Weetman AP, McGregor AM (1994) Autoimmune endocrine disease: further developments in our understanding. Endocr Rev 15:788–830
Weetman AP, McGregor AM, Ludgate M, Hall R (1984) Effect of tri-iodothyronine on normal human lymphocyte function. J Endocrinol 101:81–86
Weetman AP, Gunn C, Hall R, McGregor AM (1984b) Immunosuppression by perchlorate. Lancet i:906
Weetman AP, Bhandal SK, Burrin JM, Robinson K, McKenna W (1988) Amiodarone and thyroid autoimmunity in the United Kingdom. Br Med J 297:33
Weetman AP, Tandon N, Morgan BP (1992) Antithyroid drugs and release of inflammatory mediators by complement-attacked thyroid cells. Lancet 340:633–636
Weiner HL (1994) Oral tolerance. Proc Natl Acad Sci USA 91:10762–10765
Wenzel KW, Lente JR (1984) Similar effects of thionamide drugs and perchlorate thyroid-stimulating immunoglobulins in Graves' disease: evidence against an immunosuppressive action of thionamide drugs. J Clin Endocrinol Metab 58:62–69
Werner SC, Platman SR (1965) Remission of hyperthyroidism (Graves' disease) and altered pattern of serum-thyroxine binding induced by prednisone. Lancet ii:751–756
Wick G, Müller P-U, Schwarz S (1982) Effect of cyclosporin A on spontaneous autoimmune thyroiditis of Obese strain (OS) chickens. Eur J Immunol 12:877–881
Wick G, Hu Y, Schwarz S, Kroemer G (1993) Immunoendocrine communication via the hypothalamo-pituitary-adrenal axis in autoimmune diseases. 14:539–563
Wick G, Cole R, Dietrich H, Maczek C, Müller P-U, Hála K (1994) The Obese strain of chickens with spontaneous autoimmune thyroiditis as a model for Hashimoto disease. In: Cohen IR, Miller A (eds) Autoimmune disease models: a guidebook. Academic, San Diego, pp 107–122
Wiersinga WM (1992) Immunosuppressive treatment of Graves' ophthalmopathy. Thyroid 2:229–233
Wilder RL (1995) Neuroendocrine-immune system interactions and autoimmunity. Annu Rev Immunol 13:307–338
Wilson CA, Jacobs C, Baker P, Baskin BG, Dower S, Lernmark Å, Toivola B, Vertrees S, Wilson D (1990) IL-1β modulation of spontaneous autoimmune diabetes and thyroiditis in the BB rat. J Immunol 144:3784–3787
Yoshikawa N, Arreaza G, Mukuta T, Resetkova E, Miller N, Jamieson C, Nishikawa M, Inada M, Volpé R (1994) Effect of FK-506 on xenografted human Graves' thyroid tissue in severe combined immunodeficient mice. Clin Endocrinol (Oxf) 41:31–37

Subject Index

MIX
Papier aus verantwortungsvollen Quellen
Paper from responsible sources
FSC® C105338
www.fsc.org

If you have any concerns about our products,
you can contact us on
ProductSafety@springernature.com

In case Publisher is established outside the EU,
the EU authorized representative is:
Springer Nature Customer Service Center GmbH
Europaplatz 3, 69115 Heidelberg, Germany

Printed by Libri Plureos GmbH
in Hamburg, Germany